Stimulation of the Peripheral Nervous System
The Neuromodulation Frontier

Progress in Neurological Surgery

Vol. 29

Series Editor

L. Dade Lunsford Pittsburgh, Pa.

Stimulation of the Peripheral Nervous System

The Neuromodulation Frontier

Volume Editor

Konstantin V. Slavin Chicago, Ill.

80 figures, 46 in color, and 25 tables, 2016

KARGER Basel · Freiburg · Paris · London · New York · Chennai · New Delhi · Bangkok · Beijing · Shanghai · Tokyo · Kuala Lumpur · Singapore · Sydney

Konstantin V. Slavin, MD, FAANS
Department of Neurosurgery
University of Illinois at Chicago
Chicago, Ill., USA

Library of Congress Cataloging-in-Publication Data

Stimulation of the peripheral nervous system: the neuromodulation frontier / volume editor, Konstantin V. Slavin.
p.; cm. -- (Progress in neurological surgery, ISSN 0079-6492; vol. 29)
Includes bibliographical references and indexes.
ISBN 978-3-318-02808-9 (hard cover: alk. paper) -- ISBN 978-3-318-02809-6 (electronic version)
I. Slavin, Konstantin V., editor. II. Series: Progress in neurological surgery; v. 29. 0079-6492
[DNLM: 1. Electric Stimulation--methods. 2. Peripheral Nerves--physiology.
3. Electric Stimulation Therapy--methods.
4. Neurotransmitter Agents--physiology. W1 PR673 v.29 2016 / WL 500]
RM872
615.8'45--dc23

2015026977

Bibliographic Indices. This publication is listed in bibliographic services, including Current Contents® and PubMed/MEDLINE.

www.karger.com
Printed in Germany on acid-free and non-aging paper (ISO 9706) by Kraft Druck GmbH, Ettlingen
ISSN 0079–6492
e-ISSN 1662–3924
ISBN 978–3–318–02808–9
e-ISBN 978–3–318–02809–6

Contents

VII **Series Editor's Note**
Lunsford, L.D. (Pittsburgh, Pa.)

IX **Preface**
Slavin, K.V. (Chicago, Ill.)

1 **Technology for Peripheral Nerve Stimulation**
Parker, J.L.; Cameron, T. (Artarmon, N.S.W./Sydney, N.S.W.)

20 **Theoretical Basis of Vagus Nerve Stimulation**
Attenello, F.; Amar, A.P.; Liu, C.; Apuzzo, M.L.J. (Los Angeles, Calif.)

29 **Vagus Nerve Stimulation: Surgical Technique and Complications**
Tronnier, V.M. (Lübeck)

39 **Vagus Nerve Stimulation for Epilepsy: An Evidence-Based Approach**
Cukiert, A. (Sao Paulo)

53 **Vagus Nerve Stimulation for Major Depressive Episodes**
Eljamel, S. (Dundee)

64 **Phrenic Nerve Stimulation: Technology and Clinical Applications**
Abdunnur, S.V.; Kim, D.H. (Houston, Tex.)

76 **Trigeminal Ganglion Stimulation**
Van Buyten, J.-P. (Sint-Niklaas/Brussels)

83 **Carotid Sinus/Nerve Stimulation for Treatment of Resistant Hypertension and Heart Failure**
Yin, D.; Slavin, K.V. (Chicago, Ill.)

94 **Hypoglossal Nerve Stimulation for Obstructive Sleep Apnea**
Mwenge, G.B.; Rombaux, P.; Lengele, B.; Rodenstein, D. (Brussels)

106 **Sphenopalatine Ganglion Stimulation in Neurovascular Headaches**
Schoenen, J. (Liège)

117 **Occipital Nerve Stimulation for Migraine: Update from Recent Multicenter Trials**
Schwedt, T.J.; Green, A.L.; Dodick, D.W. (Phoenix, Ariz.)

127 **Peripheral Nerve Stimulation for Back Pain**
Verrills, P. (Melbourne, Vic.); Russo, M. (Newcastle, N.S.W.)

139 **Peripheral Nerve Stimulation for Pain in Extremities: An Update**
Pope, J.E. (Santa Rosa, Calif.); Carlson, J.D. (Phoenix, Ariz./Glendale, Ariz.);
Rosenberg, W.S. (Kansas City, Mo.); Slavin, K.V. (Chicago, Ill.); Deer, T.R. (Charleston, W.Va.)

158 **Peripheral Neuromodulation to Treat Postamputation Pain**
Soin, A. (Dayton, Ohio/Xenia, Ohio/Beavercreek, Ohio); Fang, Z.-P. (Willoughby Hills, Ohio); Velasco, J. (Kettering, Ohio)

168 **Peripheral Neurostimulation with a Microsize Wireless Stimulator**
Yearwood, T.L. (Pascagoula, Miss./Mobile, Ala.); Perryman, L.T. (Fort Lauderdale, Fla.)

192 **Sacral Neuromodulation for Genitourinary Problems**
Banakhar, M. (Jeddah); Hassouna, M. (Toronto, Ont.)

200 **Sacral Nerve Stimulation in the Treatment of Bowel Disorders**
Nordenstam, J.; Boller, A.-M.; Mellgren, A. (Chicago, Ill.)

213 **Stimulation of the Dorsal Root Ganglion**
Liem, L. (Nieuwegein)

225 **Regulation of Peripheral Nerve Stimulation Technology**
Birk, D.M.; Yin, D.; Slavin, K.V. (Chicago, Ill.)

238 **Author Index**

239 **Subject Index**

Series Editor's Note

As a series editor of *Progress in Neurological Surgery*, I would like to congratulate Dr. Slavin and the coauthors of this new update on the role of advanced stimulation technology in the management of patients with epilepsy, chronic pain, depression, treatment-resistant hypertension, obstructive sleep apnea, and other innovative indications.

The increasing adoption of peripheral nerve stimulation for a wide variety of patient conditions is a testament to the remarkable ingenuity and perseverance of this group of clinicians and investigators. Peripheral nerve stimulation techniques have continued to expand and have proven to be safe and effective for diverse conditions, often in clinical situations where virtually no other therapeutic option exists. The authors, who come from multidisciplinary backgrounds, work at centers with special expertise in the analysis and development of these technologies. The authors provide a striking example of how persistence and innovation pays off in terms of improving patient outcomes. This update on the current status of peripheral nerve stimulation should be a valuable resource to the field of neurosurgery and pain management specialists. I am sure it will become an important reference for specialists who care for these diverse patient problems that also include respiratory, gastrointestinal, genitourinary, and cardiac indications. The possibilities for neuromodulation have greatly expanded beyond its earlier role in the treatment of chronic pain and medically refractory epilepsy.

L. Dade Lunsford, MD, Pittsburgh, Pa.

Preface

In the most common impression, the term 'peripheral nerve' refers to the large nerves that travel through the trunk and extremities carrying motor, sensory, and autonomic information. These 'peripheral nerves' are then differentiated from 'cranial nerves' and used synonymously to the actual alternative of the cranial nerves, the spinal nerves. Even the most commonly used list of medical procedures, the Current Procedural Terminology (CPT) [1], differentiates interventions performed on 'peripheral' and 'cranial' nerves – thereby adding to the confusion in terminology.

Anatomy, however, is a precise science and anatomical terminology is very well defined. Even the most accepted compendium of anatomical terminology, the medical dictionary, provides clear division of the nervous system into central and peripheral parts, defining the peripheral nervous system as everything outside of the brain and spinal cord [2]. In vertebrates, mammals, primates, and humans, the central nervous system includes the brain and the spinal cord. According to the authoritative book *The Peripheral Nervous System* [3], the subject of the book's title is defined as the cranial nerves, spinal nerves, and peripheral ganglia which lie outside the brain and spinal cord. With this scheme, all nerves that originate from the cranial part of the central nervous system – the cranial nerves (with the exception of the olfactory and optic nerves which are considered parts of the central nervous system) – and all those that originate from the spinal cord – the spinal nerves – fall under the same category of the peripheral nerves, and this categorization is supported by their anatomy, histology, and physiology.

This discrepancy between a common misconception (i.e. peripheral nerves differ from cranial nerves) and the actual anatomophysiological similarity became obvious after the first volume of *Peripheral Nerve Stimulation* was published in 2011 [4]. Multiple clinical applications of cranial nerve stimulation remained omitted as most chapters concentrated on those nerves that travel through the trunk and extremities. Not surprisingly, those applications that dealt with indications other than pain (epilepsy, depression, sleep apnea, etc.) were not included in the book, as most of them specifically involve stimulation of the cranial nerves (vagus, hypoglossal). Along with these, the stimulation of the phrenic nerves used for respiratory insufficiency was left uncovered even though there is no controversy about phrenic nerve stimulation being a 'true' example of peripheral nerve stimulation (PNS). Moreover, several applications of neuromodulation that would not fall under strict definition of PNS, but instead represent so-called 'peripheral neurostimulation' – i.e. stimulation of the trigeminal ganglion, dorsal root ganglion, sacral nerves, and nerve roots – are covered in this second part of *Peripheral Nerve Stimulation* from the popular and well-established series *Progress in Neurological Surgery.*

In addition to all of these new topics, this volume includes other important chapters. One of them deals with theoretical and technical aspects of peripheral nerve interface with neurostimulation devices. Others describe principles of wireless energy transmission that are used in modern miniaturized neuromodulation devices and characteristics of high-frequency PNS that results in a block of nerve conduction. Several chapters are dedicated to in-depth updates on the most common PNS indications, such as migraines, low back pain, and pain in extremities. Not surprisingly, the field of PNS is rapidly progressing, and as our experience grows, so does our understanding of surgical indications, proper patient selection, technical nuances of operative procedures, and complication-avoidance techniques. Instead of case reports and small retrospective single-surgeon or single-institution studies, we now have multicenter prospective studies that may be used in critical analysis of clinical evidence that could justify our interventions.

The growing clinical experience is paralleled by industrial developments. Instead of routinely using devices designed for spinal cord stimulation in PNS applications, there are now more than a dozen device-manufacturing companies that dedicate themselves to the creation of a new generation of electrodes and generators specifically designed for PNS use. Miniaturization, rechargeability, wireless interfaces, and customized designs – terms that only recently were considered futuristic and not applicable to PNS – are becoming reality at a very rapid pace.

The final chapter of this volume deals with regulatory aspects of PNS and related applications since over the last few years the field of peripheral neuromodulation has enjoyed several important approvals, mainly in Europe, Canada, and Australia, making PNS, once again, a legitimate intervention in the spectrum of available interventions, alongside spinal cord stimulation and deep brain stimulation approaches.

Even though this is yet another volume in *Progress in Neurological Surgery,* not all interventions covered here are performed by the neurosurgeons. The uniqueness of the neuromodulation field is that it blossomed at the intersection of multiple medical specialties, including neurosurgery, neurology, anesthesiology, physiatry, orthopedics, cardiology, urology, gastroenterology, otolaryngology, pulmonology, psychiatry, oral surgery, colorectal surgery, and others – the field of PNS undoubtedly brings together physicians from different backgrounds. One has to keep in mind, however, that the implantable nature of neuromodulation still requires surgery, and the substrate of our interventions is still the nervous system. And who would be better qualified for surgery on the nervous system than neurosurgeons? Being a neurosurgeon myself, I can already hear the criticism from my nonneurosurgical colleagues who perform the overwhelming majority of neuromodulation procedures, including PNS and spinal cord stimulation, and who over the years have become much more comfortable with reaching the nerves all over the human body. And since I have taught hundreds of them how to make neuromodulation procedures safer, I feel confident that this volume will be of interest to the entire neuromodulation community, reflecting the interdisciplinary nature of our field and, among other things, reminding myself and other neurosurgeon readers what we may be missing!

Konstantin V. Slavin, MD, FAANS, Chicago, Ill.

References

1 AMA: CPT: 2015 Standard Edition (Current Procedural Terminology). Chicago, American Medical Association, 2014.

2 Medical Glossary.org: Peripheral nervous system. http://www.medicalglossary.org/nervous_system_peripheral_nervous_system_definitions.html (accessed on January 12, 2015).

3 Hubbard J (ed): The Peripheral Nervous System. New York, Plenum Press, 1974.

4 Slavin KV (ed): Peripheral Nerve Stimulation. Basel, Karger, 2011.

Slavin KV (ed): Stimulation of the Peripheral Nervous System. The Neuromodulation Frontier.
Prog Neurol Surg. Basel, Karger, 2016, vol 29, pp 1–19 (DOI: 10.1159/000434651)

Technology for Peripheral Nerve Stimulation

John L. Parker[a–c] • Tracy Cameron[a, b]

[a]Saluda Medical, Artarmon, N.S.W., and [b]National ICT Australia, and [c]Graduate School of Biomedical Engineering, University of New South Wales, Sydney, N.S.W., Australia

Abstract

Peripheral nerve stimulation (PNS) has been in use for over 50 years to treat patients suffering from chronic pain who have failed conservative treatments. Despite this long history, the devices being used have changed very little. In fact, current PNS technology was developed specifically for spinal cord stimulation. The use of technology developed for other applications in PNS has led to an unnecessary number of device complications and the limited adoption of this promising therapy. The following chapter provides an overview of PNS technology throughout the years, outlining both the benefits and limitations. We will briefly explore the electrophysiology of PNS stimulation, with an emphasis on technology and indication-specific devices. Finally, design and technical requirements of an ideal PNS device will be discussed.

Peripheral Nerve Stimulation Technology Throughout the Years

Compared to other types of medical devices, technological advances in peripheral nerve stimulation (PNS) have been rather few and far between. Only a few minor improvements have been made over the years and many of these improvements have been the result of the application of new technology developed in other neuromodulation therapies such as spinal cord stimulation (SCS). The following sections summarize PNS technology (fig. 1), with an emphasis on device complications and limitations.

Early Devices

The earliest recorded use of PNS was in 1962 by Shelden [1] who implanted 3 patients for the indication of pain due to trigeminal neuralgia. This was several years before the publication of the gate control theory [2] and was based on the rationale of

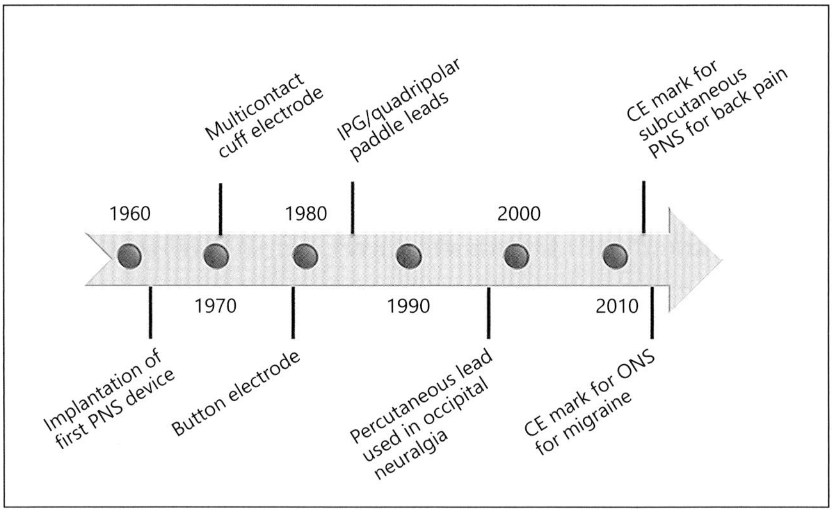

Fig. 1. Timeline of the significant technological changes since the inception of PNS. ONS = Occipital nerve stimulation.

depressing excitatory transmission by depolarization of the nerves [3]. The device was fully implantable and powered by an external radiofrequency (RF) generator. The RF device was capable of delivering 10 V at a frequency of 14.5 kHz. Shelden implanted platinum electrodes over the mandibular division of the trigeminal nerve in all 3 patients. One patient reported favorable outcomes up to 31 months after surgery. Single case reports by other researchers appearing around the same time [4] found stimulation of a variety of peripheral nerves was able to suppress chronic pain caused by complex regional pain syndrome and neural trauma.

PNS with RF generators and nerve cuff electrodes became much more common in the 1970s [5–8]. A device described by Long [5] in 1973 had the bipolar or monopolar electrodes wired directly to the RF-receiving coil. This required that the location of the receiving coil be determined by the position of the stimulating electrode. Long reported complete pain relief in 6 out of 10 patients. He found the device to be more efficacious in the upper extremities than the lower, likely due to increased difficulty in implanting electrodes in the hip area. Long did not report any complications due to the device. Patient selection was performed by a short period of percutaneous trial stimulation (in the order of minutes) with cordotomy electrodes connected to either a StimTech (StimTech Corporation, Minneapolis, Minn., USA) or Medtronic (Medtronic, Minneapolis, Minn., USA) external stimulator (1-ms pulse width, 10–25 pulses/s, 1–4 V).

Campbell and Long [6] continued to implant and reported a further 33 patients also using a bipolar nerve cuff and RF receiver. Electrodes were wrapped around the nerve corresponding to the area of the patient's pain (sciatic, brachial plexus, median, and ulnar nerves). They reported an overall success rate of 45%. Of the 17 failures, 12 were in patients with either low back pain with sciatica or pain from metastatic disease.

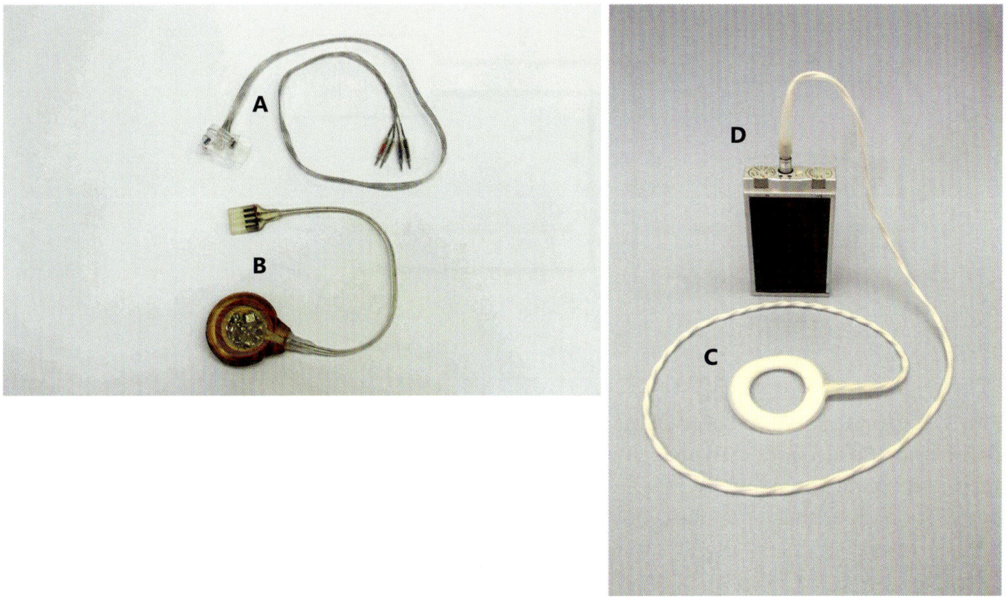

Fig. 2. Photograph of the Avery PNS system: (**A**) quadripolar cuff electrode, (**B**) radio frequency receiver, (**C**) external antenna, and (**D**) external stimulator (image courtesy of Avery Biomedical Inc., reprinted with permission).

Complications included two infections, 1 tissue reaction, 1 soreness over the receiver, 1 motor activation, and 1 wire disconnection.

In summary, the first generation of PNS devices showed the promise of peripheral stimulation to treat chronic pain, but they were limited by the hard-wired connection between the RF receiving coil and electrodes and the number of electrodes that could be stimulated at any one time.

Second-Generation PNS Devices

The next generation of devices employed quadripolar cuff electrodes developed by Avery Laboratories (Farmingdale, New York, N.Y., USA; fig. 2). As well as having multiple contact electrodes, this system had a connector between the leads and the generator, allowing greater flexibility in receiver location.

Law et al. [8] in 1980 reported on 22 chronic pain patients implanted with multiple contact cuff electrodes from Avery Laboratories. Despite the benefit of the extra contacts, the RF receiver was only capable of controlling two electrodes at a time (anode and cathode), and patients were therefore required to undergo a trial period during which the electrode lead was percutaneously passed to a switching box and the different combinations of electrodes were tested (fig. 3). When the optimal electrode configuration was determined, the switch box was disconnected and the selected

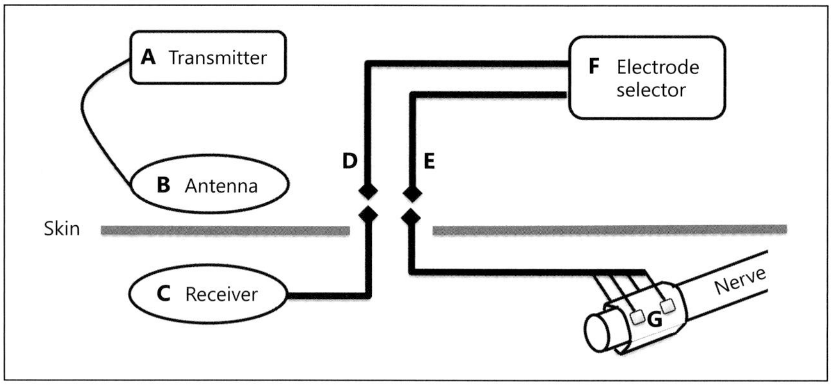

Fig. 3. Schematic representation of the components of the Avery PNS system. Before internalization of the lead, the electrodes (**G**) are connected by wires (**E**) and connectors (**D**) to the electrode selector (**F**); when the optimal electrodes are determined, they are connected to the internal receiver (**C**). Stimulation is transmitted to the receiver (**C**) via an antenna (**B**) attached to the transmitter (**A**).

electrodes were attached to the receiver and internalized. With this technique Law et al. reported a success rate of 62% for an average follow-up of 25 months. However, 50% of the patients required multiple operations to change the electrode selection. Other complications included equipment failure and repositioning of the connector, and a total of 6 patients required device removal, mainly due to lack of efficacy. It was clear from this early experience that electrode position played a critical role in the efficacy of treatment.

Waisbrod et al. in 1985 [9] reported on 19 chronic pain patients implanted with the Avery Laboratories device. Patients underwent a preimplantation trial using a percutaneous needle (stimulation 80–100 Hz, 0.3 V) for approximately 30 min. To qualify for implantation, each patient was required to have at least 50% reduction in pain. Patients were then implanted with a nerve cuff, attached to a cable buried subcutaneously. Two days later, patients returned to evaluate different electrode combinations for optimal pain relief. Waisbrod et al. reported a success rate of 84%. Complications included two skin erosions at the implant site, one necrosis of the cables, and one infection.

A series of 35 patients implanted with peripheral nerve stimulators from 1970 to 1979 was reported by Nashold et al. [10] in 1982. Electrodes were implanted on the median, ulnar, and radial nerves in the upper extremities and on the sciatic and tibial nerves in the lower extremities. Success in the upper extremities was higher (52.6%) than in the lower extremities (31%). They attributed their failures in the lower extremity to the stress of weight-bearing and anatomical positioning.

In 1979, Nashold et al. [11] replaced the cuff electrode with a newly developed PNS electrode with button contacts that could be sutured directly to the nerve. This new electrode eliminated complications associated with using a nerve cuff such as nerve compression and electrode rotation [12].

The Avery system was used for many years; however, by the mid-1980s the RF receiver began being replaced with an implantable pulse generator (IPG) [13]. The RF device provided good pain relief, but a drawback was the need to have an external coil attached to the skin to operate. This often resulted in skin irritation and the need to wear the external controller reduced patient compliance. In addition, these devices could not be used 24 h/day, e.g. during bathing or other activities that involved water. The fully implantable generator eliminated these issues.

In 1990, Racz et al. [14] also described modifications in the lead implantation technique. Most notably, the electrode was covered with a thin fibrous membrane made from intramuscular septa in order to reduce the foreign body reaction related to direct electrode contact with the nerve. The focus of PNS up to this point was targeting specific nerves and implantation of electrodes very close to the nerves.

This focus continued with clinicians exploring the use of multipolar paddle leads commercially developed by Medtronic for SCS. Strege et al. [15] in 1994 reported on their initial experience using a 4-contact paddle lead with an RF stimulator (Resume/X-trel transmitter/receiver unit, Medtronic). This system, like that of Avery Laboratories, used a polyurethane-covered receiver unit implanted subcutaneously and required that a portable transmitter unit be carried at all times to activate the receiver through an antenna placed over the skin. Strege et al. later switched to a 4-contact IPG (Itrel System, Medtronic). This IPG could be programmed through the skin using telemetry and required no external unit to maintain stimulation. Both systems provided good results with a combined success rate of 62.5%. Complications included hardware problems with the generator, electrode migration, and foreign body reaction. The above technology continued to be used through the 1990s with good success and is still an option for patients with pain generated by a single easily accessible nerve.

Introduction of Percutaneous Leads for Peripheral Nerve Stimulation

The first documented use of percutaneous leads implanted to stimulate a peripheral nerve was in 1982 by Urban and Nashold [16], who described a technique combining SCS and PNS. They placed the percutaneous lead over the peripheral nerve by first inserting the lead epidurally and then advancing it through the intervertebral foramen (fig. 4). The peripheral electrode was placed percutaneously and positioned along the course of the anterior division of the spinal nerve anterolateral to the vertebral bodies. Their patients were implanted with the Avery percutaneous electrical bipolar nerve stimulator for PNS (50–400 μs, 7–200 Hz, and 0–14 V) and the Medtronic system for SCS (monophasic square wave 0.1- to 1-ms pulse width, 1–120 Hz, 0–10 V).

Urban and Nashold's study [16] examined stimulation from both epidural and peripheral leads in 23 patients with intractable leg pain. During implantation, patients were assessed to determine the location of the paresthesia with respect to their pain. After intraoperative assessment, 16 patients proceeded to chronic stimulation.

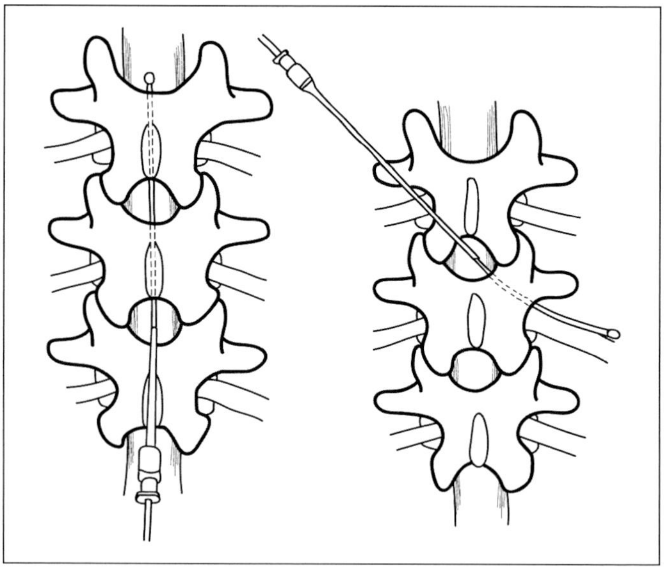

Fig. 4. Schematic illustration of the SCS (left) and PNS (right) electrode placement.

Peripheral electrodes were placed on the lumbar and first sacral nerves. The overall success rate for patients implanted with both SCS and PNS was 62.4%. One patient was lost to follow-up after 1 month. Only a few late complications of a minor nature were reported and the overall results were similar to those from conventional epidural spinal cord stimulator implantation.

Although Urban and Nashold [16] reported good success with the use of a percutaneous lead to stimulate a peripheral nerve, it did not become popular until 1999 when Weiner and Reed [17] treated occipital neuralgia by applying a percutaneous lead over the greater occipital nerves. This report prompted many clinicians to begin placing percutaneous leads in the periphery to treat a variety of disorders including trigeminal neuropathy [18], supraorbital neuralgia [19], cluster headache [20], and chronic migraine [21]. All the leads, anchors, and generators used in these studies were designed for SCS. Although there was an attempt to increase the lead spacing and development of a curved Tuohy needle [22], very little of the existing SCS device was modified for this new application. This led to a number of hardware complications related specifically to the implantation procedure including lead migration, lead breakage, pain at the lead site, and skin erosion [21, 23]. In 2007, Schwedt et al. [24] found that by 3 years all patients required revision surgery due to lead migration, and 42% also had their batteries reach end of life prematurely, likely due to higher than expected stimulation voltage requirements. This latter complication led to the adoption of rechargeable generators, but the lead migration and other lead-related issues remain open with the current technology.

In addition to the stimulation of the nerves of the head and neck, a number of researchers have placed percutaneous leads over the nerve roots using various techniques. The original transspinal approach of Urban and Nashold [16] has been modified to include simply guiding an epidurally placed lead laterally in the epidural space so that it lies over the targeted nerve roots. A transforaminal approach goes one step further by directing the lead out through the neural foramen [25]. An extraforaminal stimulation procedure avoids the spinal canal completely by placing the lead directly into the neural foramina [26]. It must be noted that all these techniques use current SCS technology and are associated with all the standard SCS complications, in addition to possible nerve root damage.

A more recent addition to the peripheral nerve approach is to not necessarily target a specific nerve, but to place leads in the periphery in the location of the pain [27]. Leads have been placed under the skin to successfully treat low back pain [28, 29], inguinal pain [30], axial neck pain [31], intractable abdominal pain [32], and postherpetic neuralgia [33]. The hardware used with all these techniques was designed for SCS. The result has been a number of complications such as lead migration, lead fracture, and connector failures, with many of these due to the high degree of motion exerted on the hardware in these locations. In addition, this technique is known to be prone to lead and anchor erosion because the location of the lead can be very superficial. To address the issue of lead migration, paddle type electrodes have been used successfully to treat migraines [34–36] and low back pain [37].

Other Devices

Some specialized devices designed specifically for peripheral nerve applications are starting to be developed. These include both percutaneous devices and fully implanted devices targeted for specific nerves.

Percutaneous electrical nerve stimulation is an approach that uses needle electrodes inserted under the skin whereby the tissue is stimulated for a period of time and then the electrodes are removed (Algotec, Crawley, UK). Percutaneous electrical nerve stimulation has been used to treat low back pain [38], diabetic neuropathy [39], and headache [40]. The therapy usually involves three 30-min treatments per week for 3 weeks. In 2000, Hamza et al. [39] found a statistically significant improvement in pain VAS scores before and after stimulation as well as improved physical activity, sense of well-being, and quality of sleep. No side effects were found with this treatment. However, this technique suffers from the same issues as RF-coupled systems in terms of diminished patient compliance and that effective pain relief requires patients to return to the clinic for multiple treatments.

An implantable device that has been developed to be used anywhere in the periphery is the microstimulator. Originally developed to be used to reanimate paralyzed muscle, this device was later redesigned by Boston Scientific to be used in the management of chronic pain conditions and renamed the Bion™ (Boston Scientific, Marlborough, Mass., USA; fig. 5). The microstimulator is a small cylindrical bipolar stimulator

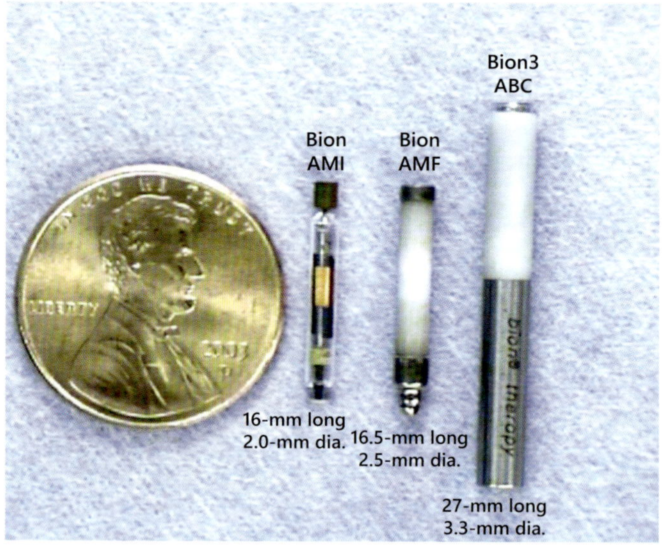

Fig. 5. Three versions of Bion™ (image courtesy of Dr. J. Loeb). dia. = Diameter.

that can be injected into a muscle or near a nerve through a 12-gauge catheter [41]. There are two versions of this device: an RF-powered version used primarily in functional electrical stimulation applications such as shoulder subluxation, knee osteoarthritis [42], hand rehabilitation [43], and foot drop [44], and a rechargeable version that has been used to treat various headache syndromes [45]. Both devices have shown promising results.

Bion™ requires no anchoring or tunneling of extensions to remote power sources; as such, complications like lead fracture or connector breakage are eliminated. However, it is possible that a foreign body such as Bion™ can migrate or become encapsulated by scar tissue. Encapsulation can increase the energy required to stimulate the target nerve, resulting in shorter battery life. Bion™ has been reported to require frequent recharges with recharging time ranging from 35 min per week to 4 h/day [45]. Finally, with only a simple bipolar pair of electrode contacts the stimulation field is limited.

An implantable device designed for a specific target location is the novel sphenopalatine ganglion (SPG) neurostimulator [Autonomic Technologies (ATI), Redwood City, Calif., USA; fig. 6). It consists of a lead with multiple contacts attached directly to a miniature neurostimulator and a fixation plate designed specifically to stimulate the SPG for cluster headaches and other indications [46]. During implantation the electrodes are positioned within the pterygopalatine fossa proximate to the SPG, with the body of the SPG neurostimulator positioned on the lateral-posterior maxilla medial to the zygoma and anchored to the zygomatic process of the maxilla using the integrated fixation plate. Patients are instructed to use the device during their cluster headache attacks by energizing the normally dormant implant with an external RF coil. A recent randomized, sham-controlled study found that 68% of patients had a clinically significant improvement [46]. The main complication was a

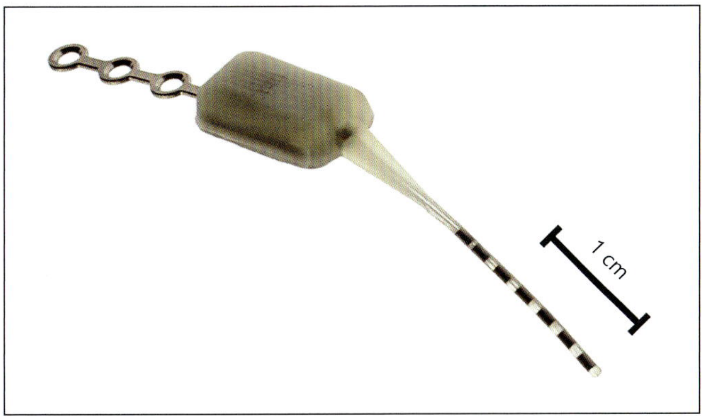

Fig. 6. ATI neurostimulator (image courtesy of Autonomic Technologies Inc., reprinted with permission).

mild-to-moderate loss of sensation within distinct maxillary nerve regions (81%); 65% of these events resolved within 3 months (for more details, see the chapter by Schoenen [this vol., pp. 106–116]).

A new device designed specifically for stimulating the dorsal nerve root ganglia is currently in clinical trials (Spinal Modulation, Menlo Park, Calif., USA). This device incorporates an introducer sheath which enables clinicians to access the dorsal root ganglia via the transforaminal (or interlaminar) approach [25]. Leads are introduced into the epidural space using a standard 14-gauge needle and a sheath is used to steer the lead laterally through the epidural space where it enters the medial aspect of the neural foramen. Deer et al. [47] in 2012 reported on the outcomes of 10 patients evaluated from 4 sites. They found that on average there was a 70% reduction in pain following stimulation ($p < 0.001$). There were some minor complications which included device malfunction due to programming error and lead migration (for more details, see the chapter by Liem [this vol., pp. 213–224]).

Finally, there is a device currently in development that incorporates high frequency nerve block for stump pain (Neuros Medical, Willoughby Hills, Ohio, USA; fig. 7). This device uses a nerve cuff attached to the nerve in a stump. A case report by Soin et al. [48] in 2011 described the evaluation and treatment of an amputee pain patient. Testing started 1 week after the surgery. Overall, the threshold and maximum tolerable amplitude were inversely correlated with frequency in the range of 5–30 kHz. At frequencies of 10 kHz, the patient reported that his pain scores dropped to 0 consistently and reproducibly (for more details, see the chapter by Soin et al. [this vol., pp. 158–167]).

Limitations with Current Technology

PNS has had a long history with limited improvements in technology. Over the years some of the early technical complications have been addressed, but many still remain. The lack of specialized tools for this approach requires clinicians to use equipment

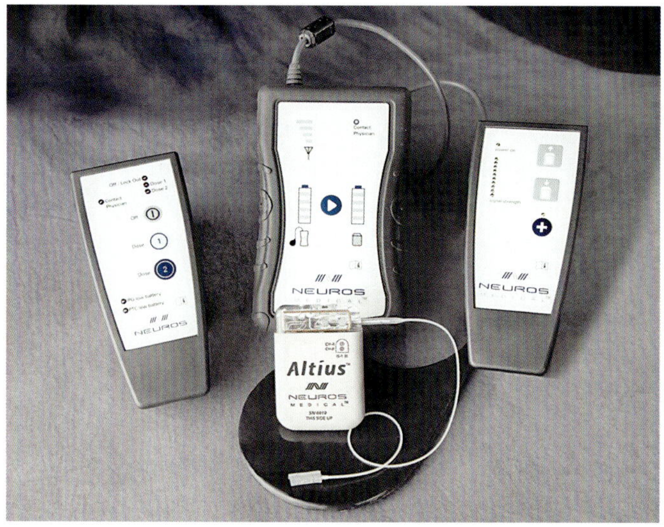

Fig. 7. Neuros Medical stimulation system: Left – physician controller; middle – charger, IPG and nerve cuff; right – patient controller (image courtesy of Neuros Medical Inc., reprinted with permission).

not designed for complex and varied anatomical locations. Some of the main complications that have been described include those related to leads, anchors, and connectors. Unlike SCS devices, leads implanted in the periphery undergo a large amount of movement, with certain areas such as the neck undergoing extensive movement. This stress on the leads can lead to mechanical failure. In addition, the relatively large diameter of the leads, approximately 1.5 mm, can be problematic when stimulating specific body areas such as the face where the skin layer is thin. This can result in complications such as skin erosion, which is further magnified by the materials used in the construction of the leads. Polyurethane, although flexible enough for use in the epidural space, is often too stiff to be used in subcutaneous locations.

Another set of complications arises because the anchors used to stabilize the lead in place were designed to be used in SCS where they are typically located deep in the soft tissues to allow suturing to the deep fascia. The size and stiffness of current anchors make them prone to erosion when used in the periphery.

The current size of IPGs limits the location where the device can be implanted. Although not an issue for SCS stimulation, this greatly limits the possible targets for PNS or requires long leads, which may be prone to breaks and migrations.

Finally, electrode size and spacing for the majority of percutaneous leads used in PNS were designed specifically to accommodate implantation in the epidural space [49, 50]. Lead design has been predominately influenced by the need to reduce activation of the dorsal root fibers while increasing activation of dorsal column fiber; in addition, SCS leads must take into consideration the role cerebral spinal fluid thickness plays in this relationship [51]. This is not an issue when it comes to PNS. However, the optimal electrodes for this indication have not yet been developed, mainly due to the lack of research and modeling in this area.

Electrical Excitation of Peripheral Nerve Fibers

The history of use of SCS devices for PNS has exposed the need for devices designed specifically for PNS. We have already mentioned mechanical aspects, but there are also electrical and stimulation requirements for PNS which differ from SCS. As stated above, the electrode spacing has been designed for SCS applications. In order to suggest areas for improvement we must first understand some of the basics of electrical stimulation.

The electrical excitation of neural tissue has been studied extensively both experimentally and with computer modeling. The physical principles are well understood in applications in the brain, spinal cord, and nerve fibers. To date there has been little published on the applications of this knowledge to PNS.

To understand how electrical stimulation affects peripheral nerves, we must begin with an understanding of the structure and density of the target fibers for electrical stimulation. The skin layers consist of epidermis (0.5–1 mm thick), dermis (2 mm), and adipose layers. The sensory nerves innervating the cutaneous layers of the skin consist of A-beta, A-delta, and C fibers. The A-beta fibers are large-diameter myelinated fibers (in humans, 8–10 μm in diameter). A-delta are myelinated fibers (3–6 μm in diameter) that lose their myelin upon entering the dermis layer, at which point they are indistinguishable from the unmyelinated and smaller (0.2–1.5 μm in diameter) C fibers [52]. Fibers branch extensively in the cutaneous layers; A-beta fibers can have approximately 60 nerve endings per mm^2 [53, 54], while A-delta fibers can have over 160 per mm^2 [55].

Most of our understanding of the electrical excitability of neurons has been derived from studies and modeling of straight fibers. These myelinated axons generate action potentials in response to electrical fields generated by flow of current through a near-by electrode. It is the relationship between current and recruited fibers (or action potential generation) which is critical to the performance of neuromodulation systems. The power requirements of the devices and the extent of coverage, or area of recruited fibers, are determined by understanding this relationship. With current technology, the extent of fiber recruitment can only be measured by subjective means. The current intensity and location is varied by the programmer and the implanted individual provides feedback describing the feeling of the stimulation.

There are many factors that influence the relationship between the current and the number of recruited fibers, including the anatomical characteristics of the fibers, the tissue between the fibers and the electrodes, and the physical characteristics of the electrode (fig. 8). The relationship between the fiber diameter and threshold is well understood. Large-diameter fibers have much lower thresholds than smaller-diameter fibers [56], and the axon branch points which occur extensively in the dermis have lower thresholds to electrical stimulation than straight fibers [57].

Simulations of Hodgkin-Huxley models of straight nerve fibers reveal the relationships between the key stimulation parameters:

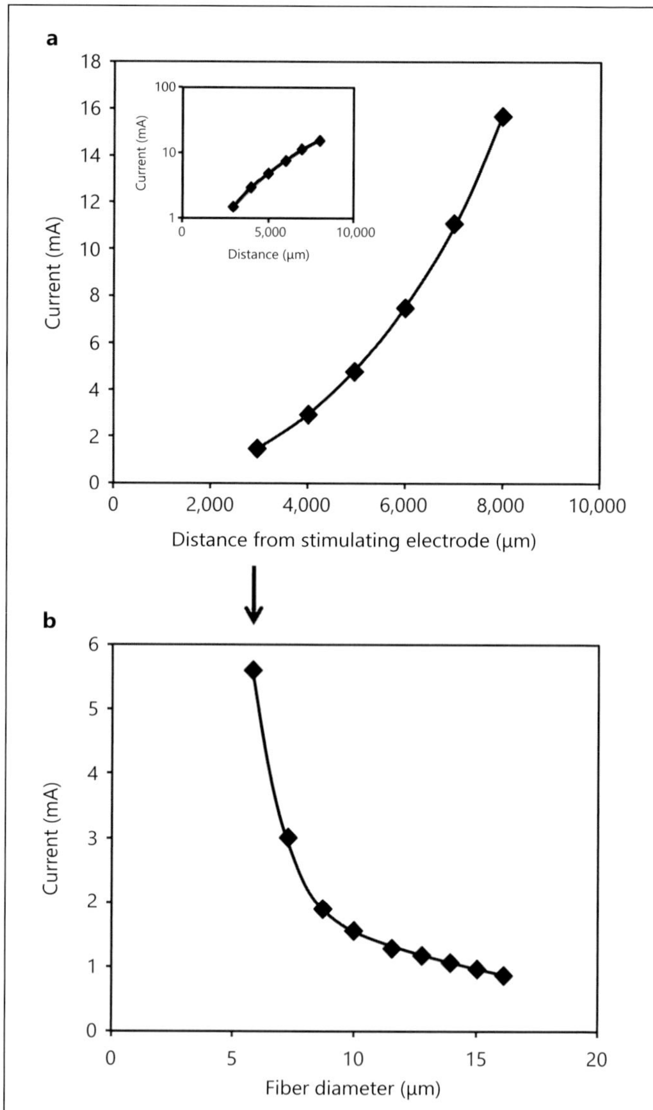

Fig. 8. The relationship between distance from an electrode to a 10-μm diameter fiber and threshold stimulation current required to depolarize and generate an action potential (**a**). The points were calculated using neurons and the model described by MacIntyre et al. [59]. The stimulation parameters were 80-μs pulse width biphasic stimuli, cathode on the first phase, and 50-μs interphase gap. **a** The stimulating electrode height above the axon was set at 3 mm and the current was adjusted to find the threshold for action potential generation. The inset displays the same data plotted on a log plot. **b** Calculated threshold for different fiber diameters at a fixed stimulation electrode fiber distance of 3 mm.

- To stimulate fibers at larger distances from the electrodes requires more charge.
- Lower charge is required as the pulse width is increased.
- Higher charge is required for smaller diameter fibers.
- Shorter pulse widths are more selective for fibers of different sizes.

There have been few experimental studies of the relationship between the electrode separation and the recruitment of the fibers. Ranck [56] has summarized the data from a large number of studies and concluded:

- Most CNS myelinated fibers have chronaxies of 50–100 μs.
- High currents (>8 times threshold) close to the cathode will block action potentials.
- The current-distance relationship follows a power law with an ~r^2 relationship.

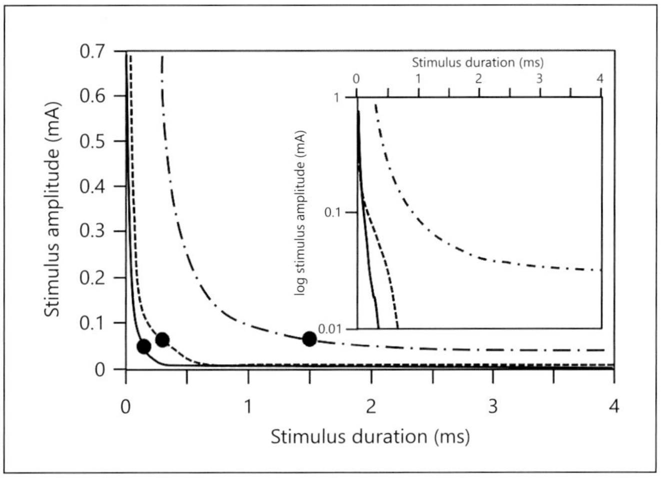

Fig. 9. Strength duration curves for A-beta (solid line), A-delta (dashed line), and C (dash-dot line) fibers. The figure was redrawn from data presented for the saphenous nerve of the cat [58]. The large dots indicate the chronaxies and the insert shows the same data presented on a logarithmic scale.

There are very few direct experimental measures of the differences in excitability of the different fiber classes. Measurements from the cat saphenous nerve have shown that the diameter of the fiber and extent of myelination effects the excitability in the way which would be expected from modeling [58] (fig. 9). C fibers required a stimulus strength of 75 times, and A-delta a stimulus strength of 3.3 times, the strength required to recruit A-beta fibers. Thus, achieving selective stimulation of A-beta fibers and not the others would appear to be achievable with such a large difference in excitability between the fibers. However, we must also take into account the field distribution.

The electric field extends from the surface of the electrode and generates an extracellular potential at each node of Ranvier:

$$V(r) = I\rho/4\pi r$$

In this equation, I is the stimulating current, ρ is the electrical resistivity, and r is the electrode to node distance. The second derivative of the extracellular field drives the membrane polarization. The net effect is that when the electrode is close to the fiber (much less than the distances between nodes of Ranvier) the relationship between the fiber separation falls with 1/r as in the equation above, but at larger separations it varies with a $1/r^2$ relationship.

For a given stimulation current, the extent of stimulation can be thought of as an area around the electrode where the field strength is sufficient to generate an action potential. This area is larger for the more excitable fibers (i.e. the A-beta fibers and smaller for the A-delta fibers). The maximal distance from a point source electrode for a fiber was calculated as a function of current for a single long axon modeled in a neuron (for details of the model see McIntyre et al. [59]).

Figure 10 shows two different axon fiber diameters (5.7 and 10 µm); the distance from the electrode to the furthest fiber, which can be stimulated, forms a radius of stimulation within which all fibers of that size or greater will be stimulated. From this radius the area

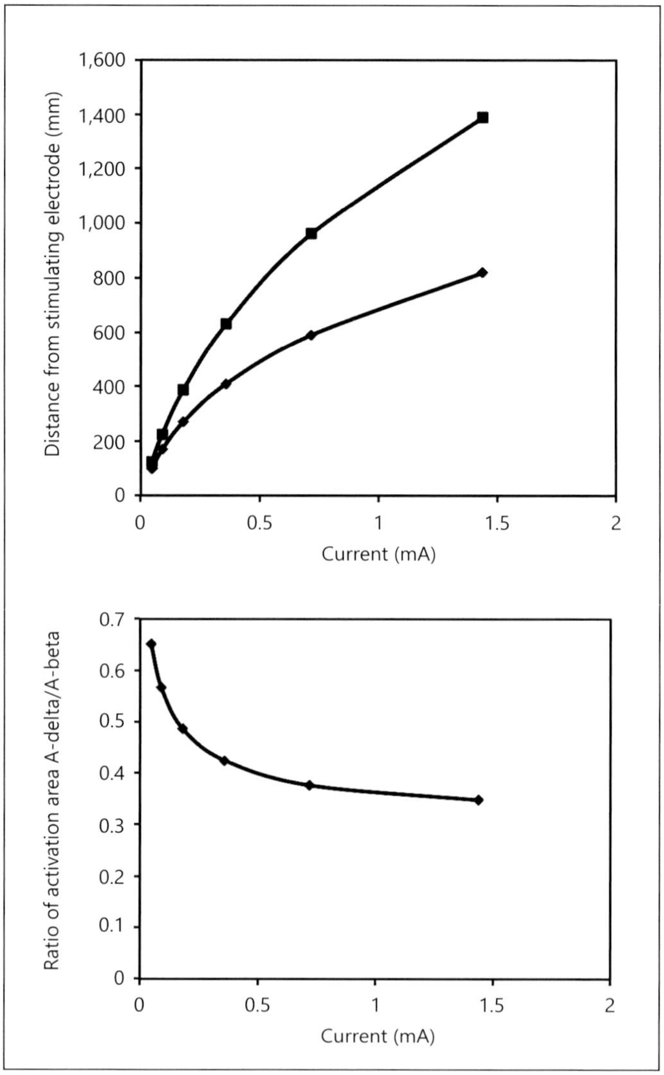

Fig. 10. The calculated current required to depolarize an axon 10 μm in diameter as a function of the separation from the electrode (upper panel). For comparison, data for a 5-μm fiber is also shown. The 5-μm fiber represents the upper bound for the size of A-delta fibers. The ratio of the area of activation (10-μm fiber/5-μm fiber) is shown in the lower panel.

can be calculated and the ratio of areas for A-beta and A-delta fibers can be determined (fig. 10). Doubling the diameter of the fiber roughly triples the area of stimulation, but one should note that it is not possible to obtain a stimulation area of A-beta fibers which is more than 3 times the area of A-delta fibers. The very simple geometry of this model is obviously a very gross approximation. It does not take into account the differences in impedance of the various layers of the skin, the boundary effects from the surface of the skin, and the three dimensional shape of the electrode and fiber branching. In order to account for these effects, more complex models should be developed.

As mentioned previously, electrodes currently used for PNS in treatment of pain have been designed primarily for use elsewhere in the body. The primary goal of PNS electrode design would be an improved selectivity between A-beta and A-delta fibers.

To date there have been some attempts to do this through programming. Reports have described increasing the field by spreading the current along a number of electrodes and across a number of leads at once [60]. However, as described above, the stimulation field falls off with the inverse square of the distance and the current electrode size and spacing between the electrode (typically 4 mm or greater) are not optimal to produce a uniform field. A more efficient way to improve selectivity and ratio of A-beta/A-delta fiber recruitment is to increase the stimulation field by increasing the surface area of the electrode. This would allow stimulation at shorter pulse widths and lower currents. Current electrode fabrication technology is not suitable for fabrication of very large surface area electrodes. The construction techniques, which rely on the use of electrode elements fabricated from bulk metal (tubes or plates) impart rigidity to the electrode array. As discussed above, since skin erosion and lead migration remain complications for PNS systems, increasing the electrode size with current technology would likely increase this complication.

The Ideal Peripheral Nerve Stimulation Device

As we have seen from our review of the technology, there is no simple single description of a PNS application. In some applications, such as PNS for migraine, the target for electrical stimulation is a specific nerve, but in others the targets are the dispersed sensory nerve endings in the region of pain. The notion that both the specific and nonspecific targets can be best stimulated with a single design of electrode is obviously erroneous. However, that is precisely what is done in clinical practice. There are unique design requirements for all the components of neuromodulation system that are application dependent. These major components are illustrated in figure 11.

The first key challenge designers of neuromodulation devices face is how to get power into the device. Transcutaneous inductive links were used in the early PNS devices but suffer from poor efficiency and the requirement that an external coil be positioned over the implant during stimulation. This led to the development of devices with implantable batteries. Currently, both primary cell and rechargeable cells are being used. However, notably in an application which does not require continuous stimulation, such as an ATI device, an inductive link is a viable option. There is a careful trade-off between the size of the battery and how long it will last, which is also dependent on the current draw from the system.

Rechargeable batteries have the advantage that they can extend the operating life of the device between replacements, but they need to be recharged at regular intervals. They are charged with the same kind of transcutaneous inductive link as the RF device and there is a limit to the amount of energy, which can be transferred across this link at a given time. Too much can cause heating of the tissue, resulting in serious complications. Too little energy extends the time that it takes to recharge the device. In order to accommodate various PNS applications, a rechargeable battery has become the

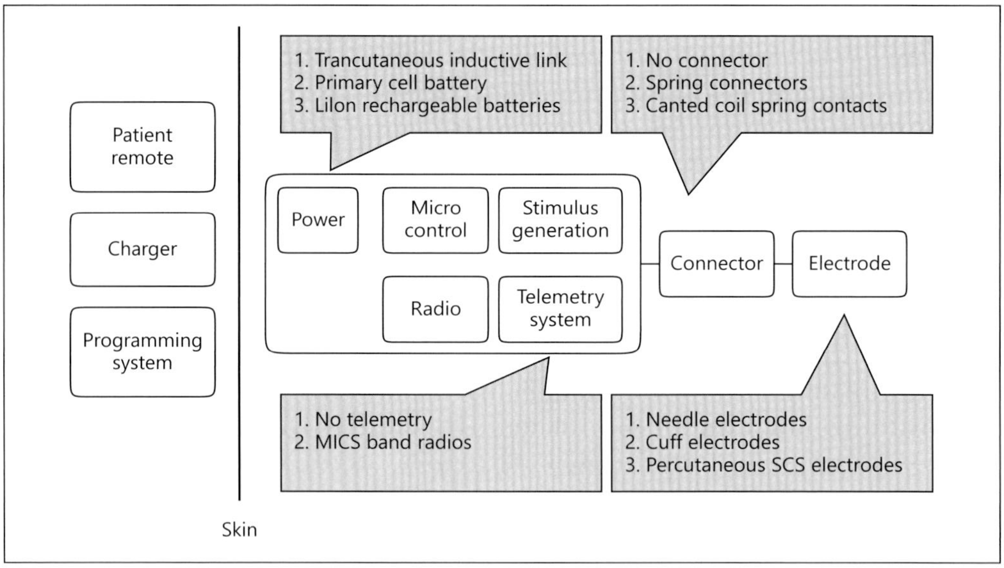

Fig. 11. Schematic diagram of the elements of PNS stimulation system. The evolution of subcomponents is detailed in the call outs. Medical Implant Communication Service (MICS) is the name of a specification for using frequencies between 402 and 405 MHz for communication with medical implants. LiIon refers to lithium ion rechargeable batteries.

power source of choice. One key advantage in using rechargeable powered devices is that they can be made smaller, and in PNS applications where the leads are placed in the region of pain, the choice of location for the generator is often limited.

Modern neurostimulation systems are highly programmable and employ low-power microcontrollers to generate timing and stimulation sequences. There have been dramatic advances in microcontroller technology over the last decade, and more and more powerful processing is available for implementation in neuromodulation systems; however, for PNS it is not yet clear how this potential translates into clear clinical benefit. The range of programming options is vast, but so far there is no clear rationale for choosing parameters.

The area that can make the biggest impact on both efficacy and safety of PNS is lead design. As mentioned previously, the major complications that occur in PNS are related to the leads, extensions, or anchors. Current leads are too stiff and large for most of the target areas where they are implanted. Lead diameters should be much smaller compared to current leads to accommodate placement in locations such as the face or periphery. A lead designed for PNS applications should have flexibility regarding the location of the electrodes as each application has unique stimulation requirements. Electrodes need to occupy a large portion of the lead while maintaining flexibility. Large electrodes will create larger fields with low currents preferentially stimulating A-beta fibers over A-delta. These requirements will require a shift in the way current leads are made and potentially new materials.

Despite the relatively limited engineering design efforts that have been made with regard to PNS, it is becoming a popular alternative therapy for patients with certain types of chronic pain. Focused efforts on PNS are needed to create specific devices for this application to increase its acceptance, improve the therapy, and reduce complications.

References

1 Shelden CH: Depolarization in the treatment of trigeminal neuralgia. Evaluation of compression and electrical methods; clinical concept of neurophysiological mechanism; in Kingston RS, Dumke PR (eds): Pain. Boston, Little Brown, 1966, pp 373–386.

2 Melzack R, Wall PD: Pain mechanisms: a new theory. Science 1965;150:971–979.

3 Fromm GH, Terrence CF, Maroon JC: Trigeminal neuralgia: current concepts regarding etiology and pathogenesis. Arch Neurol 1984;41:1204–1207.

4 Sweet WH, Wepsic JG: Treatment of chronic pain by stimulation of fibers of primary afferent neuron. Trans Am Neurol Assoc 1968;93:103–107.

5 Long DM: Electrical stimulation for relief of pain from chronic nerve injury. J Neurosurg 1973;39: 718–722.

6 Campbell JN, Long DM: Peripheral nerve stimulation in the treatment of intractable pain. J Neurosurg 1976;45:692–699.

7 Picaza JA, Cannon BW, Hunter SE, Boyd AS, Guma J, Maurer D: Pain suppression by peripheral nerve stimulation. Part II. Observations with implanted devices. Surg Neurol 1975;4:115–126.

8 Law JD, Swett J, Kirsch WM: Retrospective analysis of 22 patients with chronic pain treated by peripheral nerve stimulation. J Neurosurg 1980;52:482–485.

9 Waisbrod H, Panhans C, Hansen D, Gerbershagen HU: Direct nerve stimulation for painful peripheral neuropathies. J Bone Joint Surg Br 1985;67:470–472.

10 Nashold BS Jr, Goldner JL, Mullen JB, Bright DS: Long-term pain control by direct peripheral-nerve stimulation. J Bone Joint Surg Am 1982;64:1–10.

11 Nashold BS Jr, Mullen JB, Avery R: Peripheral nerve stimulation for pain relief using a multicontact electrode system: technical note. J Neurosurg 1979;51: 872–873.

12 Neilson KD, Watts C, Clark WK: Peripheral nerve injury from implantation of chronic stimulating electrodes for pain control. Surg Neurol 1976;5:51–53.

13 Racz GB, Browne T, Lewis R Jr: Peripheral stimulator implant for treatment of causalgia caused by electrical burns. Tex Med 1988;84:45–50.

14 Racz GB, Lewis B Jr, Heavner JE, Scott J: Peripheral nerve stimulator implant for treatment of RSD; in Stanton-Hicks MD, Jänig W, Boas RA (eds): Reflex Sympathetic Dystrophy. New York, Springer, 1990, pp 135–141.

15 Strege DW, Cooney WP, Wood MB, Johnson SJ, Metcalf BJ: Chronic peripheral nerve pain treated with direct electrical nerve stimulation. J Hand Surg 1994;19:931–939.

16 Urban BJ, Nashold BS Jr: Combined epidural and peripheral nerve stimulation for relief of pain. J Neurosurg 1982;57:365–369.

17 Weiner RL, Reed KL: Peripheral neurostimulation for control of intractable occipital neuralgia. Neuromodulation 1999;2:217–221.

18 Slavin KV, Colpan ME, Munawar N, Wess C, Nersesyan H: Trigeminal and occipital peripheral nerve stimulation for craniofacial pain: a single-institution experience and review of the literature. Neurosurg Focus 2006;21:E5.

19 Dunteman E: Peripheral nerve stimulation for unremitting ophthalmic postherpetic neuralgia. Neuromodulation 2002;5:32–37.

20 Matharu MS, Bartsch T, Ward N, Frackowiak RSJ, Weiner R, Goadsby PJ: Central neuromodulation in chronic migraine patients with suboccipital stimulators: a PET study. Brain 2004;127:220–230.

21 Silberstein SD, Dodick DW, Saper J, Huh B, Slavin KV, Sharan A, Reed K, Narouze S, Mogilner A, Goldstein J, Trentman T, Vaisman J, Ordia J, Weber P, Deer T, Levy R, Diaz RL, Washburn SN, Mekhail N: Safety and efficacy of peripheral nerve stimulation of the occipital nerves for the management of chronic migraine: results from a randomized, multicenter, double-blinded, controlled study. Cephalalgia 2012; 32:1165–1179.

22 Slavin KV, Wess C: Trigeminal branch stimulation for intractable neuropathic pain: technical note. Neuromodulation 2005;8:7–13.

23 Trentman TL, Zimmerman RS: Occipital nerve stimulation: technical and surgical aspects of implantation. Headache 2008;48:319–327.

24 Schwedt TJ, Dodick DW, Hentz J, Trentman TL, Zimmerman RS: Occipital nerve stimulation for chronic headache – long-term safety and efficacy. Cephalalgia 2007;27:153–157.
25 Aló KM, Yland MJ, Redko V, Feler C, Naumann C: Lumbar and sacral nerve root stimulation (NRS) in the treatment of chronic pain: a novel anatomic approach and neuro stimulation technique. Neuromodulation 1999;2:23–31.
26 Falco FJ, Kim D, Onyewu CO: Cervical nerve root stimulation: demonstration of an extra-foraminal technique. Pain Physician 2004;7:99–102.
27 Goroszeniuk T, Kothari S, Hamann W: Subcutaneous neuromodulating implant targeted at the site of pain. Reg Anesth Pain Med 2006;31:168–171.
28 Paicius RM, Bernstein CA, Lempert-Cohen C: Peripheral nerve field stimulation for the treatment of chronic low back pain: preliminary results of long-term follow-up: a case series. Neuromodulation 2007;10:279–290.
29 Verrills P, Mitchell B, Vivian D, Sinclair C: Peripheral nerve stimulation: a treatment for chronic low back pain and failed back surgery syndrome? Neuromodulation 2009;12:68–75.
30 Stinson LW, Roderer GT, Cross NE, Davis BE: Peripheral subcutaneous electrostimulation for control of intractable post-operative inguinal pain: a case report series. Neuromodulation 2001;4:99–104.
31 Lipov EG, Joshi JR, Sanders S, Slavin KV: Use of peripheral subcutaneous field stimulation for the treatment of axial neck pain: a case report. Neuromodulation 2009;12:292–295.
32 Paicius RM, Bernstein CA, Lempert-Cohen C: Peripheral nerve field stimulation in chronic abdominal pain. Pain Physician 2006;9:261–266.
33 Yakovlev AE, Peterson AT: Peripheral nerve stimulation in treatment of intractable postherpetic neuralgia. Neuromodulation 2007;10:373–375.
34 Kapural L, Mekhail N, Hayek SM, Stanton-Hicks M, Malak O: Occipital nerve electrical stimulation via the midline approach and subcutaneous surgical leads for treatment of severe occipital neuralgia: a pilot study. Anesth Analg 2005;101:171–174.
35 Jones RL: Occipital nerve stimulation using a Medtronic Resume II electrode array. Pain Physician 2003;6:507–508.
36 Oh MY, Ortega J, Bellotte JB, Whiting DM, Aló K: Peripheral nerve stimulation for the treatment of occipital neuralgia and transformed migraine using a c1-2-3 subcutaneous paddle style electrode: a technical report. Neuromodulation 2004;7:103–112.
37 Ordia J, Vaisman J: Subcutaneous peripheral nerve stimulation with paddle lead for treatment of low back pain: case report. Neuromodulation 2009;12: 205–209.
38 Ghoname EA, White PF, Ahmed HE, Hamza MA, Craig WF, Noe CE: Percutaneous electrical nerve stimulation: an alternative to TENS in the management of sciatica. Pain 1999;83:193–199.
39 Hamza MA, White PF, Craig WF, Ghoname ES, Ahmed HE, Proctor TJ, Noe CE, Vakharia AS, Gajraj N: Percutaneous electrical nerve stimulation: a novel analgesic therapy for diabetic neuropathic pain. Diabetes Care 2000;23:365–370.
40 Ahmed HE, White PF, Craig WF, Hamza MA, Ghoname ES, Gajraj NM: Use of percutaneous electrical nerve stimulation (PENS) in the short-term management of headache. Headache 2000;40:311–315.
41 Cameron T, Loeb GE, Peck RA, Schulman JH, Strojnik P, Troyk PR: Micromodular implants to provide electrical stimulation of paralyzed muscles and limbs. IEEE Trans Biomed Eng 1997;44:781–790.
42 Salter AD, Bagg SD, Creasy JL, Romano C, Romano D, Richmond FJR, Loeb GE: First clinical experience with BION implants for therapeutic electrical stimulation. Neuromodulation 2004;7:38–47.
43 Baker L, Palmer E, Waters R, Chun S: Rehabilitation of the arm and hand following stroke – a clinical trial with BIONs. Conf Proc IEEE Eng Med Biol Soc 2004;6:4186–4188.
44 Weber DJ, Stein RB, Chan KM, Loeb G, Richmond F, Rolf R, James K, Chong SL: BIONic WalkAide for correcting foot drop. Neural Syst Rehabil Eng IEEE Trans 2005;13:242–246.
45 Trentman TL, Rosenfeld DM, Vargas BB, Schwedt TJ, Zimmerman RS, Dodick DW: Greater occipital nerve stimulation via the Bion microstimulator: implantation technique and stimulation parameters. Clinical trial: NCT00205894. Pain Physician 2009;12:621–628.
46 Schoenen J, Jensen RH, Lantéri-Minet M, Láinez MJ, Gaul C, Goodman AM, Caparso A, May A: Stimulation of the sphenopalatine ganglion (SPG) for cluster headache treatment. Pathway CH-1: a randomized, sham-controlled study. Cephalalgia 2013;33:816–830.
47 Deer TR, Grigsby E, Weiner RL, Wilcosky B, Kramer JM: A Prospective study of dorsal root ganglion stimulation for the relief of chronic pain. Neuromodulation 2013;16:67–72.
48 Soin A, Kilgore K, Bhadra H, Fang ZP: Feasibility study on high-frequency electrical nerve block for amputation pain. Neuromodulation 2011;14:561.
49 Holsheimer J, Struijk JJ, Rijkhoff NJ: Contact combinations in epidural spinal cord stimulation. A comparison by computer modeling. Stereotact Funct Neurosurg 1991;56:220–233.
50 Law JD: Spinal stimulation: statistical superiority of monophasic stimulation of narrowly separated, longitudinal bipoles having rostral cathodes. Appl Neurophysiol 1983;46:129–137.

51 Holsheimer J, Wesselink WA: Optimum electrode geometry for spinal cord stimulation: the narrow bipole and tripole. Med Biol Eng Comput 1997;35: 493–497.
52 Gardner EP, Martin JH, Jessell TM: The bodily senses; in Kandel E, Schwartz J (eds): Principles of Neural Science, ed 4. New York, McGraw-Hill, 2000, pp 430–450.
53 Provitera V, Nolano M, Pagano A, Caporaso G, Stancanelli A, Santoro L: Myelinated nerve endings in human skin. Muscle Nerve 2007;35:767–775.
54 Nolano M, Provitera V, Crisci C, Stancanelli A, Wendelschafer-Crabb G, Kennedy WR, Santoro L: Quantification of myelinated endings and mechanoreceptors in human digital skin. Ann Neurol 2003;54:197–205.
55 Ebenezer GJ, Hauer P, Gibbons C, McArthur JC, Polydefkis M: Assessment of epidermal nerve fibers: a new diagnostic and predictive tool for peripheral neuropathies. J Neuropathol Exp Neurol 2007;66: 1059–1073.
56 Ranck JB Jr: Which elements are excited in electrical stimulation of mammalian central nervous system: a review. Brain Res 1975;98:417–440.
57 Struijk JJ, Holsheimer J, van der Heide GG, Boom HB: Recruitment of dorsal column fibers in spinal cord stimulation: influence of collateral branching. IEEE Trans Biomed Eng 1992;39:903–912.
58 Li CL, Bak A: Excitability characteristics of the A- and C-fibers in a peripheral nerve. Exp Neurol 1976; 50:67–79.
59 McIntyre CC, Richardson AG, Grill WM: Modeling the excitability of mammalian nerve fibers: influence of afterpotentials on the recovery cycle. J Neurophysiol 2002;87:995–1006.
60 Falco FJ, Berger J, Vrable A, Onyewu O, Zhu J: Cross talk: a new method for peripheral nerve stimulation. An observational report with cadaveric verification. Pain Physician 2009;12:965–983.

Tracy Cameron, PhD
18 Norma Crescent
Toronto, Ont. M6P 3H1 (Canada)
E-Mail tcameron086@gmail.com

Slavin KV (ed): Stimulation of the Peripheral Nervous System. The Neuromodulation Frontier.
Prog Neurol Surg. Basel, Karger, 2016, vol 29, pp 20–28 (DOI: 10.1159/000434652)

Theoretical Basis of Vagus Nerve Stimulation

Frank Attenello · Arun Paul Amar · Charles Liu · Michael L.J. Apuzzo

Department of Neurological Surgery, University of Southern California, Los Angeles, Calif., USA

Abstract

Despite a myriad of medical and surgical treatments for epilepsy developed over the past few decades, a large subset of patients remains refractory to treatment. Over this time period, vagus nerve stimulation (VNS) has become an accepted and viable treatment modality for this population. Since the earliest report of VNS implantation in 1988, tens of thousands of patients worldwide have received VNS therapy, and >100,000 patient-years of experience have been accrued. The mechanisms underlying the response to VNS therapy continue to be elucidated. As understanding of the VNS mechanisms of action continues to grow, more pathologies will arise as potential treatment indications. Furthermore, current treatment populations with refractory epilepsy, depression, and inflammatory diseases may enjoy improved response to stimulation.

Despite a myriad of medical and surgical treatments for epilepsy developed over the past few decades, a large subset of patients remains refractory to treatment. Over this time period, vagus nerve stimulation (VNS) has become an accepted and viable treatment modality for this population. The stimulator system is comprised of the Neurocybernetic Prosthesis (NCP) from Cyberonics Inc. (Houston, Tex., USA), with the earliest report of VNS implantation performed in 1988. Since then, tens of thousands of patients worldwide have received VNS therapy, and >100,000 patient-years of experience have accrued (Cyberonics, data on file).

The system relies on a mechanism that delivers electrical stimulation to the left cervical vagus nerve trunk, activating axons of afferent neurons, and subsequent changes to neuronal excitability throughout the central nervous system (CNS). Despite widespread use and clinical success in the implementation of the VNS system, the target(s) within the brain and exact mechanism by which VNS modulates seizure activity remain unclear [1]. Here, we review the theoretical rationale of VNS for a variety of CNS disorders. Additional details can be found in our previous publications [1–5].

Historical Basis for Vagus Nerve Stimulation Therapy

Pelops, often cited as a teacher of Galen, was the first to note the concept of external modulation for seizure treatment in the second century AD. His writings refer to aborting continued progression or generalization of a partial seizure via use of ligatures applied to the seizing limb. J.L. Corning, in the 1880s, believed seizures to be the product of alterations in blood flow in the brain. He employed an 'electrocompressor', targeting the vagus nerve at the cervical trunk using transcutaneous stimulation [6]. Due to inconsistent outcomes, however, the pursuit of the vagus nerve as a target of seizure therapy remained limited.

In 1938, it was reported that VNS induced synchronized activity in the motor cortex of cats [7]. Subsequent work in 1952 by Zanchetti et al. [8] revealed electroencephalographic desynchronization in response to VNS ranging from 2 to 300 Hz. These effects were blocked with ligature of the proximal vagus nerve trunk.

More recent work has confirmed theories that stimulation of multiple sensory pathways, including cutaneous afferent fibers and the cervical vagus nerve, shows profound effect on both electroencephalogram (EEG) synchronization and sleep cycle.

As seizure activity also exhibits these specific synchronized patterns, it is hypothesized that appropriately timed stimulation of the vagus nerve may interfere and thus prevent epileptiform activity. However, it was not until 1988 that VNS implantation for drug-resistant epilepsy was reported as an implantable system in humans [9].

Vagus Nerve Anatomy and Physiology

To understand the theory and rationale behind VNS, the underlying function of the vagus nerve must be understood and considered. Arising from the medulla, the paired vagus nerves exit the jugular foramen and extend via the nodose ganglia into the neck, following the esophagus and entering the abdomen as a dorsal and ventral trunk [10].

The vagus nerve is most commonly viewed as a primary efferent nerve, due to well-documented efferent tracts innervating striated muscle of the larynx and parasympathetic projections controlling the heart, lungs, and gastrointestinal tract. It is important to note, however, that up to 80% of vagal fibers project as general somatic afferents and visceral afferent fibers towards the brain [11].

The nerve is composed of A-, B-, C-, and A-delta fibers, designated by conduction velocity, size, and myelination status. A-fibers are large, myelinated fibers carrying afferent visceral information. B-fibers are small and myelinated, and carry parasympathetic signals. C-fibers are the most numerous, comprising up to 80% of fibers; these small unmyelinated fibers carry afferent visceral signals to the brain [12].

Of note, early theories suggesting that VNS relied on recruitment of sensory afferent C-fibers and A-delta fibers were put into question by studies showing that the antiepileptic effects of VNS were retained following selective inactivation of these small unmyelinated fibers by capsaicin treatment. Because destruction of C-fibers does not alter VNS seizure suppression in rats, A- and B-fibers are now suspected as the activated groups [13].

The somatic sensory afferents, representing a small fraction of the vagus, transmit sensation from the concha of the ear. The visceral afferent fibers, comprising a larger fraction of the nerve, originate from multiple receptors in the aorta, heart, lungs, and gastrointestinal tract, mediating digestive reflexes [11]. These afferent vagal tracts then project to multiple sites of potential seizure genesis throughout the brain, including the diencephalon, amygdala, hippocampus, and insular cortex, as well as the cerebellum and brainstem centers. The majority of these projections pass through the nucleus tractus solitarius (NTS), the entry level of peripheral vagal nerve afferents [14]. The NTS then projects sensory information to the forebrain via the parabrachial nucleus and also has direct output to the amygdala and hypothalamus.

The NTS is hypothesized as a central mediator of VNS action, as afferent polysynaptic pathways project to widespread cortical regions, increasing activity in thalamocortical projection pathways and decreasing activity in the amygdala and hippocampus [15].

A smaller subset of fibers forms direct monosynaptic connection with targets in the medial reticular formation of the medulla, the dorsal motor nucleus of the vagus, the area postrema, and the nucleus cuneatus. Studies in animal models suggest that the locus coeruleus and raphe nucleus may mediate the most important of these other pathways, as bilateral chemical lesions of these centers abolish the seizure-suppressing effects of VNS therapy [16]. Furthermore, rat models treated with VNS show increased *c fos* expression, representing increased neuronal activity, in the locus coeruleus [17].

The importance of the locus coeruleus and raphe nucleus suggests a central role for their respective neurotransmitter products, norepinephrine and serotonin, in the antiepileptic mechanism of VNS.

Norepinephrine and serotonin are further noted to induce interneurons to release gamma-amino butyric acid (GABA) in the brain, potentially increasing seizure threshold. However, evaluation of cerebrospinal fluid levels of GABA and serotonin metabolites in VNS-treated patients has suggested an inverse correlation with efficacy, providing continued ambiguity regarding the role of neurotransmitters in the antiepileptic function of VNS therapy [1].

The VNS stimulation settings commonly used in patient care are insufficient to produce any effect on the overall background of EEG rhythms [18]. However, multiple cortical, subcortical, and other forebrain structures have been implicated as pivotal in VNS therapy. Regions including the cerebral cortex, hippocampus, brainstem, thalamus, and cerebellum have shown reported effects from VNS therapy. The response of these disparate regions has prompted authors to propose that its antiepileptic actions relate to effects on the brainstem reticular activating system, which projects to these forebrain structures [4].

Studies employing positron emission tomography (PET) have further elucidated the cortical regions associated with VNS treatment by measuring regional cerebral blood flow during treatment. Rapid changes in regional cerebral blood flow are thought to reflect transsynaptic neurotransmission [19]. These studies suggest changes in several regions, including the ipsilateral anterior thalamus and cingulate gyrus, contralateral thalamus, and ipsilateral cerebellum, or bilateral activation of the hypothalami and insular cortices [1, 4]. PET scans demonstrating increases in thalamic blood flow during VNS therapy have shown positive correlations with improved seizure responsiveness [20].

In addition to the disparate regions activated, variation is noted following short- and long-term phases of VNS treatment, possibly reflecting the effects of attenuated response to individual VNS impulses following chronic adaptation to central processing. Functional imaging has noted longer-term changes in regions with vagal nerve projections including the thalamus, cerebellum, orbitofrontal cortex, limbic system, hypothalamus, and medulla [21]. Studies have been further confounded by limitations of the study populations, including effects of prior cranial surgery and seizures during PET scanning [1].

With the option of two separate vagus nerve targets for stimulation, the symmetry of vagal nerve response to stimulation has been investigated. Right- versus left-sided vagal stimulation is equally effective in controlling seizures in animal models, and bilateral stimulation produces no measurably greater effect than unilateral stimulation [1]. Using techniques such as EEG and immunolabeling against *fos*, these studies suggest that unilateral afferent vagal impulses generate bilaterally symmetric responses in the cerebral cortex and subcortical structures [1].

In contrast, vagal efferent innervation appears asymmetric. In some species, the right vagus nerve innervates the sinoatrial node (primarily affecting the pacemaker of the heart), while the left one preferentially supplies the atrioventricular node, primarily affecting contractility alone [1]. Canine studies have shown that stimulation of the right vagus nerve produces greater cardiac slowing than similar stimulation of the left vagus. For these reasons, the NCP VNS system is generally inserted on the left side, although anecdotal experience with right-sided VNS in humans has been well tolerated [12].

Some animal studies have shown that cardiac and respiratory function are adversely affected by VNS while others have not, depending on the species used, the stimulation parameters applied, and other variables [1]. Such side effects do not occur in humans because stimulation can be performed distant from the site at which the cardiac branches originate from the cervical vagus trunk [22].

Alternative Uses of Vagus Nerve Stimulation

In the course of studying VNS for the treatment of epilepsy, a number of serendipitous effects have been observed. For instance, many patients have reported an improvement in mood, cognition, and well-being not related to seizure control per se [1].

Stimulation of the vagus nerve has been shown to enhance retention in verbal learning tasks, confirming the hypothesis that vagus nerve activation modulates memory formation similarly to influence of arousal. In addition, VNS has been shown to exert an antinociceptive effect in rats.

As a result of these fortuities, VNS has been proposed as a treatment for medically refractory depression [23]. Studies have noted substantial improvements in mood during VNS trials for epilepsy that were not attributable to seizure control alone. Furthermore, neuroanatomic studies of vagal afferent connections suggest that the NTS and locus coeruleus project to the amygdala, stria terminalis, and other limbic structures involved in mood regulation [11]. During VNS trials for epilepsy, PET studies incidentally noted decreased blood flow to the hippocampus, amygdala, and cingulate gyrus reminiscent of the effects of selective serotonin reuptake inhibitors and other antidepressant drugs [23]. Functional magnetic resonance imaging (MRI) studies in depressed patients show VNS-induced increases in blood oxygen level-dependent activity in multiple regions associated with mood disorders [21].

Depression has been hypothesized to result from imbalances in cerebral metabolism characterized by frontal hypometabolism and limbic hypermetabolism [24]. MRI and PET studies have revealed correction specific to this imbalance when VNS is employed: stimulation results in enhanced blood flow to frontal regions including the orbitofrontal cortex, and decreased blood flow to the subgenual cingulate cortex, hippocampus, insula, amygdala, and temporal and parietal regions [25].

In addition, many anticonvulsant medications have mood-stabilizing effects and are useful treatments for the depressive phase of bipolar affective disorder [23]. Conversely, electroconvulsive therapy, an effective antidepressant therapy, has been noted to exert anticonvulsant effects. Finally, VNS alters the CNS concentrations of multiple neurotransmitters noted in the pathogenesis of major depression, including norepinephrine, serotonin, glutamate, and other monoamine neurotransmitters [23].

Other hints suggest that VNS may have utility for additional neuropsychiatric illnesses. For instance, several theories of anxiety purport faulty or erratic interpretation of peripheral information that flows into the CNS [23]. By affecting the flux of this information, VNS might have therapeutic potential in treating anxiety disorders. Similarly, the vagus nerve is known to transmit signals pertaining to hunger, satiety, and pain. For those reasons, potential applications for obesity, addiction, and pain syndromes seem plausible.

The effects of VNS on feeding behavior were investigated in a canine model [26]. Six dogs underwent bilateral VNS at parameters similar to those used for epilepsy. Feeding times, amount consumed, and weight were serially monitored and compared with baseline. In response to VNS, feeding behavior changed following a variable period of latency. Both the rate of consumption and the amount consumed decreased, leading to weight loss. When stimulation was suspended, eating returned to baseline in 3–5 days, but resuming the stimulation reproduced the initial dietary changes.

The NTS sends fibers to the dorsal raphe and other areas of the reticular formation known to control levels of consciousness [11]. Thus, VNS has been considered as a potential treatment for disorders of sleep or alertness such as narcolepsy and coma. VNS is also a possible treatment for additional conditions such as movement disorders, migraine, and others. Preliminary results in patients suffering from both epilepsy and autism suggest that VNS may exert beneficial effects in treatment of the latter condition alone.

More recent evidence has suggested a significant role for the vagus nerve in maintenance of homeostasis via activation of a cholinergic anti-inflammatory pathway through afferent and efferent projections [27]. Circulating proinflammatory cytokines normally released from the intestine including interleukin-1β, interleukin-6, and tumor necrosis factor (TNF), locally stimulate vagus afferents, leading to activation of the hypothalamic-pituitary-adrenal axis.

Vagal efferents then activate a cholinergic anti-inflammatory pathway, through acetylcholine released at the nerve terminal, activating macrophages via the α_7-nicotinic acetylcholine receptor. Activated macrophages then inhibit release of pro-inflammatory cytokines [28]. The spleen, a major source of TNF-α in endotoxemia [29], is thought to be another major end effector in these anti-inflammatory effects, as VNS during endotoxemia attenuates TNF-α release by spleen macrophages [30].

Impairment of this pathway is associated with multiple inflammatory pathologies including rheumatoid arthritis, inflammatory bowel disease, pancreatitis, colitis, multiple sclerosis, asthma, and dermatitis [31, 32].

Subsequent VNS employment in animal models has shown decreased macrophage activation [33] as well as an increase in anti-inflammatory ACTH and corticosterone plasma levels [34]. Furthermore, colonic inflammation and weight loss are decreased in rats with colitis during VNS therapy [35]. The efferent limb of the vagus is noted to be the necessary effector, as ligation of proximal vagus does not decrease the anti-inflammatory effect [33, 36].

Vagus Nerve Stimulation Amplitudes and Frequency Modification for Site-Specific Cerebral Modulation

The NCP device permits the delivery of VNS at different amplitudes, frequencies, pulse widths, and duty cycles [1]. At present, these settings are titrated empirically according to the desired effect and tolerability. Varying these parameters in different combinations affects different regions of the brain, subsequently influencing distinct pathologic conditions.

The pulse frequency of stimulation for activation of the vagal nerve fibers occupies a critical role in the function of various therapies. While high-frequency stimulation (20–30 Hz) is employed most commonly in VNS treatment for epilepsy and depression, lower frequencies (1–10 Hz) are noted to select for vagal efferents and the above-noted cholinergic anti-inflammatory pathway through α_7-nicotinic acetylcholine receptors [33, 36]. Low-frequency stimulation specificity for the efferent vagus results from slow natural pacemaker activity (1–2 Hz) of signals emitted from the dorsal motor nucleus of the vagus that are observed in projections to the digestive tract [37].

The following differential effects were demonstrated in a population of depressed adults. Blood oxygen level-dependent functional MRI showed increased brain activity in the orbitofrontal cortex, frontal pole, hypothalamus, left pallidum, and thalamus with 20-Hz VNS, while decreased brain activity was noted with a 5-Hz frequency. A more subtle frequency and dose effect of stimulation on resulting cerebral blood flow was further noted [21].

Furthermore, a rat model has quantified *c fos* reactivity in response to isolated afferent VNS stimulation after vagotomy. At frequencies of 10 Hz, a significant dose-dependent increase in *c fos* expression was noted when compared to lower frequencies [38].

Low-frequency stimulation at 1–10 Hz by VNS in animal models has suggested activation of vagal efferents and subsequent anti-inflammatory effects in response to endotoxin-induced TNF-mediated shock [36] and macrophage activation [33]. The anti-inflammatory effects of efferent VNS stimulation have generated interest in trials targeting rheumatoid arthritis and Crohn's disease using VNS therapy.

Conclusion

The mechanisms underlying the response to VNS therapy continue to be elucidated more than a quarter century after the first-reported VNS implantation in 1988. As understanding of the VNS mechanisms of action continues to grow, more pathologies will arise as potential treatment indications. Furthermore, current treatment populations with refractory epilepsy, depression, and inflammatory diseases may enjoy improved response to stimulation.

References

1 Amar AP, Heck CN, Levy ML, Smith T, DeGiorgio CM, Oviedo S, Apuzzo ML: An institutional experience with cervical vagus nerve trunk stimulation for medically refractory epilepsy: rationale, technique, and outcome. Neurosurgery 1998;43:1265–1276, discussion 1276–1280.

2 Amar AP, Apuzzo ML, Liu CY: Vagus nerve stimulation therapy after failed cranial surgery for intractable epilepsy: results from the vagus nerve stimulation therapy patient outcome registry. Neurosurgery 2004;55:1086–1093.

3 Amar AP, DeGiorgio CM, Tarver WB, Apuzzo ML: Long-term multicenter experience with vagus nerve stimulation for intractable partial seizures: results of the XE5 trial. Stereotact Funct Neurosurg 1999;73: 104–108.

4 Amar AP, Heck CN, DeGiorgio CM, Apuzzo ML: Experience with vagus nerve stimulation for intractable epilepsy: some questions and answers. Neurol Med Chir (Tokyo) 1999;39:489–495.

5 Amar AP, Levy ML, McComb JG, Apuzzo ML: Vagus nerve stimulation for control of intractable seizures in childhood. Pediatr Neurosurg 2001;34:218–223.

6 Lanska DJ: J.L. Corning and vagal nerve stimulation for seizures in the 1880s. Neurology 2002;58:452–459.
7 Bailey H, Bremer F: Sensory cortical representation of the vagus nerve. J Neurophysiol 1938;1:405–412.
8 Zanchetti A, Wang SC, Moruzzi G: Effect of afferent vagal stimulation on the electroencephalogram of the cat in cerebral isolation. Boll Soc Ital Biol Sper 1952;28:627–628.
9 Penry JK, Dean JC: Prevention of intractable partial seizures by intermittent vagal stimulation in humans: preliminary results. Epilepsia 1990;31(suppl 2):S40–S43.
10 Berthoud HR, Neuhuber WL: Functional and chemical anatomy of the afferent vagal system. Auton Neurosci 2000;85:1–17.
11 Rutecki P: Anatomical, physiological, and theoretical basis for the antiepileptic effect of vagus nerve stimulation. Epilepsia 1990;31(suppl 2):S1–S6.
12 Woodbury DM, Woodbury JW: Effects of vagal stimulation on experimentally induced seizures in rats. Epilepsia 1990;31(suppl 2):S7–S19.
13 Krahl SE, Senanayake SS, Handforth A: Destruction of peripheral C-fibers does not alter subsequent vagus nerve stimulation-induced seizure suppression in rats. Epilepsia 2001;42:586–589.
14 Cheng G, Zhou X, Qu J, Ashwell KW, Paxinos G: Central vagal sensory and motor connections: human embryonic and fetal development. Auton Neurosci 2004;114:83–96.
15 Beekwilder JP, Beems T: Overview of the clinical applications of vagus nerve stimulation. J Clin Neurophysiol 2010;27:130–138.
16 Krahl SE, Clark KB, Smith DC, Browning RA: Locus coeruleus lesions suppress the seizure-attenuating effects of vagus nerve stimulation. Epilepsia 1998;39:709–714.
17 Naritoku DK, Terry WJ, Helfert RH: Regional induction of fos immunoreactivity in the brain by anticonvulsant stimulation of the vagus nerve. Epilepsy Res 1995;22:53–62.
18 Salinsky MC, Burchiel KJ: Vagus nerve stimulation has no effect on awake EEG rhythms in humans. Epilepsia 1993;34:299–304.
19 Henry TR: Therapeutic mechanisms of vagus nerve stimulation. Neurology 2002;59(6 suppl 4):S3–S14.
20 Henry TR, Votaw JR, Pennell PB, Epstein CM, Bakay RA, Faber TL, Grafton ST, Hoffman JM: Acute blood flow changes and efficacy of vagus nerve stimulation in partial epilepsy. Neurology 1999;52:1166–1173.
21 Lomarev M, Denslow S, Nahas Z, Chae JH, George MS, Bohning DE: Vagus nerve stimulation (VNS) synchronized BOLD fMRI suggests that VNS in depressed adults has frequency/dose dependent effects. J Psychiatr Res 2002;36:219–227.
22 Amar AP, Levy ML, Apuzzo ML: Vagus nerve stimulation for intractable epilepsy; in Rengachary S (ed): Neurosurgical Operative Atlas. Chicago, American Association of Neurological Surgeons, 2000, pp 179–188.
23 George MS, Sackeim HA, Rush AJ, Marangell LB, Nahas Z, Husain MM, Lisanby S, Burt T, Goldman J, Ballenger JC: Vagus nerve stimulation: a new tool for brain research and therapy. Biol Psychiatry 2000;47:287–295.
24 Mayberg HS: Positron emission tomography imaging in depression: a neural systems perspective. Neuroimaging Clin N Am 2003;13:805–815.
25 Conway CR, Sheline YI, Chibnall JT, George MS, Fletcher JW, Mintun MA: Cerebral blood flow changes during vagus nerve stimulation for depression. Psychiatry Res 2006;146:179–184.
26 Reddy R, Horovitz J, Roslin M: Chronic bilateral vagal nerve stimulation (VNS) changes eating behavior resulting in weight loss in a canine model. J Am Coll Surg 2000;191:S27–S28.
27 Dantzer R, Konsman JP, Bluthe RM, Kelley KW: Neural and humoral pathways of communication from the immune system to the brain: parallel or convergent? Auton Neurosci 2000;85:60–65.
28 de Jonge WJ, Ulloa L: The alpha7 nicotinic acetylcholine receptor as a pharmacological target for inflammation. Br J Pharmacol 2007;151:915–929.
29 Huston JM, Ochani M, Rosas-Ballina M, Liao H, Ochani K, Pavlov VA, Gallowitsch-Puerta M, Ashok M, Czura CJ, Foxwell B, Tracey KJ, Ulloa L: Splenectomy inactivates the cholinergic antiinflammatory pathway during lethal endotoxemia and polymicrobial sepsis. J Exp Med 2006;203:1623–1628.
30 Rosas-Ballina M, Ochani M, Parrish WR, Ochani K, Harris YT, Huston JM, Chavan S, Tracey KJ: Splenic nerve is required for cholinergic antiinflammatory pathway control of TNF in endotoxemia. Proc Natl Acad Sci U S A 2008;105:11008–11013.
31 Bonaz BL, Bernstein CN: Brain-gut interactions in inflammatory bowel disease. Gastroenterology 2013;144:36–49.
32 The FO, Boeckxstaens GE, Snoek SA, Cash JL, Bennink R, Larosa GJ, van den Wijngaard RM, Greaves DR, de Jonge WJ: Activation of the cholinergic antiinflammatory pathway ameliorates postoperative ileus in mice. Gastroenterology 2007;133:1219–1228.
33 de Jonge WJ, van der Zanden EP, The FO, Bijlsma MF, van Westerloo DJ, Bennink RJ, Berthoud HR, Uematsu S, Akira S, van den Wijngaard RM, Boeckxstaens GE: Stimulation of the vagus nerve attenuates macrophage activation by activating the Jak2-STAT3 signaling pathway. Nat Immunol 2005;6:844–851.

34 Hosoi T, Okuma Y, Nomura Y: Electrical stimulation of afferent vagus nerve induces IL-1beta expression in the brain and activates HPA axis. Am J Physiol Regul Integr Comp Physiol 2000;279:R141–R147.
35 Meregnani J, Clarencon D, Vivier M, Peinnequin A, Mouret C, Sinniger V, Picq C, Job A, Canini F, Jacquier-Sarlin M, Bonaz B: Anti-inflammatory effect of vagus nerve stimulation in a rat model of inflammatory bowel disease. Auton Neurosci 2011;160:82–89.
36 Borovikova LV, Ivanova S, Zhang M, Yang H, Botchkina GI, Watkins LR, Wang H, Abumrad N, Eaton JW, Tracey KJ: Vagus nerve stimulation attenuates the systemic inflammatory response to endotoxin. Nature 2000;405:458–462.
37 Fogel R, Zhang X, Renehan WE: Relationships between the morphology and function of gastric and intestinal distention-sensitive neurons in the dorsal motor nucleus of the vagus. J Comp Neurol 1996;364:78–91.
38 Osharina V, Bagaev V, Wallois F, Larnicol N: Autonomic response and Fos expression in the NTS following intermittent vagal stimulation: importance of pulse frequency. Auton Neurosci 2006;126–127:72–80.

Arun Paul Amar, MD
Department of Neurological Surgery
University of Southern California
1520 San Pablo Street, Suite 3800
Los Angeles, CA 9033 (USA)
E-Mail amar@aya.yale.edu

Slavin KV (ed): Stimulation of the Peripheral Nervous System. The Neuromodulation Frontier.
Prog Neurol Surg. Basel, Karger, 2016, vol 29, pp 29–38 (DOI: 10.1159/000434653)

Vagus Nerve Stimulation: Surgical Technique and Complications

Volker M. Tronnier

Department of Neurosurgery, University of Lübeck, Germany

Abstract

Chronic stimulation of the left vagus nerve (VNS) is commonly performed for different clinical conditions such as refractory epilepsy in children and adults, and major and bipolar depression. Despite more than 20 years of cumulative experience with VNS implantation, various surgery- and modality-related complications continue to occur in a sizable percentage of patients. A clear understanding of surgical anatomy and following standard operating protocol may, at least theoretically, reduce the number of complications. Here we present our way to perform VNS implantation and discuss different kinds of complications that each implanter should be aware of. Technical details of revision surgery are also presented.

Chronic stimulation of the left vagus nerve (VNS) is performed for different clinical conditions like refractory epilepsy in children and adults [1, 2], different pain syndromes [3, 4], depression [5], atrial fibrillation and chronic heart failure [6, 7], and morbid obesity [8, 9].

Experimental studies in animals and humans have demonstrated clinical efficacy of VNS in different acute and chronic pain models [10, 11]. Small clinical series of VNS alone [12–14] or in combination [15] have been successful in alleviating different headache syndromes often combined with the anticonvulsant effect. The central mechanisms [16, 17] responsible for the alleviation of different symptoms are beyond the scope of this chapter.

Surgical Technique

Anesthesiological Considerations

Anesthesia-related considerations are especially important in patients with refractory epilepsies. In these patients antiepileptic drugs should be given on the morning of surgery. The anesthesiologist should be aware that cytochrome p450 induction by many antiepileptic drugs may alter the metabolism of anesthetic drugs leading to higher consumption of opioids or muscle relaxants. Normocarbia should be pursued because hyperventilation may precipitate seizures. Propofol, midazolam, and thiopental have seizure-depressant effects, while ketamine may trigger seizure activity and should be avoided. During intraoperative trial stimulation, asystole or significant bradycardia can occur. Therefore, atropine and catecholamines should be immediately available. Postoperative hypoxic situations can occur (postoperative hemorrhage with airway obstruction, sleep apnea caused by stimulation) and should be taken into consideration. Careful monitoring of the patient in the recovery room and the ward is essential. Therefore, VNS should not be performed as an outpatient procedure.

Ear, Nose, and Throat Considerations
A pre- and postoperative laryngoscopy is recommended. Especially after surgery when intermittent or permanent hoarseness occurs, the cause should be diagnosed (vocal cord paresis, glottis edema, etc.). In case of dysphagia, a barium swallow might be necessary.

Skin-to-Skin Procedure
Informed consent should include possible complications:
- Infection (ca. 8–10%)
- Hemorrhage (<1%)
- Vocal cord paralysis (ca. 1–2%)
- Lead fracture or generator malfunction (1.0%)
- Bradycardia and asystole (<0.1%)
- Voice alteration, hoarseness, dysphonia during stimulation (ca. 40%)
- Horner's syndrome, facial weakness
- Hypertrophic scars
- Generator migration
- Painful muscle stimulation or muscle spasm (sternocleidomastoid)
- Shortness of breath, sleep apnea

Perioperative antibiotic prophylaxis with a second-generation cephalosporin is given (e.g. 3 doses of 1.5 g cefuroxime in adults or weight-adjusted in children). After induction of general anesthesia, the patient is positioned supine with the head turned slightly to the right (ca. 30°) and the neck extended with a shoulder roll (fig. 1). This facilitates passage of the tunneling rod. A 5-cm curved incision is made medially to the shoulder joint over the pectoral muscle below the clavicle (anterior fold of the axilla).

We prefer a transverse incision at the level of the 5th or 6th cervical vertebra of about 3–4 cm, crossing the ventral border of the sternocleidomastoid muscle pointing to the midline (fig. 2).

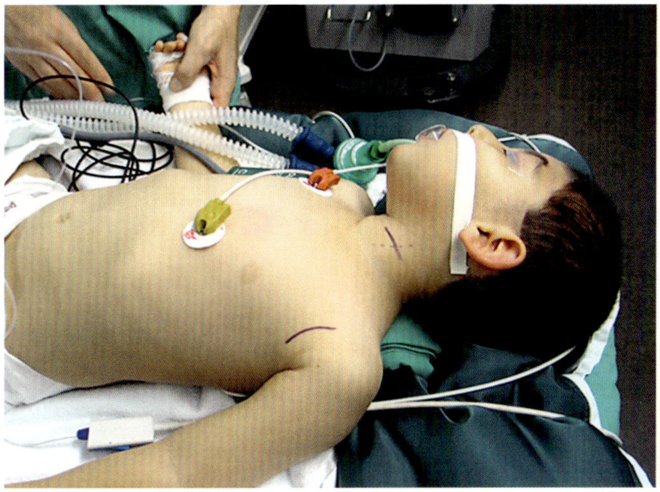

Fig. 1. Patient positioning with head turned to the opposite site and shoulder roll.

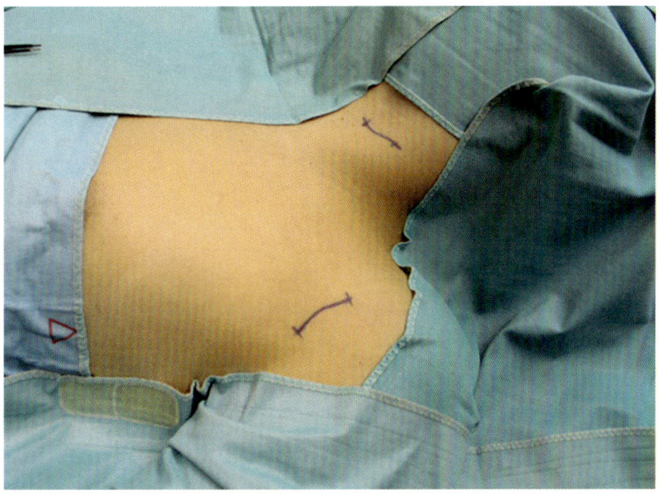

Fig. 2. Transverse skin incision at the anterior border of the sternocleidomastoid muscle and curved incision medially of the shoulder joint slightly above the anterior axillary fold.

The platysma is bluntly divided and retracted. The deep cervical fascia is opened at the anterior border of the sternocleidomastoid muscle (fig. 3).

Palpating the pulse of the carotid artery is essential before blunt dissection (with fingers) down to the neurovascular sheath. Sometimes the ventral part of the omohyoid muscle hinders exposure. Veins of the common facial vein complex can be coagulated and divided.

The sheath is then opened sharply with identification of the carotid artery medially and the internal jugular vein laterally. The vagus nerve is usually found in between in the depth. Sometimes a nerve is identified superficially of the carotid artery. This structure usually is part of the ansa cervicalis and should not be misinterpreted as the vagus nerve (fig. 4, 5).

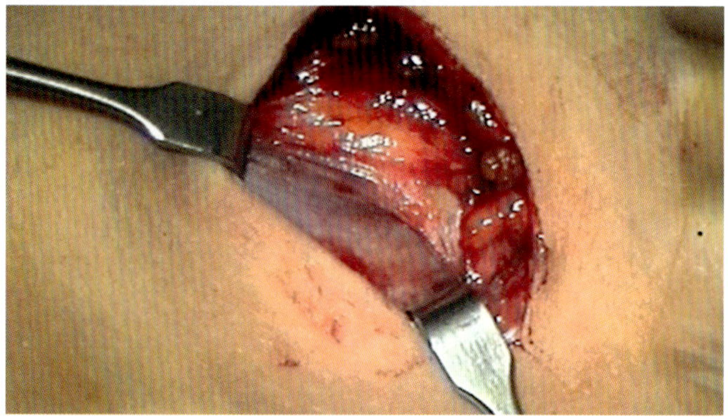

Fig. 3. Opening of the deep cervical fascia and blunt dissection medially of the sternocleidomastoid muscle.

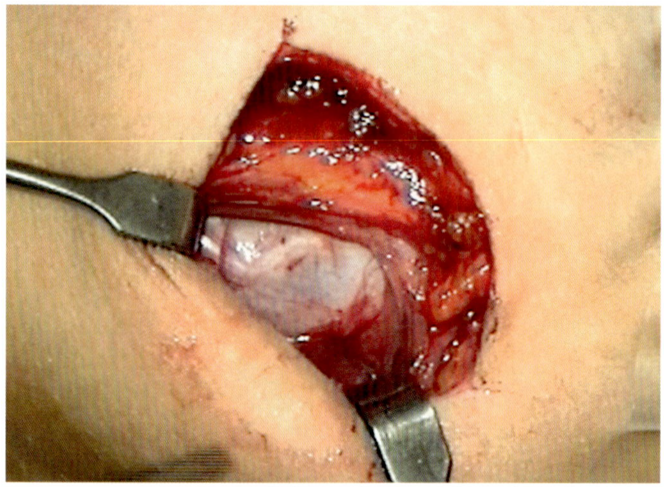

Fig. 4. A neural structure is seen under the neurovascular sheath superficially to the carotid artery (ansa cervicalis).

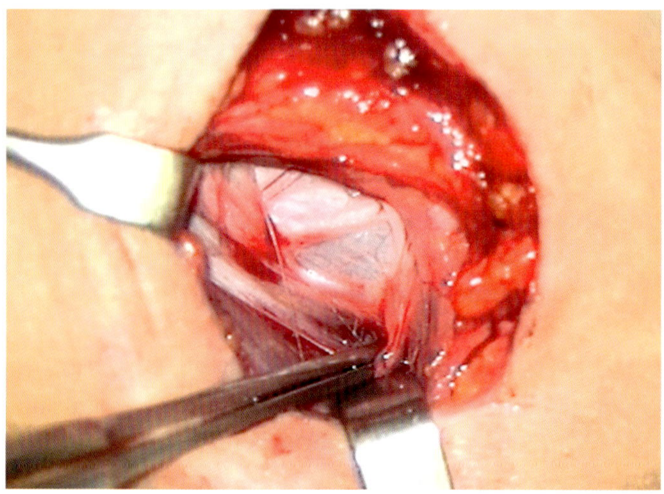

Fig. 5. Dissection of the ansa.

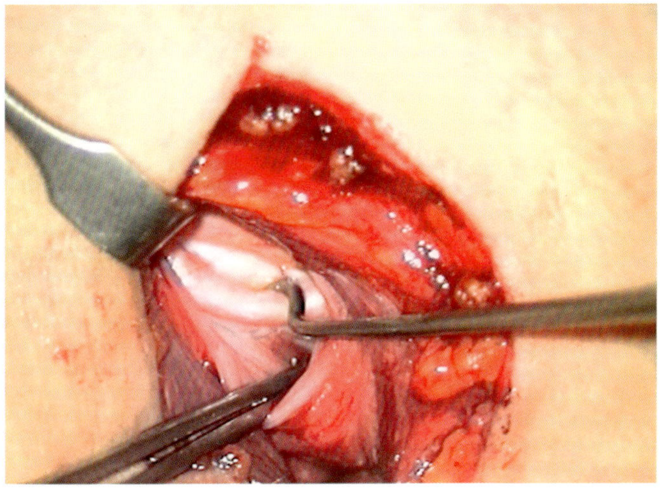

Fig. 6. Careful dissection of the nerve from the carotid artery with a blunt hook. The ansa is retained with a forceps.

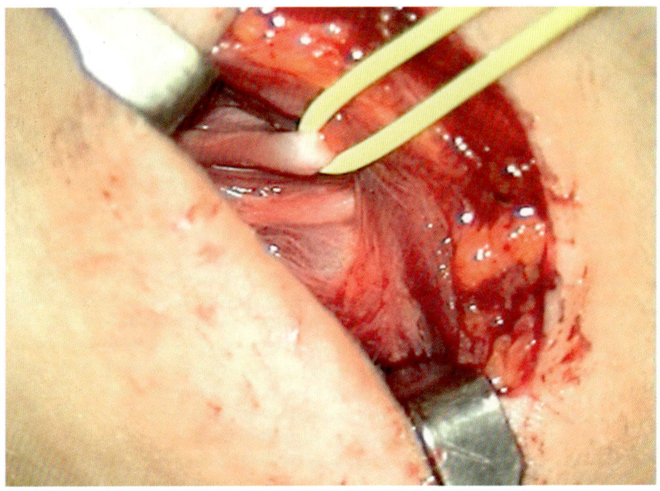

Fig. 7. The vagus nerve is carefully dissected with the help of a loop.

The nerve is dissected carefully using nerve loops and blunt hooks to hold the vascular structures away. To facilitate the application of the electrode, 3–4 cm of the nerve should be freed from the surrounding tissue (fig. 6, 7). Care has to be taken to keep the vasculature (vasa nervorum) intact.

In children, usually a 2-mm diameter helical coil electrode is used (3 mm in male adults). The electrode should fit snugly around the nerve and allow minimal motions without compressing the nerve or causing abrasions of perineural tissue. With anatomical grasping forceps, the suture tail is grasped at either end. The electrode should be placed perpendicular to the nerve and the suture ends at both sides stretched in order to bring the convolutions around the nerve and redirect the electrode along the nerve. Because of the narrow surgical place, this may be challenging to accomplish.

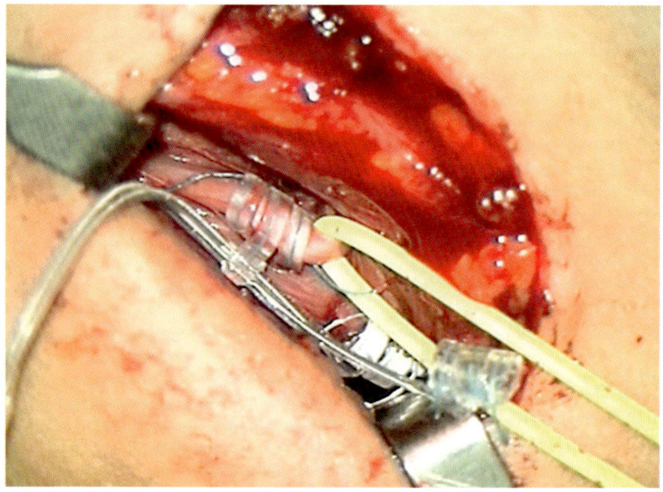

Fig. 8. The tether is distally fixed to the dissected vagus nerve.

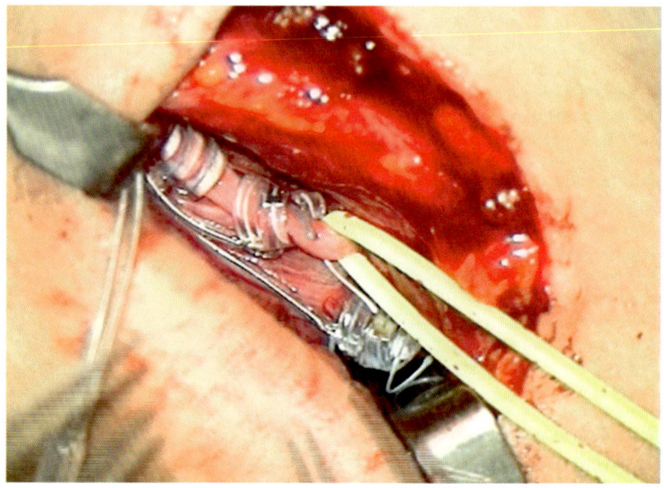

Fig. 9. The center cathode is fixed around the nerve.

Therefore, we start with the anchoring tether first, followed by the center cathode and finally the distal electrode (anode) (fig. 8, 9).

The lead is then tunneled to the subclavicular wound and connected to the generator. The electrode resistance (impedance) is then tested along with the function of the generator. A relaxing loop is then formed underneath the platysma and secured to the strap muscles with silastic tabs (fig. 10).

The lead connector pins are inserted into the generator and secured with set screws. In dual pin connectors, the white connector with the serial number is the positive connector which should be placed in the lower cavity.

The wounds are closed in layers. We prefer to perform an intracutaneous suture with 3-0 or 4-0 Vicryl and glue the wound. This makes removal of stitches in children or developmentally delayed people unnecessary.

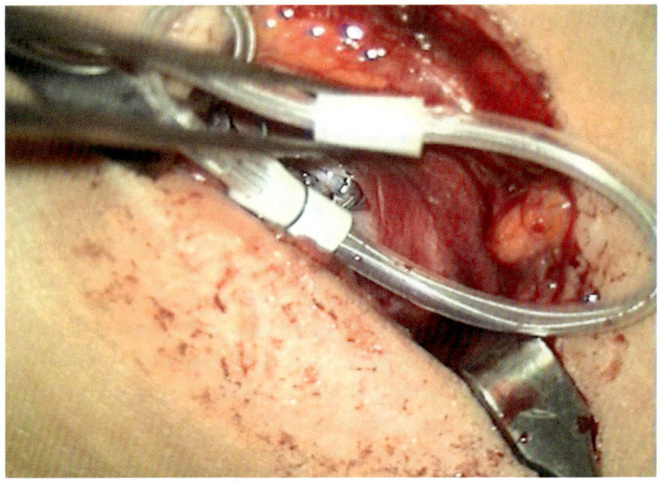

Fig. 10. Two silastic tins fix the lead to the strap muscles.

Revisions: Problems and Pitfalls
Revisions of VNS can be very difficult or even impossible. In cases of lead fracture as demonstrated by high impedances and loss of therapeutic effect, a revision of VNS might be necessary.

After opening the scar, the lead wire with its silicon ties is usually identified in the subplatysmal plane. Careful preparation along the wire is necessary. In these cases we prefer to use the microscope. After retracting the sternocleidomastoid muscle laterally, the lead has to be followed to the neurovascular complex. Dense scar tissue is often found around the carotid artery, jugular vein, and vagus nerve, making sharp dissection under magnification necessary. Monopolar cautery close to the electrode is strictly forbidden in order to prevent heating damage to the nerve. Electrode removal should occur in a caudal-to-cranial direction. The helical anchoring loops can carefully be twisted around the nerve or cut with straight microscissors and removed. Neurolysis of the nerve can be performed, but usually it is preferable to dissect the nerve more cephalad and to place a new electrode proximal to the old electrode site. The old site can be tried if the distance is too small, but it is absolutely necessary to perform impedance measurements in order to rule out epi- or endoneural scarring.

Right-Sided Implantation
Right-sided VNS sometimes has to be considered in revision surgery or due to other surgical reasons. Several cases have been reported in literature. However, the question of cardiac interference has not been solved yet [18–20]. It seems that right-sided VNS is just as or less effective, it possibly acts via different mechanisms, and can have cardiac or respiratory interferences. Therefore, implantation and initial follow-up should be carefully monitored by ECG.

Complications

There are three parts of this section that have to be discussed separately: surgical complications and avoidance strategies, hardware-related complications and avoidance strategies, and stimulation-induced complications and avoidance strategies.

Postoperative infections occur in 3–8% of patients [21–23]. Since small children or children with epilepsy and mental retardation are prone to infection due to excoriation of their wounds [24], surgery always has to be performed under the highest aseptic conditions with perioperative antibiotics. While superficial wounds often can be treated conservatively, a pocket empyema or deep infection of the wound in the neck area requires a removal of the complete system or its parts [25, 26]. Subpectoral implantation, especially for very thin children, is described [27]. However, the skin-to-generator distance should not exceed 3 cm in order to guarantee good telemetry of the device.

Left cord paralysis, usually temporary, as a result of direct manipulation to the laryngeal nerves has been described in 1.4–2.7% of patients in larger series [23, 26, 28–30]. There has also been a report of vocal cord paralysis after twisting of the electrodes by generator rotation [31]. Therefore, the stimulator has to be stitched to the underlying muscle fascia and additional loops of the extension cable should be laid underneath the platysma to reduce the traction forces by movements of the shoulder or neck and underneath the implantable pulse generator.

Hardware-related complications occurred in our series in 9.5% of the patients [23]. The major technical problem was lead fracture (7.6%) that was detected by either radiographs or by increased impedance, device malfunction, and lead displacement (0.95% each). In another recent publication [32] with 251 procedures in 143 patients, hardware-related complications were reported in 16.8% of the patients, with lead fractures in 11.9%, disconnection in 2.8%, and implantable pulse generator malfunction in 2.8%.

Stimulation-induced side effects are more challenging. Stimulation-induced cough, hoarseness, or voice alteration (up to 60%) and dyspnea are initially often observed side effects which subside in the long term, resulting in a frequency in one study of 1.5% for cough, 18.7% voice alteration, and 2.3% dyspnea after 5 years of stimulation [33]. Cardiac symptoms (bradycardia or asystole) have been reported mainly in adults [30, 34–36]. This age-dependent effect is not clear. During intraoperative testing, atropine should be available; in the long term this side effect has not been reported. Other stimulation-induced effects are paresthesia, pain, and sternocleidomastoid activation [23, 28, 37].

According to the literature, no increased incidence of sudden unexpected, unexplained deaths in epilepsy has occurred in the VNS [21].

References

1 Binnie CD: Vagus nerve stimulation for epilepsy: a review. Seizure 2000;9:161–169.
2 Elliott RE, Rodger SD, Bassani L, Morsi A, Geller EB, Carlson C, Devinsky O, Doyle WK: Vagus nerve stimulation for children with treatment-resistant epilepsy: a consecutive series of 141 cases. J Neurosurg Pediatr 2011;7:491–500.
3 Lange G, Janal MV, Maniker A, FitzGibbons J, Fobler M, Cook D, Natelson BH: Safety and efficacy of vagus nerve stimulation in fibromyalgia: a phase I/II proof of concept trial. Pain Med 2011;12:1406–1413.
4 Mauskop A: Vagus nerve stimulation relieves chronic refractory migraine and cluster headaches. Cephalalgia 2005;25:82–86.
5 Berry SM, Broglio K, Bunker M, Jayewardene A, Olin B, Rush AJ: A patient-level meta-analysis of studies evaluating vagus nerve stimulation therapy for treatment-resistant depression. Med Devices (Auckl) 2013;6:17–35.
6 Brack KE, Winter J, Ng GA: Mechanisms underlying the autonomic modulation of ventricular fibrillation initiation – tentative prophylactic properties of vagus nerve stimulation on malignant arrhythmias in heart failure. Heart Fail Rev 2013;18:389–408.
7 Park H-W, Shen MJ, Lin S-F, Fishbein MC, Chen LS, Chen P-S: Neural mechanisms of atrial fibrillation. Curr Opin Cardiol 2012;27:24–28.
8 Burneo JG, Faught E, Knowlton R, Morawetz R, Kuzniecky R: Weight loss associated with vagus nerve stimulation. Neurology 2002;59:463–464.
9 Greenway F, Zheng J: Electrical stimulation as treatment for obesity and diabetes. J Diabetes Sci Technol 2007;1:251–259.
10 Bohotin C, Scholsem M, Bohotin V, Franzen R, Schoenen J: Vagus nerve stimulation attenuates heat- and formalin-induced pain in rats. Neurosci Lett 2003;351:79–82.
11 Kirchner A, Stefan H, Bastian K, Birklein F: Vagus nerve stimulation suppresses pain but has little effects on neurogenic inflammation in humans. Eur J Pain 2006;10:449–455.
12 Cecchini AP, Mea E, Tullo V, Curone M, Franzini A, Broggi G, Savino M, Bussone G, Leone M: Vagus nerve stimulation in drug-resistant daily chronic migraine with depression: preliminary data. Neurol Sci 2009;30(suppl 1):S101–S104.
13 Kirchner A, Birklein F, Stefan H, Handwerker HO: Vagusstimulation – eine Behandlungsoption für chronische Schmerzen? Schmerz 2001;15:272–277.
14 Sadler RM, Purdy Ra, Rahey S: Vagal nerve stimulation aborts migraine in patients with intractable epilepsy. Cephalalgia 2002;22:482–484.
15 Franzini A, Messina G, Leone M, Cecchini AP, Broggi G, Bussone G: Feasibility of simultaneous vagal nerve and deep brain stimulation in chronic cluster headache: case report and considerations. Neurol Sci 2009;30(suppl 1):S137–S139.
16 Fanselow EE: Central mechanisms of cranial nerve stimulation for epilepsy. Surg Neurol Int 2012; 3(suppl 4):S247–S254.
17 Krahl SE, Clark KB: Vagus nerve stimulation for epilepsy: a review of central mechanisms. Surg Neurol Int 2012;3(suppl 4):S255–S259.
18 McGregor A, Wheless J, Baumgartner J, Bettis D: Right-sided vagus nerve stimulation as a treatment for refractory epilepsy in humans. Epilepsia 2005;46: 91–96.
19 Navas M, Navarrete EG, Pascual JM, Carrasco R, Núñez JA, Shakur SF, Pastor J, Sola RG: Treatment of refractory epilepsy in adult patients with right-sided vagus nerve stimulation. Epilepsy Res 2010;90: 1–7.
20 Spuck S, Nowak G, Renneberg A, Tronnier V, Sperner J: Right-sided vagus nerve stimulation in humans: an effective therapy? Epilepsy Res 2008;82: 232–234.
21 Ben-Menachem E: Vagus nerve stimulation, side effects, and long-term safety. J Clin Neurophysiol 2001;18:415–418.
22 Patel NC, Edwards MS: Vagal nerve stimulator pocket infections. Pediatr Infect Dis J 2004;23:681–683.
23 Spuck S, Tronnier V, Orosz I, Schönweiler R, Sepehrnia A, Nowak G, Sperner J: Operative and technical complications of vagus nerve stimulator implantation. Neurosurgery 2010;67(2 suppl operative):489–494.
24 Le H, Chico M, Hecox K, Frim D: Interscapular placement of a vagal nerve stimulator for prevention of wound tampering. Technical note. Pediatr Neurosurg 2002;36:164–166.
25 Air EL, Ghomri YM, Tyagi R, Grande AW, Crone K, Mangano FT: Management of vagal nerve stimulator infections: do they need to be removed? J Neurosurg Pediatr 2009;3:73–78.
26 Smyth MD, Tubbs RS, Bebin EM, Grabb PA, Blount JP: Complication of chronic vagus nerve stimulation for epilepsy in children. J Neurosurg 2003;99:500–503.
27 Baumann JA, Ridgeway EB, Devinsky O, Doyle WK: Subpectoral implantation of the vagus nerve stimulator. Neurosurgery 2006;58(4 suppl 2):ONS-322–ONS-325.
28 Rychlicki F, Zamponi N, Cesaroni E, Corpaci L, Trignani R, Ducati A, Scerrati M: Complication of vagal nerve stimulation for epilepsy in children. Neurosurg Rev 2006;29:103–107.

29 Spuck S, Nowak G, Sperner J, Tronnier V: Implantation und Komplikation der Vagusnervstimulation. J Neurol Neurosurg Psychiatr 2007;8:16–20.
30 Zalvan C, Sulica L, Wolf S, Cohen J, Ginzalez-Yanes O, Blitzer A: Laryngopharyngeal dysfunction from the implant vagal stimulator. Laryngoscope 2003; 113:221–225.
31 Kalkanis JG, Krishna P, Espinosa JA, Naritoku DK: Self-inflicted vocal cord paralysis in patients with vagus nerve stimulators. Report of two cases. J Neurosurg 2002;96:949–951.
32 Kahlow H, Olivecrona M: Complications of vagal nerve stimulation for drug-resistant epilepsy: a single center longitudinal study of 143 patients. Seizure 2013;22:827–833.
33 Ben-Menachem E, Hellström K, Waldton C, Augustinsson LE: Evaluation of refractory epilepsy treated with vagus nerve stimulation up to 5 years. Neurology 1999;52:1265–1267.
34 Asconape JJ, Moore DD, Zipes DP, Hartmann LM, Duffell WH Jr: Bradycardia and asystole with the use of vagus nerve stimulation for the treatment of epilepsy. A rare complication of intraoperative device testing. Epilepsia 1999;40:1452–1454.
35 Ronkainen E, Korpelainen JT, Heikkine E, Myllylä VV, Huikuri HV, Isojärvi JI: Cardiac autonomic control in patients with refractory epilepsy before and during vagus nerve stimulation treatment. A one-year follow-up study. Epilepsia 2006;47:556–562.
36 Tatum WO 4th, Moore DB, Stecker MM, Baltuch GH, French JA, Ferreira JA, Carney PM, Labar DR, Vale FL: Ventricular asystole during vagus nerve stimulation for epilepsy in humans. Neurology 1999; 52:1267–1269.
37 Iriarte J, Artieda J, Alegre M, Schlumberger E, Urrestarazu E, Pastor MA, Vitor C: Spasm of the sternocleidomastoid muscle induced by vagal nerve stimulation. Neurology 2001;57:2319–2320.

Volker M. Tronnier, MD, PhD
Department of Neurosurgery
University Hospital Lübeck
Ratzeburger Allee 160, DE–23538 Lübeck (Germany)
E-Mail volker.tronnier@uksh.de

Slavin KV (ed): Stimulation of the Peripheral Nervous System. The Neuromodulation Frontier.
Prog Neurol Surg. Basel, Karger, 2016, vol 29, pp 39–52 (DOI: 10.1159/000434654)

Vagus Nerve Stimulation for Epilepsy: An Evidence-Based Approach

Arthur Cukiert

Epilepsy Surgery Program, Clinica de Epilepsia de Sao Paulo and Department of Neurology and Neurosurgery, ABC Faculty of Medicine, Sao Paulo, Brazil

Abstract

Medical treatment of seizures yields a satisfactory response in 75–80% of the patients; resective epilepsy surgery is a therapeutic option for those patients who are refractory to drug therapy, but there is still a considerable portion (20–30%) of patients who are ineligible for surgery or failed surgery. Vagus nerve stimulation (VNS) might be an option for these very refractory patients. We carried out an evidence-based search to identify the best evidence presently available related to the use of VNS. We used multiple searchable databases (primary: PubMed-MEDLINE, EMBASE, LILACS, and SciELO; secondary: Cochrane Library) and a standard structured approach know as the PICO scheme: P (patient), I (intervention), C (comparison), and O (outcome). Publications were selected based on study design, PICO components, language, and availability of full text. For study design, we included papers designed as 'randomized controlled trials'; these trials were evaluated according to the Jadad score; the type II error was not used while selecting studies to avoid further limitations. Twenty-eight papers were selected, all from PubMed-MEDLINE. The search results showed that patients older than 12 years with refractory partial seizures (with or without generalization) may benefit from VNS. Children might also benefit, but might need different stimulation parameters. We also noted that higher stimulation settings are associated with increased occurrence of hoarseness, throat pain, cough, and dyspnea. The available randomized controlled trials and cohorts made it clear that VNS is a useful palliative procedure in adult patients with partial epilepsy, and a 50–60% reduction in seizure frequency might be expected in at least 50% of the patients. VNS is a useful palliative procedure in patients with refractory epilepsy. As our practical experience and understanding of the mechanism of action of VNS increase, more homogeneous patient populations that might respond better to VNS are being recognized, such as children with secondary generalized epilepsy and some types of reflex epilepsy.

Medical treatment for seizures yields a satisfactory response in 75–80% of the patients; however, a portion of them presents with refractory epilepsy. Resective epilepsy surgery is a therapeutic option for those patients who are refractory to drug therapy, but there are still many patients (20–30%) who are ineligible for surgery or failed surgery, or who would not benefit from this option. These patients have frequent seizures that limit their ability to work and participate in everyday activities. Many also suffer from the effects of high doses and long duration of chronic drug therapy. Seizures not adequately controlled often lead to a lower quality of life (QOL) and secondary psychiatric symptoms, and are associated with a higher prevalence of sudden unexpected death. On the other hand, seizure control leads to improved QOL, decreased risk of sudden unexpected death, use of lower doses or discontinuation of anticonvulsants, and a decrease or cessation of use of emergency or intensive care units (ICUs). Patients who do not respond to standard anticonvulsant medications might benefit from new therapeutic strategies such as vagus nerve stimulation (VNS) [1].

The mechanisms for the antiepileptic effects of VNS are not completely understood but are possibly related to the effects on the reticular activating system. The nucleus of the solitary tract, the main termination of vagal afferents, has direct and indirect projections to the locus coeruleus, raphe nucleus, reticular formation, and other brainstem nuclei that are known to modulate the epileptic threshold [2].

The VNS procedure consists of the implantation of a programmable pulse generator connected to electrodes implanted around the left cervical vagus nerve. Being an extracranial procedure, VNS carries lower surgical and anesthetic morbidity, especially compared to classic resective surgery. Stimulus characteristics may vary. Usual programmable parameters include stimulation current (mA), pulse duration (μs), frequency (Hz), the 'on' period (s), and the 'off' period (min) [3]. The possible effects, beneficial or not, are fully reversible when the device is turned off.

The Search for Clinical Evidence

To identify the best evidence presently available related to the use of VNS in patients with epilepsy, we asked the question, 'Do patients with epilepsy benefit from vagus nerve stimulation?', as a clinical query in a multiple searchable databases (primary: PubMed-MEDLINE, EMBASE, LILACS, and SciELO; secondary: Cochrane Library). We also used a standard structured approach known as the PICO scheme: P (patient), I (intervention), C (comparison), and O (outcome).

For PubMed-MEDLINE, the search terms were as follows:

- Search 1: (Vagus Nerve Stimulation) OR (Vagus Nerve AND Electric Stimulation Therapy) OR (Vagus Nerve AND Electric Stimulation) AND (Random).
- Search 2: (Epilepsy OR Seizure OR Lennox-Gastaut Syndrome OR Epileptogenic Disorder OR Epilepsies OR Partial Seizures OR Epilepsy OR Complex Partial)

Table 1. Number of papers recovered using the search strategy described in the text

Info base	Papers, n
Primary	
PubMed-Medline	846
EMBASE	61
Secondary	
Cochrane Library	1

AND (Vagus Nerve Stimulation OR Electric Vagus Nerve Stimulation Therapy) OR (Vagus nerve AND Electric Stimulation) AND (Random).

- Search 3: (Epilepsy OR Seizure OR Lennox-Gastaut Syndrome OR Epileptogenic Disorder OR Epilepsies OR Partial Seizures OR Seizures OR Complex Partial) AND (Vagus Nerve Stimulation OR Vagus Nerve) AND (Electric Stimulation Therapy OR Vagus Nerve) AND (Electric Stimulation) AND (Therapy/broad[filter] OR Comparative Study OR Comparative Studies).

For EMBASE/Cochrane, the search terms were as follows:

- (Epilepsy) AND (Vagus nerve stimulation).

The results of our search are listed in table 1. From these, we narrowed our inclusion criteria based on several principles: the publications were selected based on study design, PICO components, language, and availability of full text. For study design, we included papers designed as 'randomized controlled trials'. These trials were evaluated according to the score designed by Jadad et al. [4]; the type II error was not used while selecting studies to avoid further limitations. For PICO components we chose: patients with epilepsy for 'patients', VNS for 'intervention', VNS or medical managent for 'comparison', and clinical outcome for 'outcome'. In terms of language, we analyzed papers in English, Portuguese, and Spanish. Finally, for publication availability, we considered for critical evaluation only those papers where the full text was available.

Based on our inclusion criteria, 28 studies were included – all from PubMed-MEDLINE. No papers were selected using a manual search. In tune with the history of this clinical application, the assessment period include papers published between 1992 and 2012. Finally, if the selected evidence was defined as a randomized controlled trial, it was subjected to a check-list for an appropriate critical evaluation (table 2). A critical evaluation of the randomized controlled trial allowed us to classify it according to the Jadad score; we considered those scored <3 as inconsistent (grade B), and those with scores ≥ 3 as consistent (grade A). Prior to individual discussion of selected papers, we listed the main reasons for exclusion of selected studies (table 3).

Table 2. Roadmap for critical evaluation of randomized controlled trials (checklist)

Study data	
	Reference, study design, Jadad score, and strength of evidence
Patient selection	
	Inclusion and exclusion criteria
Randomization	
	Blinding description and allocation
Treatment protocol	
	Intervention, control, and blinding
Outcomes	
	Primary, secondary, and instrument for measuring the outcome
Sample calculation	
	Estimated differences, power, significance level, and number of patients
Patients	
	Recruited, randomized, and prognostic differences
Patient follow-up	
	Time, lost, and migrated
Analysis	
	Intention to treat (intervention and control)
Results	
	Absolute benefit or harm, mean benefit or harm

Table 3. Number of papers included/excluded in the analysis

Primary search	Included	Excluded	Reasons for exclusion
28	8	20	Not a randomized controlled trial; a technique comparison; uncontrolled trial; open follow-up; no primary outcome outlined; post hoc analysis

Do Patients with Epilepsy Benefit from Vagus Nerve Stimulation?

In a study by Holder et al. [3], high-intensity VNS (table 4) resulted in seizure frequency reduction of 33% ($p < 0.001$) compared to 12 weeks of observation before VNS implantation (baseline) in patients who were 12–60 years of age with refractory seizures (6 or more simple or complex partial seizures per month for a period of 3 months with or without secondary generalization). The group with low-intensity stimulus showed no reduction in seizure frequency (8.4%, $p = 0.223$) compared to baseline. Results were different when comparing the high versus low-intensity groups ($p = 0.025$). There was no difference between different seizure types.

Two reports from the VNS First International Study Group [5, 6] described a cohort of patients of 12–60 years of age with refractory seizures (6 or more simple or complex partial seizures with or without generalization per month for a period of 3 months) that received VNS using high- or low-intensity parameters. Seizure

Table 4. Stimulation parameters used in published studies of VNS for epilepsy

Author/ reference/year	Intensity	Current, mA	Frequency, Hz	Pulse duration, µs	Time 'on', s	Time 'off', min	Manual activation
Holder [3], 1992	High		30 (20–50)	500	30–90	5–10	
	Low		1 (1–2)	130	30	60–80	
Ben-Menachem [5], 1994; Ramsay [6], 1994	High	1.5 (0.25–3)	30 (20–50)	500	30–90	5 (5–10)	
	Low	1.25 (0.25–3)	1 (1–2)	130	30	90 (60–180)	
VNS study group [1], 1995	High	1.5 (0.25–3)	30 (20–50)	500	30–90	5–10	Allowed
	Low	1.25 (0.25–3)	1 (1–2)	130	30	60–180	Disabled
Handforth [2], 1998	High	≤3.5	30	500	30	5	
	Low	≤3.5	1	130	30	180	
Amar [8], 1998	High	≤3.5	30 (20–50)	500	30	5	Allowed
	Low	perception point	1 (1–2)	130	30	180	Disabled
Klinkenberg [9, 10], 2012, 2013	High	0.25–1.75	30	500	30	5	
	Low	0.25	1	100	14	60	

frequency decreased >50% in 38.7% of the patients during high-intensity stimulation and in 19.4% during low-intensity stimulation; this difference was significant (p = 0.03). The mean reduction in seizure frequency in the high-intensity stimulation group was 30.9% (p = 0.0001) and 11.3% in the low-intensity stimulation (not significant, p = 0.072) when compared to baseline. The difference between the means was significant (p = 0.029) [5]. Manual activation of the generator after simple partial seizures reduced seizure frequency by 20.7 and 8.8% after high- and low-intensity stimulation, respectively [number needed to treat (NNT) = 8, p = 0.036] [5].

Hoarseness and other adverse effects were noted in 25.8% of the patients. These occurred in 35.5% of the patients in the high-intensity group and in 13.9% in the group stimulated with lower intensity. There was no difference between the high- versus low-intensity group: local pain, sore throat, and other local changes, including a feeling of inflammation, occurred in 12.9% of the patents in the high-intensity group and in 13.9% of the patients in the low-intensity group. Cough was present in both groups, but was significant only in the high-intensity group (12.9%). Paresthesia (numbness in the throat and chin) was observed in 9.7% of the patients in the high-intensity group and in 8.3% of the patients in the low-intensity group. Muscle pain was directly associated with stimulus intensity and was present in 9.7% of the patients in the high-intensity group [6]. Other adverse effects were reported, such as abdominal pain, nausea, restriction of breathing, and chest pain, and were associated with high-intensity stimuli, although statistical significance was not reached [6].

In a subsequent report of a randomized controlled trial of chronic VNS for treatment of medically intractable seizures by the VNS Study Group [1], patients undergoing high-intensity VNS presented significant reduction in seizure frequency when compared to low-intensity stimulation (24.5 vs. 6.1%, $p = 0.01$; NNT = 6). Patients in the high-intensity group showed a significant reduction in seizure frequency (95%, $p < 0.01$) when compared to baseline, but there was no difference in the low-intensity group. In the high-intensity group, 31.0% of patients achieved a ≥50% reduction in seizure frequency, but only 13.0% of the patients in the low-intensity group experienced this. The difference between these groups was significant ($p = 0.02$) [7]. The most frequent side effects were hoarseness and other voice changes, which were directly associated with stimulation intensity; they were present in 37.2% of the patients in the high-intensity group and in 13.3% of the patients in the low-intensity group [$p < 0.01$; number needed to inflict harm (NNH) = 4]. Sore throat and cough were present in 12% of the patients. Other less frequent adverse effects were dyspnea, paresthesia, muscle pain, and headache [1].

In 1998, Handforth et al. [2] reported the results of a randomized active-control trial of VNS therapy for partial-onset seizures. Patients 12–65 years of age with medically refractory epilepsy (6 or more complex partial seizures with or without generalization per month, with a seizure-free interval shorter than 21 days) were studied. High-intensity VNS showed an average reduction in seizure frequency of 27.9%; this was also the case in 15.2% of the patients in the low-intensity group (NNT = 8). There was a significant difference between the groups (aligned ranks test, $p = 0.04$; t test, $p = 0.02$). In the high-intensity group, a ≥75% reduction in seizure frequency was noted in 10.6% of patients ($p = 0.015$, Fisher's exact test). There was no significant difference between the groups when considering a ≥50% reduction in seizure frequency ($p = 0.172$, χ^2). Both groups showed a significant reduction in the overall frequency of complex partial seizures when compared to baseline.

Voice changes were the most common adverse event and were present in 66.3% of the patients in the high-intensity group and in 30.1% of the patients in the low-intensity group; this difference was significant ($p = 0.001$; NNT = 3). Cough (45.3% of the patients in the high-intensity group vs. 42.7% in the low-intensity group, $p < 0.0001$), dyspnea (25.3% of the patients in the high-intensity group vs. 10.7% of the patients in the low-intensity group, $p = 0.007$, NNH = 7), and paresthesia (19.7% of the patients in the high-intensity group vs. 25.2% of the patients in the low-intensity groups, $p < 0.0001$, NNH = 6) were less frequent but significantly more prevalent when compared to baseline. Other less frequent adverse effects were pharyngitis, pain, headache, dyspepsia, vomiting, and nausea [2].

Also in 1998, Amar et al. [8] reported their institutional experience with VNS for medically refractory epilepsy. Patients 12–65 years of age with 6 or more complex partial seizures with or without generalization per month, with seizure-free intervals shorter than 21 days, were studied. High-intensity VNS showed an average reduction in seizure frequency of 71.0%, compared to 6.0% in the low-intensity group (NNT = 2). The difference between groups was significant ($p = 0.004$).

In the latest randomized controlled trial, Klinkenberg et al. [9, 10] studied children aged 4–18 years with medically refractory epilepsy. There was no difference in seizure frequency reduction between the high- and low-intensity groups, although both groups compared favorably to baseline. The most common side effects were changes in the voice, cough, and sore throat. There was no significant difference after VNS regarding mood, depression, or cognitive changes among the high- and low-intensity groups.

Summary of the Evidence in Refractory Epilepsy

Patients older than 12 years with refractory partial seizures (with or without generalization) may benefit from VNS. Children might also benefit, but might need different stimulation parameters. However, higher stimulation settings are associated with increased occurrence of hoarseness, throat pain, cough, and dyspnea.

Present and Future

The available randomized controlled trials and cohorts made it clear that VNS is a useful palliative procedure in adult patients with partial epilepsy, and a 50–60% reduction in seizure frequency might be expected in at least 50% of the patients. Although widely used in children and in patients with generalized epilepsy, high-level evidence of VNS efficacy is still lacking in this patient population. Progressive improvement over time has been noted, but the open-label nature of these cohorts and observations could not provide adequate information regarding this. This also holds true for the use of the manual activation feature that allows the patient to use the provided magnet to acutely activate the generator previously to or during a seizure. Presently, standard stimulus parameters include: 30 Hz, 500 μs, current ranging from 1 to 2.5 mA, 30 s 'on' and 5 min 'off'. Over the years, we have been trying to define a patient population that would be better candidates for VNS. We describe some of these efforts below.

Vagus Nerve Stimulation in Children with Lennox-Gastaut or Lennox-Like Syndrome

We studied 24 consecutive children under the age of 12 years by the time of surgery who were implanted with VNS and had at least 2 years of postimplantation follow-up [11]. They had secondary generalized epilepsy of the Lennox-Gastaut (LGS) or Lennox-like (LLS) type, including multiform (atonic, myoclonic, tonic-clonic, tonic, atypical absence) daily seizures, mental retardation, and generalized EEG findings. The generator was turned on using 0.25 mA, 30 Hz, 500 μs, 30 s 'on', and 5 min 'off' stimulation parameters; the current was then increased by 0.25 mA every 2 weeks until 3.5 mA was reached or adverse effects were noted. Stimulation parameters and anticonvulsant drugs were kept stable during the follow-up. Patients who showed at least a 50% reduction in any specific seizure type were considered responders.

Age ranged from 5 to 12 years (mean = 8.4) by the time of surgery (19 males). Age of seizure onset varied from 1 day of life to 10 years (mean = 2.8 years). Follow-up time ranged from 24 to 53 months (mean = 32). Six children had been previously submitted to extended (90%) callosotomy, and 4 to frontal lobe resection. One child was taking a single antiepileptic drug, 9 were taking two, 12 were taking three, 2 were taking four, and 1 was taking five different antiepileptic drugs. Fourteen children were diagnosed as having LGS and 10 with LLS (Lennox-Gastaut phenotype without the recruiting rhythm during sleep). MRI was normal in 9 children, showed nonspecific gliosis in 4, diffuse cortical dysplasia in 4, diffuse atrophy in 3, tuberous sclerosis in 2, cytomegalovirus sequelae in 1, and septo-optic dystrophy in 1 [11].

Only 1 child was formally testable from a neuropsychological point of view, and rated as mentally retarded. The other 23 children were more severely impaired. After VNS, an additional child turned out to be testable, but the rest remained untestable. Sixteen children were unable to speak and 3 were unable to walk. QOL and health measures improved in up to 50% (mean = 25%) of the scale's items in 20 children, including 4 nonresponders to VNS in terms of seizures (see below). There was no worsening in QOL measures. Attention was noted to improve in 21 out of 24 children, in up to 92% (mean = 58%) of the scale's items [11].

Frequency and pulse duration were kept stable during the study (30 Hz and 500 μs, respectively). Final intensity parameters ranged from 2 to 3.5 mA (mean = 3.1). Eleven children were stimulated using 3.5 mA: 4 with 3.0 mA, 3 with 2.75 mA, 4 with 2.5 mA, 1 with 2.25 mA, and 2 with 2.0 mA. A 'honeymoon effect', characterized by at least 50% seizure frequency reduction immediately after implantation and with the generator off, was noted in 14 out of the 24 children and lasted a mean of 20.2 days (range: 5–45). We could not evaluate different stimulation settings since duration and frequency were kept constant, and intensity was maximized up to the highest tolerated level or until 3.5 mA was reached [11].

All patients had more than one seizure type; at presentation, atypical absence was present in 15 children: tonic seizures in 5, myoclonic seizures in 10, atonic seizures in 4, and generalized tonic-clonic seizures in 13. A reduction of seizure frequency of at least 50% was noted in 35 seizure types: 32 seizure types improved more than 60%, 26 seizure types improved more than 70%, 24 seizure types improved more than 80%, 21 seizure types improved more than 90%, and 17 seizures types disappeared after VNS (generalized tonic-clonic, n = 9; myoclonic, n = 3; atonic, n = 1; atypical absence, n = 4). Twenty out of the 24 children had a 50% improvement in at least one seizure type and in 4 children there was no worthwhile improvement. Atypical absence frequency dropped from 15.5/day at baseline to 7.6/day after 24 months of VNS ($p < 0.05$), tonic seizure frequency went from 8.6 to 7.8/day (nonsignificant), myoclonic seizures frequency went from 27.8 to 5.3/day ($p < 0.05$), atonic seizures frequency from 9.3 to 11.6/day (nonsignificant), and generalized tonic-clonic seizure frequency from 8.3 to 2.0/day ($p < 0.05$). No seizure frequency worsening was noted at the final optimal stimulation parameters. Within the nonresponder group (n = 4), there were 2 children with tuberous sclerosis: 1 with diffuse cortical dysplasia and 1 with diffuse gliosis. Of 6 children who had been previously submitted to callosotomy, 5 were good responders and 1 did not respond to VNS. Additionally, 4 children had been previously submitted to frontal lobe resection, and all were good responders. Evaluating the average seizure frequency for the whole series alone would not be that useful, but one has to look into the number of patients who had a specific seizure type abolished [11].

Transient seizure frequency worsening potentially related to stimulation intensity increase was noted in 10 of the 24 children, at a mean of 3.1 mA (range: 2.25–3.5). In all, seizure frequency came back to the previous one after a 0.5-mA decrease in stimulation intensity. Persistent hoarseness was noted in 1 child and 1 child had to be discontinued after the occurrence of parkinsonian symptoms related to VNS [11].

This experience showed that VNS was effective in reducing atypical absence and generalized tonic-clonic and myoclonic seizures in children with LGS or LLS. A concomitant improvement in attention level and QOL and health was also noted. No worthwhile improvement occurred in the frequency of tonic and atonic seizures in the studied patient population. Measuring outcome is critical in this type of patient population with multiform seizures, and would depend on which seizure type was the prevailing or more disabling one, as well as how that seizure type responded to treatment. Since VNS is a palliative treatment, outcome measures should include not only raw seizure frequency reduction rates, but also QOL and general health evaluations. Each seizure type has both a clinical and an electroencephalographic definition, and is homogeneous among the studied patients. Total seizure counts might not reflect clinical improvement in this patient population since the different seizure types are not equally disabling. Thus, atonic seizures are usually more disabling then myoclonic seizures, although the latter might be more frequent. As in other palliative procedures, we chose to report on the outcome of each seizure type [11].

Vagus Nerve Stimulation versus Callosotomy in Children with Lennox-Gastaut or Lennox-Like Syndrome

We studied 44 consecutive patients with refractory generalized epilepsy [12]. Twenty-four patients were submitted to callosotomy from 2006 to 2007 (group 1), and 20 additional patients underwent VNS implant from 2008 to 2009 (group 2). All of them had generalized epilepsy of LGS or LLS type, including multiform daily seizures, mental retardation, and generalized EEG findings.

Table 5. Seizure types in patients with LGS and LLS undergoing callosotomy (group 1, n = 24) and VNS (group 2, n = 20)

Seizure type	Tonic	Atonic	Myoclonic	Generalized tonic-clonic	Atypical absence
Incidence in group 1, %	55	75	50	55	75
Incidence in group 2, %	20	20	40	55	60
Daily frequency in group 1 before surgery	8.4±4.9	10.0±5.7	37.0±18.0	7.0±3.5	25.0±9.7
Daily frequency in group 1 after surgery	6.9±2.3	**1.2±1.2**	26.0±16.8	**2.9±2.4**	**4.2±2.4**
Daily frequency in group 2 before surgery	8.6±6.1	9.3±5.2	27.0±18.2	8.0±6.2	15.0±8.1
Daily frequency in group 2 after surgery	7.8±5.9	11.6±3.8	**5.3±5.1**	**2.0±0.3**	**7.6±7.2**

Frequencies are presented as means ± SD. Bold font indicates significant improvement in frequency of a particular seizure type after the intervention.

The mean age of seizure onset was 2.8 ± 1.6 and 2.88 ± 1.4 years for groups 1 (55% males) and 2 (80% males), respectively. The mean age at surgery was 11.2 ± 3.3 and 8.6 ± 3.2 years for groups 1 and 2, respectively. Fifteen and 12 patients were diagnosed as having LGS in groups 1 and 2, respectively; the remaining patients in each group were diagnosed as having LLS. MRI showed cortico-subcortical atrophy in 70% of group 1 and 62.5% of group 2 patients; nonspecific gliosis was present in the remaining patients [12].

Group 1 patients were submitted to a maximized callosal section (90%), which was performed as a one-stage procedure under general anesthesia. Group 2 patients underwent left VNS implantation under general anesthesia. The generator was turned on using the parameters of 0.25 mA, 30 Hz, 500 μs, 30 s 'on', and 5 min 'off'; the current was then increased by 0.25 mA every 2 weeks until 3.5 mA was reached or adverse effects were noted [12].

All patients had multiple seizure types: 15 and 55% had two seizure types in groups 1 and 2, respectively, 30 and 20% had three seizure types in groups 1 and 2, respectively, and 55 and 25% had 4 seizure types in groups 1 and 2, respectively. Incidences of seizure types and changes in their frequency due to surgical intervention are listed in table 5 [12].

Seizure-free patients accounted for 10% of group 1 and none of group 2. Ten and sixteen percent of the group 1 and 2 patients, respectively, were complete nonresponders [12].

Improvements in attention and QOL were noticed in 85% of the patients in both groups 1 and 2. Rupture of secondary bilateral synchrony was noted in 85% of group 1 patients, and there was no EEG modification after VNS in group 2 [12].

All but one group 1 patient disclosed acute callosal disconnection syndrome immediately after the operation, consisting of apathy, urinary incontinence, and nondominant hemineglect, and lasting for up to 3 weeks; one Group 2 patient presented hoarseness after VNS activation. No major long-lasting morbidity or mortality occurred in either group 1 or 2. The mean hospital stay was 7.5 ± 1.2 (mean ± SD) and 2.0 ± 0.3 days in groups 1 and 2, respectively. The mean stay in the ICU was 2.7 ± 0.3 days in group 1; the group 2 patients only stayed overnight in the ICU. Forty-five percent of the group 1 patients received at least 250 ml of blood transfusion; no blood was transfused in the group 2 patients [12].

Our data showed that both procedures were effective regarding the control of atypical absences and generalized tonic-clonic seizures, although there was a trend towards better results regarding atypical absences after callosotomy. Both procedures were not effective in controlling tonic seizures. Callosotomy was very effective in reducing the frequency of atonic seizures, but VNS was ineffective. In contrast, callosotomy was not effective in reducing myoclonic seizures, whereas VNS was. We tried to homogenize our patient population. We included only children with normal MRI results or diffuse cortico-subcortical atrophy to avoid the possible confounding effects of different etiologies that might be associated with LGS [12].

Our findings reinforce previous beliefs. However, even though the present study design has certain pitfalls, the data presented carry a higher level of evidence than our basic clinical feelings (beliefs). We did not have higher morbidity in the callosotomy series, but this procedure does have higher potential morbidity compared with VNS surgery. Longer hospital stays (including ICU stays), transient acute disconnection syndrome, and blood transfusions were characteristics of group 1 patients only. Additionally, adequate microsurgical training and technique is necessary to safely perform extended callosal sections, whereas the training requirements for VNS are much lower. Although complications are rare with both procedures, callosotomy carries a much higher risk for severe morbidity and mortality, which might explain the 'VNS first' choice currently preferred in some centers, although there is a limited technical basis for doing so. We do have to note, however, that from a practical point of view, we have been very successful in convincing patients/families/caregivers to go ahead with VNS after being submitted to callosotomy, but have very rarely succeeded the other way around ('the first procedure did not work, why should we go ahead with a more dangerous one?') [12].

Both therapeutic options are presently available in our center. Our data suggested that in children with LGS and no specific findings on MRI (such as cortical dysplasia and tuberous sclerosis), if atonic seizures prevail in the patient's clinical picture, callosotomy might be a good option as the primary treatment, whereas when myoclonic seizures prevail, this same might hold true in favor of VNS. When atypical absence or generalized tonic-clonic seizures are the main concern, although both procedures carry similar effectiveness, VNS might be considered as the initial approach, taking into account the adverse event profile. Patients should be advised that both procedures are not very effective in the treatment of tonic seizures [12].

Vagus Nerve Stimulation in Reflex Eating Seizures

Reflex eating seizures are rare, usually complex partial, and represent a disabling seizure type. Although there might be patients with reflex eating seizures alone, the majority of these patients present with both reflex and nonreflex seizures and have focal epilepsy. The trigger event might be related to many aspects of the alimentary behavior; no single relay has been specifically implicated and a multifactorial hypothesis has been postulated. The vagus nerve includes widespread visceral afferent and efferent fibers. We studied the effects of VNS on eating seizures, which theoretically would be triggered by neural activity and signaling from organs innervated by the vagus nerve [13].

Three adult patients with reflex eating seizures were studied. We considered eating seizures as those which occurred during actual food intake (not before or after). All patients had reflex and nonreflex complex partial seizures, but reflex eating seizures was the most frequent seizure type in all of them.

The first patient, a 34-year-old man, had experienced seizures since the age of 16. The seizures occurred daily, especially during meals (98% of all episodes). Interictal EEG showed bitemporal independent midtemporal spiking, and ictal recordings disclosed bilateral independent temporal lobe seizure onset. MRI showed bilateral perisylvian polymicrogyria. He received VNS at the age of 26 (final settings: 2.0 mA, 500 μs, 30 Hz, 30 s 'on', 5 min 'off'). There was a 95% reflex-seizure frequency reduction. Nonreflex seizures remain sporadic (1 every 4 months). He gained weight since meals were not interrupted anymore. After 6 years, his battery went off and the reflex-seizure frequency increased, but did not reach the preimplantation level (1 per 2–3 days).

The second patient, a 40-year-old woman, had experienced seizures since the age of 13. These were reflex eating and hot water seizures. She had daily reflex (80% of all ictal events) and nonreflex ictal events. She had interictal bilateral independent temporal lobe spiking and normal MRI. Prior to her presentation, she underwent a right temporo-occipital resection in another institution that had no effect on seizure frequency, but which left her with severe memory deficit and contralateral homonymous hemianopsia. Repeat video EEG at our institution showed seizures coming from the nonoperated left temporal lobe. She received VNS at the age of 38 (final settings: 2.5 mA, 500 μs, 30 Hz, 30 s 'on', 5 min 'off'). After 2 years of follow-up, there was a marked decrease in reflex eating seizure frequency (85%), but daily nonreflex seizures and reflex hot water seizures remained unchanged; for this she is considered a candidate for deep brain stimulation.

The third patient, a 37-year-old man, had experienced seizures since the age of 4. He had daily reflex eating seizures (65% of all ictal events). He had left hemisphere interictal discharges and was submitted to left frontal resection at our institution after a subdural electrode recording that resulted in 60% seizure frequency reduction, but frequent daily nonreflex and reflex seizures (70% of all ictal events) remained. Repeat video EEG showed residual interictal and ictal activity over the left frontocentral convexity and this right-handed man was not considered a candidate for additional cortical resection. He received VNS at the age of 35 (final settings: 2.5 mA, 500 μs, 30 Hz, 30 s 'on', 5 min 'off'). After 2 years of follow-up, there was marked reduction of reflex eating seizures (70%) and a less prominent (40%) reduction in nonreflex seizure frequency.

We used standard adult VNS parameters and the results presented here were obtained under this conventional paradigm. No other stimulation parameters were tried. Reflex eating seizures improved dramatically in all 3 of our patients (70–95%). A less impressive reduction in nonreflex seizure frequency was also noted in 2 of the patients (5–40%). This was especially true in the second patient, in whom only reflex eating seizures improved after VNS, while reflex hot water and nonreflex seizures remained unchanged. This selective reduction in reflex eating seizure frequency was very likely related to modulation of the incoming visceral neural activity being transferred to CNS through the vagus nerve. Temporolimbic and insular areas might be crucial in generating eating seizures at the cortical level, but these episodes are triggered by peripheral input from organs innervated by the vagus nerve. It is not clear how such a global effect could be obtained after unilateral VNS; theoretically, the nonstimulated right vagus nerve would possibly continue to trigger ictal events. It is possible that unilateral VNS would be modulating bilaterally the ascending activity at the brainstem level, after going through the tractus solitarius complex. Battery depletion in one patient led to an increase in seizure frequency, although not to pre-VNS baseline, suggesting that there was a long-term suppressive effect on epileptogenesis after prolonged (6 years) VNS. The fact that patients get worse after battery depletion, but not back to baseline seizure frequency, is usual in patients submitted to neuromodulatory techniques (VNS or deep brain stimulation). This is very likely related to delayed neuroplasticity induced by these techniques [13].

References

1 A randomized controlled trial of chronic vagus nerve stimulation for treatment of medically intractable seizures. The Vagus Nerve Stimulation Study Group. Neurology 1995;45:224–230.

2 Handforth A, DeGiorgio CM, Schachter SC, Uthman BM, Naritoku DK, Tecoma ES, et al: Vagus nerve stimulation therapy for partial-onset seizures: a randomized active-control trial. Neurology 1998; 51:48–55.

3 Holder LK, Wernicke JF, Tarver WB: Treatment of refractory partial seizures: preliminary results of a controlled study. Pacing Clin Electrophysiol 1992; 15:1557–1571.

4 Jadad AR, Moore RA, Carroll D, Jenkinson C, Reynolds DJ, Gavaghan DJ, et al: Assessing the quality of reports of randomized clinical trials: is blinding necessary? Control Clin Trials 1996;17:1–12.

5 Ben-Menachem E, Mañon-Espaillat R, Ristanovic R, Wilder BJ, Stefan H, Mirza W, et al: Vagus nerve stimulation for treatment of partial seizures: 1. A controlled study of effect on seizures. Vagus Nerve Stimulation First International Study Group. Epilepsia 1994;35:616–626.

6 Ramsay RE, Uthman BM, Augustinsson LE, Upton AR, Naritoku D, Willis J, et al: Vagus nerve stimulation for treatment of partial seizures: 2. Safety, side effects, and tolerability. Vagus Nerve Stimulation First International Study Group. Epilepsia 1994;35: 627–636.

7 Aaronson ST, Carpenter LL, Conway CR, Reimherr FW, Lisanby SH, Schwartz TL, et al: Vagus nerve stimulation therapy randomized to different amounts of electrical charge for treatment-resistant depression: acute and chronic effects. Brain Stimul 2013;6:631–640.
8 Amar AP, Heck CN, Levy ML, Smith T, DeGiorgio CM, Oviedo S, et al: An institutional experience with cervical vagus nerve trunk stimulation for medically refractory epilepsy: rationale, technique, and outcome. Neurosurgery 1998;43:1265–1276.
9 Klinkenberg S, Aalbers MW, Vles JS, Cornips MS, Rijkers K, Leenen L, et al: Vagus nerve stimulation in children with intractable epilepsy: a randomized controlled trial. Dev Med Child Neurol 2012;54: 855–861.
10 Klinkenberg S, van den Bosch CN, Majoie HJ, Aalbers MW, Leenen L, Hendriksen J, et al: Behavioural and cognitive effects during vagus nerve stimulation in children with intractable epilepsy – a randomized controlled trial. Eur J Paediatr Neurol 2013;17:82–90.
11 Cukiert A, Cukiert CM, Burattini JA, Lima AM, Forster CR, Baise C, Argentoni-Baldochi M: A prospective long-term study on the outcome after vagus nerve stimulation at maximally tolerated current intensity in a cohort of children with refractory secondary generalized epilepsy. Neuromodulation 2013;16:551–556.
12 Cukiert A, Cukiert CM, Burattini JA, Lima AM, Forster CR, Baise C, Argentoni-Baldochi M: Long-term outcome after callosotomy or vagus nerve stimulation in consecutive prospective cohorts of children with Lennox-Gastaut or Lennox-like syndrome and non-specific MRI findings. Seizure 2013;22:396–400.
13 Cukiert A, Mariani PP, Burattini JA, Cukiert CM, Forster CR, Baise C, Argentoni-Baldochi M, Mello V: Vagus nerve stimulation might have a unique effect in eating reflex seizures. Epilepsia 2010;51:301–303.

Arthur Cukiert, MD, PhD
Epilepsy Surgery Program, Clinica de Epilepsia de Sao Paulo and
Department of Neurology and Neurosurgery, ABC Faculty of Medicine
R Dr. Alceu de Campos Rodrigues 247, #121
CEP 04544-000 São Paulo, SP (Brazil)
E-Mail acukiert@uol.com.br

Slavin KV (ed): Stimulation of the Peripheral Nervous System. The Neuromodulation Frontier.
Prog Neurol Surg. Basel, Karger, 2016, vol 29, pp 53–63 (DOI: 10.1159/000434655)

Vagus Nerve Stimulation for Major Depressive Episodes

Sam Eljamel

Department of Neurosurgery, Centre for Neurosciences, The University of Dundee, Dundee, Scotland, UK

Abstract

Stimulation of the left vagus nerve is a novel antidepressive therapy that relies upon the vagal projections to the brain stem to modulate brain circuits involved in mood regulation. There is cumulative evidence from prospective and long-term studies that has demonstrated tolerability and effectiveness of vagus nerve stimulation (VNS) in major depressive episodes (MDE). VNS in MDE has the following advantages: symptomatic response (defined as at least a 50% improvement in MDE severity) occurs in at least 15–17% of patients after 10 weeks of VNS treatment and in at least 22–37% of patients after 12 months of VNS treatment, remissions are observed in at least 15–17% of patients after 12 months of treatment, there is a sustained response in 13–27% of patients during 12 months of VNS, and successful maintenance of the initial improvement is observed in a high percentage of patients (73–77% of patients who had meaningful or greater benefit after 3 months of treatment maintained at least meaningful benefit after 12 months of treatment). VNS is a well-tolerated treatment as indicated by the high continuation rates of VNS therapy in the D01 and D02 studies after 12 months of therapy (90–98%) and the low rate of adverse event-related study discontinuations through 12 months or more in these studies (3%). Adverse effects are characterized by the absence of systemic effects associated with drug therapy and are primarily limited to those related to stimulation of the vagus nerve; many of the common adverse effects only occurred when VNS was on with the ability to stop acute stimulation-related adverse effects immediately through the use of magnet deactivation of the VNS device. More importantly, there were no adverse cognitive and psychomotor effects observed with antidepressant drugs and electroconvulsive therapy, no overdose toxicity observed with antidepressant drugs, favorable findings in animal reproductive studies, and an ability to add VNS therapy to antidepressant drug therapy without producing drug-drug interactions. Finally, VNS has high treatment compliance because VNS therapy is programmed to work automatically without the need for action on the patient's part (no pills to swallow).

Major depressive episodes (MDE), including major depressive disorders and bipolar disorders (BPD), present a major health burden to societies worldwide [1, 2] and the World Health Organization statistics predict MDE will be the leading cause of disease burden by 2030, in front of stroke, heart disease, and cancer. Treatment resistance and treatment refractoriness (TR) in patients treated for MDE are more common than previously thought [3], and generate significant financial burden as measured by patient treatment costs, disability claims, decreased productivity, and missed work [1, 4–6]. TR in MDE is generally defined as failure to respond to at least 2 adequate antidepressant drug trials from 2 different classes of antidepressants [7]. Up to 30% of MDE is refractory to treatment [8]; as a result of this high TR rate, several investigators were prompted to explore alternative therapies. Vagus nerve stimulation (VNS) for TR-MDE was one of the new therapies that has attracted attention over the last 2 decades [9].

The rationale for investigating VNS therapy as a potential treatment for depression was derived from three observations. First, during clinical trials that evaluated VNS in epilepsy, improvements in the depression scores were reported in patients receiving VNS therapy for the treatment of epilepsy. These improvements were independent of improvement in the patients' seizures [10, 11]. Second, antiepileptic drugs are prescribed as mood stabilizers in BPD to enhance the effectiveness of antidepressant drugs. Third, electroconvulsive therapy (ECT), which is often regarded as the most efficacious acute treatment for depression, exerts a marked anticonvulsant effect. Studies examining the central nervous system effects of VNS also contributed to the rationale for VNS as an antidepressant treatment. Based on the vagus nerve projections within the brain and preliminary work examining the effects of VNS on neurotransmitters, it appears that stimulating the vagus nerve produces effects on norepinephrine and serotonin, the two principal neurotransmitters implicated in the therapeutic effect of antidepressant drugs [12]. Finally, functional brain imaging has demonstrated VNS therapy modulates activity in regions of the brain believed to be involved in mood regulation, including the limbic system [13].

Clinical Issues

The main issues to discuss when VNS is considered for TR-MDE include:

- When can MDE be considered refractory or resistant to treatment?
- What is the optimal dosing of VNS in TR-MDE?
- How can responders be identified prior to VNS implantation?
- Can a TR-MDE patient give informed consent?

In MDE, treatment resistance or TR was defined as failure of at least 4 adequate antidepressive therapies, including psychotherapy and ECT [14]; out of 4 trials from 2 different classes of antidepressants, 2 must show failure to respond despite adequate antidepressant drug doses [7].

The optimal dosing of VNS in TR-MDE is currently undefined [15]. However, the treating physician must identify the optimum settings for each patient while balancing the goals of maximizing efficacy, minimizing side effects, and preserving battery life. Output current is gradually increased from 0.25 mA to the maximum tolerable level (maximum = 3.5 mA); typical therapeutic settings range from 1.0 to 1.5 mA. Greater output current is associated with increased side effects, including hoarseness of voice, tickly cough, a feeling of throat tightening, and sometimes dyspnea. Frequency is typically programmed at 20 Hz and pulse width is typically set at 250 or 500 μs. The recommended initial 'on' time is 30 s, followed by 5 min 'off' time; it is recommended that the 'off' time be greater than the 'on' time.

There are no preimplantation parameters that can reliably predict the efficacy of or response to VNS [16]. However, patients with mild-to-moderate MDE are more likely to respond to VNS therapy than those with extreme MDE [17].

Informed consent was and remains a major concern of any form of neurosurgery for mental disorders (NMD) including VNS for TR-MDE, e.g. there is the question of whether an appropriate candidate for VNS can give valid consent or can a third party, family, or society who might benefit give consent on behalf of a patient. Some have argued that NMD might produce irreversible changes in behavior, self, or mind of the consenting individual on the same bar as mutilation or disfigurement. However, with stringent and rigorous consenting processes, patients deemed to be candidates for any form of NMD should be evaluated by experienced dedicated psychiatrists at specialized (academic) centers and referred to an independent mental healthcare committee that has the authority to review the diagnosis, its refractoriness, the proposed NMD procedure, and whether the sufferer is able to give informed consent. The consenting process requires several consultations with the sufferer and his/her caregiver, and the NMD procedure is carried out only after the referring psychiatrist and mental healthcare committee are satisfied that the sufferer understands the pros and cons of the proposed procedure and the aftercare that is required. It is also to note that NMD should only be offered to patients who can give informed consent [14].

Indications of Vagus Nerve Stimulation in Major Depressive Episodes

VNS should only be considered in patients who fulfill the following criteria:

- The subjects had to be diagnosed as being in a MDE according to *Diagnostic and Statistical Manual of Mental Disorders IV* (DSM-IV) criteria ascertained from a structured interview by an expert psychiatrist.
- The subjects' depression is chronic (≥2 years' duration) and/or recurrent (≥4 lifetime episodes).
- Failed at least 2 adequate trials of 2 different classes of antidepressants.
- Failed at least one trial of ECT.
- Failed at least one trial of psychotherapy.

- The subjects had to have at least a minimum level of depression as defined by a score on the Hamilton Rating Scale for Depression (HRSD-24) of 20 or greater.
- Able to give informed consent.

Patient Selection

It has been suggested that VNS may be more effective in patients with less treatment-resistant forms of depression, at least as defined by numbers of failed 'adequate' antidepressant treatment trials [18]. This early study described a 50% response rate to VNS in patients failing 2 or 3 trials of antidepressants and a 29% response in those failing to respond to 4–7 trials. Those failing 7 or more previous antidepressant trials showed no response to VNS at all. Therefore, it has been suggested that VNS therapy is more likely to be successful if used in patients with lower degrees of pharmacological treatment resistance.

All patients considered for VNS therapy should be examined by an expert psychiatrist in depression who should conduct a detailed clinical assessment including structured clinical interview to confirm the diagnosis and the presence of comorbid conditions. Validated depression severity rating scales should be completed and a formal assessment of the patient's ability to provide informed consent should be conducted. Crucially, VNS should not be considered the only therapeutic option available to the patient, but should be considered as one option among a number of nonoperative and operative interventions. To facilitate consideration of all reasonable treatment options applicable, the input of a multidisciplinary team whose members have complementary expertise is essential. In particular, assessment of adequacy of previous trials of psychological therapies and ECT should be performed. These assessments and treatment discussions must be conducted before VNS is considered.

Outcome

The effectiveness of VNS for the treatment of depression was based primarily on analyses comparing the 12-month efficacy results from the D02 study participants treated with VNS plus standard of care with the 12-month efficacy results from the D04 study participants who were treated with standard-of-care treatment alone. Additional supportive evidence for a VNS-antidepressant effect was drawn from the efficacy results of the randomized phase of D02 study, the durability of the responses demonstrated during the long-term phase of both the D02 and D01 studies, and an indirect comparison of the D02 study's 12-month outcomes with the outcomes from a matched group of subjects in a multicenter study of ECT. The larger-scale two-part study (D02) was a randomized controlled trial of the acute effects of VNS, which recruited a total of 235 participants: 210 with major depressive disorders and

25 with BPD. These patients received either masked active or sham VNS over 10 weeks. Participants in the D02 study were adults who met DSM-IV criteria for MDE; participants could have had underlying major depressive disorders or BPD. The participants' MDE had to be chronic or recurrent. In addition, participants had to have failed in the current episode a minimum of 2 – but not more than 6 – adequate antidepressant treatments from different categories. The adequacy of prior treatment was determined using a modified version of a published scoring system developed to assess the adequacy of antidepressant treatments; a prior treatment was judged to be adequate if it received an antidepressant resistance rating of 3 or more (referred to as the Antidepressant Treatment History Form guidelines) [18]. The participants also had to have a baseline score of at least 20 on the 24-item HRSD (HRSD-24). All patients had a VNS system implanted and were then randomized to have stimulation turned on or left off for the 12-week acute treatment phase. The acute phase consisted of a 2-week recovery period following surgery during which stimulation remained off for all subjects, followed by a 2-week stimulation adjustment period for those subjects randomized to active VNS therapy (the sham-control group underwent identical procedures as did the active VNS therapy group, but had their output current set at 0 mA), followed by an 8-week period of treatment at the level of stimulation determined during the aforementioned stimulation adjustment period. Various clinical assessments, including depression ratings using standardized scales, were performed throughout the acute phase. Both the participants and the study personnel performing the depression ratings were blinded to treatment group allocation. The protocol-specified primary efficacy outcome for the acute phase was the percentage of treatment responders determined from the HRSD-24 ratings; response was defined a priori as a 50% or greater improvement in HRSD-24 score from baseline. The protocol permitted participants to continue antidepressant treatments they were receiving prior to the study, but participants could not increase antidepressant medication or add new ones. Subsequently, in a second phase of D02, 205 members of the original cohort were evaluated at 12 months after either 9 or 12 months of open-label VNS. In the first 10 weeks of the extension phase, stimulation parameter adjustments and weekly or every-other-week clinic visits and assessments were undertaken. Otherwise, the protocol specified monthly clinic visits for both groups through 12 months of active VNS therapy. Various assessments, including depression ratings, were performed throughout this period. During the long-term extension phase, investigational site programmers were allowed to adjust stimulation parameters as clinically indicated. Additionally, concomitant antidepressant treatments could be added, removed, or adjusted as clinically deemed necessary. In this naturalistic study, VNS was well tolerated and 27% of patients appeared to improve, with 16% achieving remission [10, 19–26].

Another observational study (D04) compared long-term outcomes of patients enrolled in the D02 study with a matched VNS-naïve TR-MDE population receiving 'treatment as usual'. The D04 study was conceived to collect long-term clinical and health economic outcomes from patients receiving standard antidepressant therapies without VNS for the treatment of depression. Because the study was observational in nature, the protocol did not specify specific therapies for the treatment of depression; instead, the physician managing the study participant's depression selected therapy according to his or her clinical judgment. The physician had the ability to select any antidepressant therapy available, except investigational treatments. Thus, antidepressant therapy in the D04 study comprised 'standard of care' or 'treatment as usual'. The specific assessments included the Inventory of Depressive Symptomatology Self-Report (IDS-SR), HRSD-24, Clinical Global Impressions (CGI), and Medical Outcomes Survey 36-Item Short Form Health Survey (SF-36), which were in common to D02. The IDS-SR is a 30-item, multidimensional patient self-report rating of the symptoms of mood and depression. This well-validated scale is becoming more widely used in clinical studies for assessing depression symptoms. The HRSD is the rating scale most widely used in clinical trials to assess symptoms of depression; it is a multidimensional observer-rated scale for assessing overall depression severity. There are several versions of HRSD, including ones with 28, 24, 21, and 17 items. The 28-item version of the scale was administered in the D02 and D04 studies. The CGI includes two 7-point scales completed by the clinician rater to assess a subject's condition regarding severity of illness (CGI-S) and global improvement (CGI-I). The CGI was developed by the National Institute of Mental Health to provide a standardized assessment with clinically relevant anchors; it is one of the most widely used brief assessment tools in psychiatry. The SF-36 is a widely used quality-of-life scale that assesses multiple domains. Over 12 months, 27% of VNS patients showed significant improvements as compared to 15% of the matched controls. According to an intention-to-treat analysis of the primary efficacy model (n = all 235 implanted D02 participants with VNS and all 127 D04 controls), the mean difference between the D02 and D04 groups in the estimated mean change from baseline in IDS-SR scores continued to show a superior outcome in the D02 group at the same level of significance as shown in the evaluable population analysis ($p < 0.001$; fig. 1). Ten percent (20/205) of the D02 and 12% (15/124) of the D04 participants had a diagnosis of BPD. Analyses were performed to compare the efficacy outcomes in the BPD subgroups. The results in the BPD subjects were similar to those in the overall groups. For example, the 12-month HRSD-24 response rate in the D02 evaluable population was 29% (5/17) for BPD (vs. 30% for the overall D02 evaluable population). Owing to the small sample sizes, differences between D02 and D04 were not statistically significant. The combined data prompted the FDA to approve VNS as an adjunctive treatment of TR-MDE in 2005.

Prior to D02, an open-label study (D01) was carried out; it was a prospective, open-label, nonrandomized, uncontrolled clinical study. It initially enrolled 30 patients and was reported in 2000 [16]. The results suggested that VNS provided symptom relief in 40% of the patients with MDE and that an additional 16% of the patients had remission of symptoms following VNS. The study limitations included lack of a control group, small sample size, lack of power analysis, and 10-week follow-up. An additional

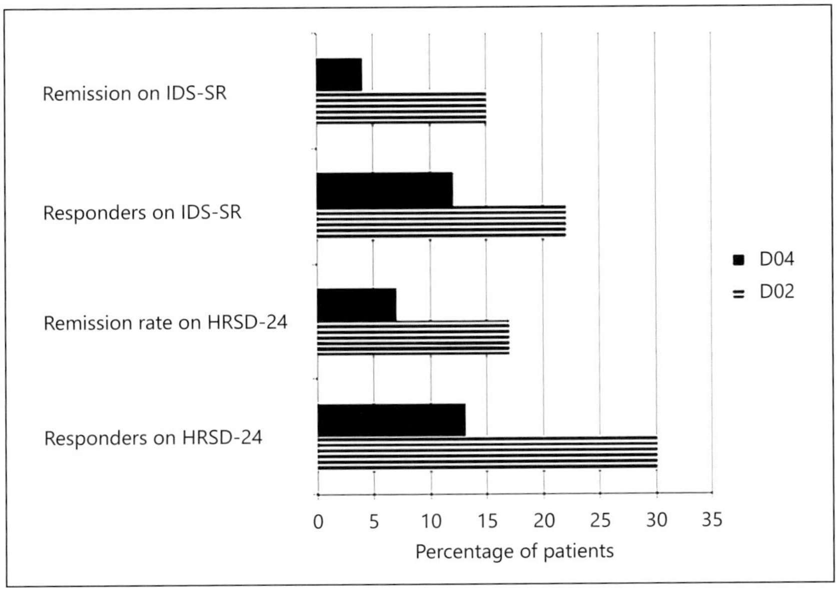

Fig. 1. Comparison of D02 and D04 outcome data.

group of 30 patients was enrolled and the results were reported in 2001 [17]. The investigators concluded that mean time from response to treatment was 48.1 days. Based on the HDRS and the Montgomery-Åsberg Depression Rating Scale (MADRS), the results were 30.5–34.0% at the 10-week follow-up. Remission was reported in 15.3% of the patients.

Subsequently, an open-label multicenter study of VNS for chronic, medication-refractory MDE was conducted in Europe (D03). Of the 74 subjects recruited, data for 70 participants were reported at 3 months, for 61 at 12 months, and for 49 at 2 years [27, 28]. As in previous studies, an increase in benefit in response (42% or 25/59) and remission (22%) rates was observed over time. Another study of VNS for the treatment of MDE was a phase IV clinical trial (D21; registered as NCT 00305565) that aimed to recruit 330 participants diagnosed with either chronic or recurrent MDE. This study commenced recruiting in January 2006 and the last participant completed the study in February 2010. The protocol required participants to have three successive randomly assigned stimulation settings. Further outcome data of this study are awaited. Though some have suggested that VNS is less effective in patients diagnosed with very resistant MDE, a recent study compared the 12-month outcome of D03 (28 patients) and 13 extremely resistant patients from the Dundee Advanced Interventions Centre (Scotland): the response rate at 12 months of the D03 patients was 35.7% and the Dundee cohort was 30.8% [29]. In 2005, a 2-year outcome study of 60 patients with VNS for MDE was published. The results indicated that remission occurred in 15% at 3 months, 27% after 12 months, and 22% after 2 years. Response rates were 31, 44, and 42% at 3, 12, and 24 months,

Table 1. Potential side effects following left VNS in MDE

Patient-reported side effects	Related to surgery, %	Stimulation related, %
Surgical site pain	30	0
Headaches	7	24 (only 7% definite)
Chest pain	3	13 (only 3% definite)
Infection	7	0
Hoarseness of voice	7	53 (only 40% definite)
Dyspnea	3	20 (only 3% definite)
Coughing	0	13 (only 10% definite)
Dysphagia	3	13 (only 10% definite)
Twitching	0	7 (none definite)

respectively. The authors concluded that VNS in TR-MDE was durable with long-term benefit [30]. In 2012, a systematic review and meta-analysis of studies to determine the efficacy of VNS MDE was published. Fourteen studies met the selection criteria and were included in the review. The meta-analysis of efficacy for uncontrolled studies showed a significant reduction in scores using the HRSD endpoint and the percentage of responders was 31.8%. To study the cause of heterogeneity in studies, a meta-regression analysis was performed. The adjusted coefficient of determination was 0.84, which implies that an 84% variation in effect size across the studies was explained by baseline severity of depression [31]. Generally, VNS is reported to be a safe and feasible procedure in MDE.

Although VNS in MDE is safe and appears to be effective in a significant number of patients, the UK National Institute for Health and Care Excellence (NICE) published a technology appraisal guideline which concluded that a total of 1,251 VNS procedures had been carried out by 2009. NICE went on to conclude that the mechanism of action, predictors of outcome, differential responses, and optimal stimulation parameters remain unknown [32].

Potential Complications of Vagus Nerve Simulation in Major Depressive Episodes

Left VNS therapy in MDE is associated with a similar side-effect profile as those observed with VNS therapy in epilepsy. These potential complications are divided into those associated with the surgical procedure to implant the VNS system, reversible side effects of electric stimulation of the left vagus nerve, and hardware related complications. The most common side effect of the procedure remains infection (5–7%). While it can be treated with antibiotics, one study showed that infection led to lead or generator removal in 1.5% of patients [33]. In this setting, reimplantation of the device is technically much more challenging. While vocal cord paralysis occurs in around 1% of patients, hoarseness of voice is much more common, but is reversible following switching the device off or changing the stimulation parameters. There is a concern about cardiac side effects, and while bradycardia and asystole have been reported intraoperatively in 0.1% of patients, this is possibly due to incorrect electrode placement, indirect cardiac nerve stimulation, accidental polarity, or device malfunction. These cardiac effects are not usually seen postoperatively [34, 35]. Other side effects include throat pain, cough, vomiting, paresthesias, and dysphagia. Dyspnea remained commonly reported in 3.2% of patients, but was classed as relatively mild by patients [33]. Table 1 summarizes potential side effects of left VNS in MDE (adopted from George et al. [19]).

Conclusions

In summary, left VNS therapy in MDE has the following advantages:

- Response (at least a 50% improvement) in at least 15–17% of patients after 10 weeks of treatment.
- Response in at least 22–37% of patients after 12 months of treatment.
- Remission rate in at least 15–17% of patients after 12 months of treatment.
- Sustained response in 13–27% of patients during 12 months of treatment.
- Successful maintenance of the initial improvement in a high percentage of patients (73–77% of patients who had meaningful or greater benefit after 3 months of treatment maintained at least meaningful benefit after 12 months of treatment).
- Safe and well-tolerated treatment as indicated by the high continuation rates of VNS therapy in the D01 and D02 studies after 12 months of therapy (90–98%) and the low rate of adverse event-related study discontinuations through 12 months or more in these studies (3%).
- Adverse effects essentially limited to those related to stimulation of the vagus nerve; absence of systemic effects associated with antidepressive drug therapy; many of the common adverse effects only occurred when stimulation of the vagus nerve was on.
- The ability to stop acute stimulation-related adverse effects immediately through the use of magnet deactivation of the VNS device.
- Absence of adverse cognitive and psychomotor effects associated with antidepressant drugs and ECT.
- Absence of the overdose toxicity observed with antidepressant drugs.
- Favorable findings in animal reproductive studies.
- Ability to add VNS therapy to antidepressant drug therapy without producing drug-drug interactions.
- High treatment compliance because VNS therapy is programmed to work automatically without the need for patient's action (no tablets, capsules, or pills to take).

References

1 Birnbaum HG, Kessler RC, Kelley D, Ben-Hammadi R, Joish VN, Greenberg PE: Employer burden of mild, moderate, and severe major depressive disorder: mental health services utilization and costs, and work performance. Depress Anxiety 2010;27:78–89.

2 Patten SB, Kennedy SH, Lam RW, O'Donovan C, Filteau MJ, Parikh SV, Ravindran AV; Canadian Network for Mood and Anxiety Treatment (CANMAT): Canadian Network for Mood and Anxiety Treatment (CANMAT) clinical guidelines for the management of major depressive disorder in adults. I. Classification, burden, and principles of management. J Affect Disord 2009;117(suppl 1):S5–S14.

3 Thase ME: STEP-BD and bipolar depression: what have we learned? Curr Psychiatry Rep 2007;9:497–503.

4 Gibson TB, Jing Y, Smith Carls G, Kim E, Bagalman JE, Buton WN, Tran QV, Pikalov A, Goetzel RZ: Cost burden of treatment resistance in patients with depression. Am J Manag Care 2007;16:370–377.

5 Fostick L, Silberman A, Beckman M, Spivak B, Amital D: The economic impact of depression: resistance or severity. Eur Neuropsychopharmacol 2010;20:671–675.

6 Hoffman DL, Dukes EM, Wittchen HU: Human and economic burden of generalized anxiety disorder. Depress Anxiety 2008;25:72–90.

7 Thase ME, Rush AJ: When at first you don't succeed: sequential strategies for antidepressant nonresponders. J Clin Psychiatry 1997;58(suppl 13):23–29.

8 Trivedi MH, Fava M, Wisniewski SR, Thase ME, Quitkin F, Warden D, Ritz L, Nierenberg AA, Lebowitz BD, Biggs MM, Luther JF, Shores-Wilson K, Rush AJ: Medication augmentation after the failure of SSRIs for depression. N Engl J Med 2006;354:1243–1252.

9 Kennedy SH, Giacobbe P: Treatment resistant depression – advances in somatic therapies. Ann Clin Psychiatry 2007;19:279–287.

10 Nahas Z, Burns C, Foust MJ, Short B, Herbsman T, George MS: Vagus nerve stimulation (VNS) for depression: what do we know now and what should be done next? Curr Psychiatry Rep 2006;8:445–451.

11 Marangell LB, Martinez M, Martinez JM, George MS, Sackeim HA: Vagus nerve stimulation: a new tool for treating depression. Prim Psychiatry 2005;12:40–43.

12 Nierenberg AA, Alpert JE, Gardner-Schuster EE, Seay S, Mischoulon D: Vagus nerve stimulation: 2-year outcomes for bipolar versus unipolar treatment-resistant depression. Biol Psychiatry 2008;64:455–460.

13 Chae JH, Nahas Z, Lomarev M, Denslow S, Lorberbaum JP, Bohning DE, George MS: A review of functional neuroimaging studies of vagus nerve stimulation (VNS). J Psychiatr Res 2003;37:443–455.

14 Eljamel S: Strategies for the return of behavioral surgery. Surg Neurol Int 2012;3(suppl 1):S34–S39.

15 Rush AJ, Siefert SE: Clinical issues in considering vagus nerve stimulation for treatment-resistant depression. Exp Neurol 2009;219:36–43.

16 Rush AJ, George MS, Sackeim HA, Marangell LB, Husain MM, Giller C, Nahas Z, Haines S, Simpson RK Jr, Goodman R: Vagus nerve stimulation (VNS) for treatment-resistant depressions: a multicenter study. Biol Psychiatry 2000;47:276–286.

17 Sackeim HA, Rush AJ, George MS, Marangell LB, Husain MM, Nahas Z, Johnson CR, Seidman S, Giller C, Haines S: Vagus nerve stimulation (VNS) for treatment-resistant depression: efficacy, side effects, and predictors of outcome. Neuropsychopharmacology 2001;25:713–728.

18 Dew RE, Kramer SI, McCall WV: Adequacy of antidepressant treatment by psychiatric residents: the antidepressant treatment history form as a possible assessment tool. Acad Psychiatry 2005;29:283–288.

19 George MS, Sackheim HA, Rush AJ, Marangell LB, Nahas Z, Husain MM: Vagus nerve stimulation: a new tool for brain research and therapy. Biol Psychiatry 2000;47:287–295.

20 Sackeim HA, Brannan SK, Rush AJ, George MS, Marangell LB, Allen J: Durability of antidepressant response to vagus nerve stimulation (VNS). Int J Neuropsychopharmacol 2007;10:817–826.

21 George MS, Rush AJ, Marangell LB, Sackeim HA, Brannan SK, Davis SM: A one-year comparison of vagus nerve stimulation with treatment as usual for treatment-resistant depression. Biol Psychiatry 2005;58:364–373.

22 Nierenberg AA, Alpert JE, Gardner-Schuster EE, Seay S, Mischoulon D: Vagus nerve stimulation: 2-year outcomes for bipolar versus unipolar treatment-resistant depression. Biol Psychiatry 2008;64:455–460.

23 Burke MJ, Husain MM: Concomitant use of vagus nerve stimulation and electroconvulsive therapy for treatment-resistant depression. J ECT 2006;22:218–222.

24 Carpenter LL, Moreno FA, Kling MA, Anderson GM, Regenold WT, Labiner DM, Price LH: Effect of vagus nerve stimulation on cerebrospinal fluid monoamine metabolites, norepinephrine, and gamma-aminobutyric acid concentrations in depressed patients. Biol Psychiatry 2004;56:418–426.

25 Conway CR, Sheline YI, Chibnall JT, George MS, Fletcher JW, Mintun MA: Cerebral blood flow changes during vagus nerve stimulation for depression. Psychiatry Res 2006;146:179–184.
26 Pardo JV, Sheikh SA, Schwindt GC, Lee JT, Kuskowski MA, Surerus C, Lewis SM, Abuzzahab FS, Adson DE, Rittberg BR: Chronic vagus nerve stimulation for treatment-resistant depression decreases resting ventromedial prefrontal glucose metabolism. Neuroimage 2008;42:879–889.
27 Schlaepfer TE, Frick C, Zobel A, Maier W, Heuser I, Bajbouj M, O'Keane V, Corcoran C, Adolfsson R, Trimble M, Rau H, Hoff HJ, Padberg F, Müller-Siecheneder F, Audenaert K, Van den Abbeele D, Matthews K [removed], Christmas D [removed], Stanga Z, Hasdemir M: Vagus nerve stimulation for depression: efficacy and safety in a European study. Psychol Med 2008;38:651–661.
28 Bajbouj M, Merkl A, Schlaepfer TE, Frick C, Zobel A, Maier W, O'Keane V, Corcoran C, Adolfsson R, Trimble M, Rau H, Hoff HJ, Padberg F, Müller-Siecheneder F, Audenaert K, van den Abbeele D, Matthews K, Christmas D, Eljamel S, Heuser I: Two-year outcome of vagus nerve stimulation in treatment-resistant depression. J Clin Psychopharmacol 2010;30:273–281.
29 Christmas D, Steele JD, Tolomeo S, Eljamel MS, Matthews K: Vagus nerve stimulation for chronic major depressive disorder: 12-month outcomes in highly treatment-refractory patients. J Affect Disord 2013;150:1221–1225.
30 Nahas Z, Marangell LB, Husain MM, Rush AJ, Sackeim HA, Lisanby SH, Martinez JM, George MS: Two-year outcome of vagus nerve stimulation (VNS) for treatment of major depressive episodes. J Clin Psychiatry 2005;66:1097–1104.
31 Martin JL, Martín-Sánchez E: Systematic review and meta-analysis of vagus nerve stimulation in the treatment of depression: variable results based on study designs. Eur Psychiatry 2012;27:147–155.
32 Vagus Nerve Stimulation for Treatment-Resistant Depression. IPG330. London, National Institute for Health and Care Excellence, 2009.
33 Ben-Menachem E: Vagus-nerve stimulation for the treatment of epilepsy. Lancet Neurol 2002;1:477–482.
34 Tatum WO 4th, Moore DB, Stecker MM, Baltuch GH, French JA, Ferreira JA, Carney PM, Labar DR, Vale FL: Ventricular asystole during vagus nerve stimulation for epilepsy in humans. Neurology 1999;52:1267–1269.
35 Asconape JJ, Moore DD, Zipes DP, Hartman LM, Duffell WH Jr: Bradycardia and asystole with the use of vagus nerve stimulation for the treatment of epilepsy: a rare complication of intraoperative device testing. Epilepsia 1999;40:1452–1454.

Prof. Sam Eljamel, MBBCh, MD, FRCSIr, FRCSEd, FRCS(SN)
Neurosurgery, HTNMS
22 Trophichen Street
Edinburgh, EH3 8JB (UK)
E-Mail sameljamel@doctors.net.uk

Slavin KV (ed): Stimulation of the Peripheral Nervous System. The Neuromodulation Frontier.
Prog Neurol Surg. Basel, Karger, 2016, vol 29, pp 64–75 (DOI: 10.1159/000434657)

Phrenic Nerve Stimulation: Technology and Clinical Applications

Shane V. Abdunnur • Daniel H. Kim

Department of Neurosurgery, University of Texas Health Science Center at Houston, Houston, Tex., USA

Abstract

Phrenic nerve stimulation is a technique used to reanimate the diaphragm of patients with central nervous system etiologies of respiratory insufficiency. Current clinical indications include congenital central hypoventilation syndrome, spinal cord injury above C4, brain stem injury, and idiopathic severe sleep apnea. Presurgical evaluation ensures proper patient selection by validating the intact circuit from the phrenic nerve through alveolar oxygenation. The procedure involves placing leads around the phrenic nerves bilaterally and attaching these leads to radio receivers in a subcutaneous pocket. The rate and amplitude of the current is adjusted via an external radio transmitter. After implantation, each patient progresses through a conditioning phase that strengthens the diaphragm and progressively provides independence from the mechanical ventilator. Studies indicate that patients and families experience an improved quality of life and are satisfied with the results. Phrenic nerve stimulation provides a safe and effective means for reanimating the diaphragm for certain patients with respiratory insufficiency, providing independence from mechanical ventilation.

History

In 1777, Cavallo was the first physician to claim that an electrical current could be used as a mechanism for artificial respiration. The modern-day concept of phrenic nerve stimulation began to take shape in 1818 when Andre Ure claimed to be able to restore ventilation in cases of suffocation, drowning, and hanging by direct stimulation of the phrenic nerve [1]. In 1872, Duchenne's seminal work on phrenic nerve stimulation in a patient showed that it was technically possible to conduct an electrical current through the phrenic nerve as a means of stimulating the diaphragm into a physiologically significant contraction [2]. Little technological advance with the

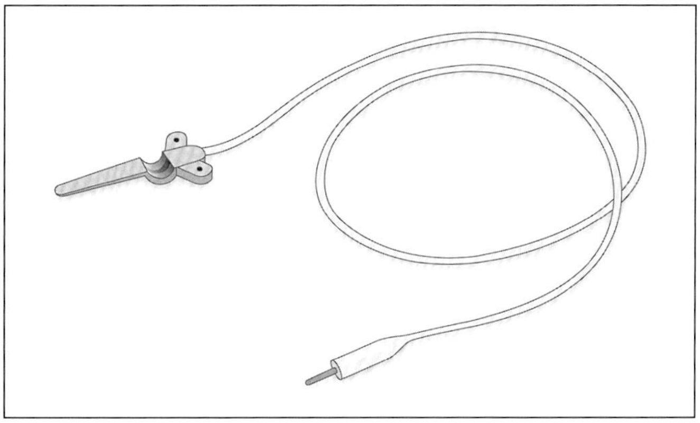

Fig. 1. Avery Mark IV Breathing Pacemaker System™ electrode lead and wire. The platinum lead is housed in silastic tubing that can be secured around the phrenic nerve. It is connected to a stainless steel wire with a connector terminus at the distal end (with permission from Avery Biomedical Devices).

technique was made over the following 150 years due to the advent and application of positive pressure ventilation or mechanical ventilation. Although the physiological aspects of electrical stimulation, muscle contraction, oxygenation, and carbon dioxide tension pressures were being elucidated, it was not until the pioneering work of William Glenn at Yale University that the intricacies of pacing and modulation began to be worked out. Meanwhile, battery technology improved, and the first implanted cardiac pacemaker was inserted in 1960. William Glenn used this newfound technology to stimulate the phrenic nerve in a patient on a long-term basis with much success [3]. Glenn partnered with Roger Avery to develop the first prototype that was brought to commercial distribution by Avery Laboratories Inc. (Commack, N.Y., USA) in the early 1970s [4].

Current Technology

Three major companies distribute phrenic nerve pacers throughout the world. Avery Laboratories distributes a pacemaker in the United States, the European Union, and several other countries. The Atrostim Phrenic Nerve Stimulator (PNS) V2.0 (Atrotech, Tampere, Finland) and Vienna Phrenic Pacemaker (MedImplant Biotechnisches Labor, Vienna, Austria) are the other two commercially available devices. Because the Avery Mark IV Breathing Pacemaker System™ is the only device approved for use in the United States and the European Union, it will be the focus of this discussion. The other systems differ from each other and the one discussed below, but these differences are not critical to the surgeon.

The Avery Mark IV Breathing Pacemaker System™ is comprised of two internally implanted electrodes and two radio receivers. The electrodes are manufactured from flexible stainless steel wire insulated by a silastic coating. The stainless steel wire is connected to a platinum nerve contact at the proximal end, and the distal end connects easily to the radio receiver (fig. 1, 2). An alternative configuration that contains

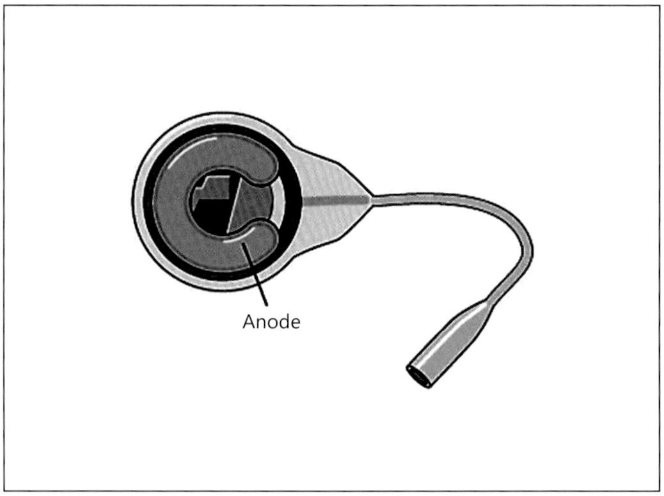

Fig. 2. Avery Mark IV Breathing Pacemaker System™ radio receiver. This internally implanted radio receiver connects to the lead and wire depicted in fig. 1. When connected, the radio receiver captures radiofrequency data that are sent by the radio transmitter and converts the data into an electrical signal that is propagated to the platinum lead connected to the phrenic nerve (with permission from Avery Biomedical Devices).

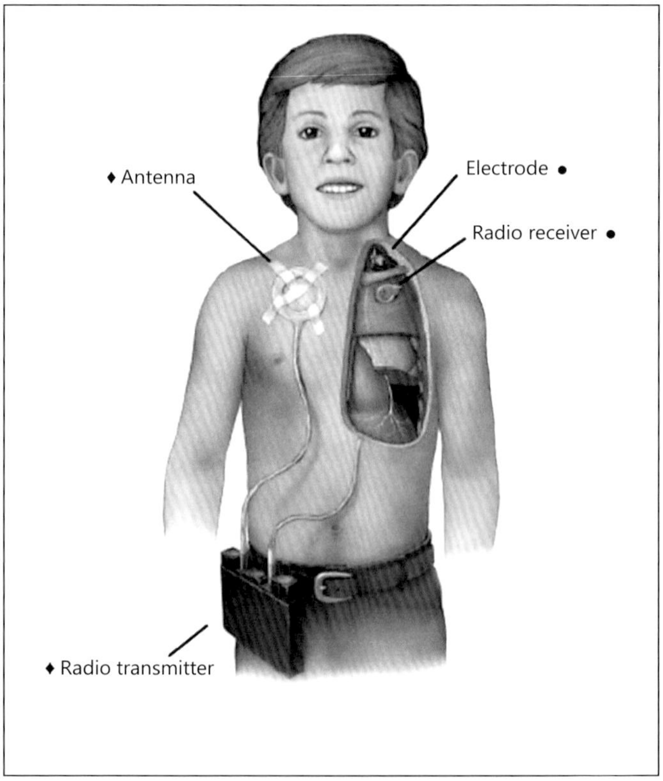

Fig. 3. Internal and external components that comprise the Avery Mark IV Breathing Pacemaker System™. This sketch depicts all components of the system, both internal (●) and external (◆) (with permission from Avery Biomedical Devices).

twin platinum contacts that connect directly to one receiver is also available. The smallest receiver has a 2.5-cm diameter and 0.55-cm thickness. All implanted elements are coated in silicon. An external antenna and radio transmitter are applied to the patient, as shown in figure 3. The manufacturer suggests that the antenna be replaced regularly every 6 months to avoid failure.

Fig. 4. Avery Mark IV Breathing Pacemaker System™ superior view radio transmitter. The external radio transmitter contains power-hungry battery functions, such as adjustment dials for the amplitude and rate output. Battery and antenna indicators help alert the patient or caregiver to impending maintenance that must occur for proper functioning (with permission from Avery Biomedical Devices).

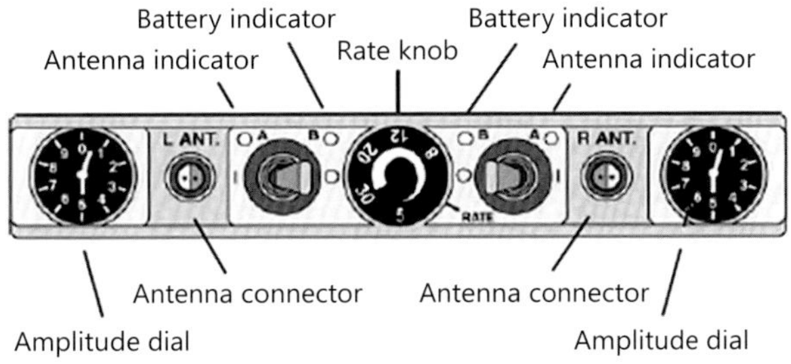

The radio transmitter is the programmable element in the circuit and consumes standard alkaline batteries. Because surgically implanted materials do not contain power-hungry programmable components, patients can typically go for many years without needing revision surgery for impulse generator purposes. Figure 4 depicts the relevant components of the radio transmitter. The radio transmitter can be adjusted with respect to the amplitude and rate. That information is transmitted to the implanted radio receivers bilaterally, and electrical stimulation of the phrenic nerve ensues. With an intact nerve and diaphragm, simultaneous right- and left-sided contraction of the diaphragm takes place and a negative inspiratory pressure ensues, providing the force needed to expand the thoracic cavity and oxygenate the alveoli.

Clinical Indications

Phrenic nerve pacers are implantable devices that provide an electrical current to the nerve, resulting in diaphragmatic contraction. This mechanism contributes support for patients with chronic ventilatory insufficiency whose phrenic nerve, diaphragm, and lungs demonstrate adequate independent function. To meet these requirements, patients need to have intact C4 anterior horn cells, phrenic nerves, diaphragm, and alveolar function. While C3, C4, and C5 all contribute to the phrenic nerve, C4 forms the largest contribution. Thus, patients with a central lesion above the C4 anterior horn cells comprise the majority of the patients who can currently benefit from the procedure. Alternatively, patients with lesions that include the C4 anterior horn cells may be candidates for direct diaphragmatic pacing or the other procedures discussed at the conclusion of this chapter. Although not the focus of this chapter, it should be noted that there are similar methods for direct pacing of the diaphragm. However, properties of the muscular contraction will differ when compared to physiological stimulation via an intact phrenic nerve.

Physicians have attempted to place stimulators in conjunction with phrenic nerve grafts in the setting of spinal cord stimulation [spinal cord injury (SCI)] below C3 and in cases of phrenic nerve injury from prior radiation or other causes. Although there are case reports of successful pacing and subsequent diaphragm conditioning, these are not typical indications. The current clinical indications include congenital central hypoventilation syndrome, SCI rostral to C4, brain stem injury, and idiopathic severe sleep apnea.

To date, congenital central hypoventilation syndrome and SCI comprise more than 75% of the patients who have received phrenic nerve pacers. Both populations, when appropriately selected, appear to benefit equally from the device. Patients have had phrenic nerve pacers placed for other indications with varying success, which is primarily due to patient selection. Patients with stroke, encephalitis, meningitis, and Shy-Drager syndrome may thus be candidates, although clinical decisions have to be strictly individualized in these cases.

Presurgical Evaluation

Candidates for the procedure must be carefully evaluated to ensure they meet the indications for implantation and successful pacing. Patients must be diagnosed with severe chronic respiratory insufficiency requiring mechanical ventilation or significant positive pressure support for more than 3 months. The viability of motor neurons should be confirmed prior to the procedure. Failure of diaphragmatic contraction after electrical stimulation is a contraindication. There may be exceptions to this dictum, as discussed in the last section of this chapter.

The viability of the phrenic nerve is critical and deserves a bit more attention. The best current means of testing its viability is by percutaneous electrical stimulation under fluoroscopy. The nerve is accessed in the neck where it passes over the anterior scalene muscle. When some axons in the nerve are viable, a brief low-amplitude contraction will occur. This is quite similar to a hiccup. A stronger contraction is desirable, and a more vigorous contraction will take place when all axons in the nerve are properly functioning [5]. The best means of assessing the strength of the contraction is on fluoroscopy. The unaided eye is not reliable due to patient factors such as age and body habitus.

The timing of these electrodiagnostic evaluations are critical and still a matter of controversy. A study in 2007 found that when tested in the acute phase after injury or insult, phrenic nerves tended to be responsive, although this response to external stimulus was not necessarily enduring. Conversely, the study also showed that patients whose phrenic nerves were not responsive in the subacute phase could become responsive to external stimulus up to a year later [6]. The current best recommendation is to perform percutaneous phrenic nerve electrical stimulation trials under fluoroscopy at 3 months after injury. Because some patients can recover phrenic nerve function after 3 months, it is reasonable to repeat the study at 12 months if the first trial did not show intact phrenic nerve conduction.

Surgical Technique

The cervical technique first described by Glenn et al. in 1976 [7] has undergone minor modifications over the last 40 years. The thoracic approach was initially developed for children whose necks were too small to accommodate the leads. With the size and technology of the current devices, this is rarely a concern. The following section will review both the thoracic and cervical approaches. It should be noted that both approaches are described for completeness, although the authors utilize the cervical technique due to its overall simplicity and excellent results.

Thoracoscopic Technique

Shaul et al. [8] were one of the first to describe the thoracoscopic approach, which is preferred over open thoracotomy. A patient older than 10 years should be prepared by establishing single-lung ventilation via a dual-lumen endotracheal tube. In a younger patient, it is sometimes possible to use a contralateral main stem intubation using a small cuffed endotracheal tube. The patient is then positioned on a bean bag so that the chest is almost full lateral while the hips are flatter, allowing for the abdomen to be in the semilateral position. Preoperative antibiotics are administered and surgical antiseptic techniques are utilized. The spare wire connecting the internal platinum electrode to the receiver is coiled upon itself and loosely held together with a nonabsorbable suture so that the appropriate length of wire unravels as the child grows. With the establishment of single contralateral ventilation, 0.5% bupivacaine is infiltrated into the subcutaneous tissue and a 5-mm trocar is introduced at the seventh intercostal space in the posterior axillary line. To inflate the chest and speed lung deflation, 5-mm Hg pressure is used. Two additional 5-mm trocars are inserted, one at the ninth intercostal space and the other at the fifth intercostal space, all in the posterior axillary line. A fourth trocar can be placed at the discretion of the surgeon if a lung retraction is required. The phrenic nerve is located and identified at the cephalad aspect of the pericardium. The nerve will overlie the mediastinal pleura. Two small incisions are made on either side of the phrenic nerve in a parallel trajectory to the nerve. Attention is then turned to implanting the device. A small subcostal incision is made, and a subcutaneous pocket is formed to house the radio receiver and excess wire. A 10-cm Penrose drain is placed over the male end of the connector and tied in place with a heavy suture. The opposite end of the Penrose drain is inserted through the ninth intercostal space trocar, and the drain, wire, and electrode are placed into the chest. A small tunnel is then created with a tonsil clamp, which is inserted into the chest through the anterolateral aspect of the diaphragm. The male end of the Penrose drain is brought through the chest into the subcutaneous pocket through the fifth intercostal space trocar. The phrenic nerve lead is then passed under the mediastinal pleura so that the nerve lies over the groove in the lead. This is sutured in place using a 4-0 silk suture. The lead is attached to the receiver, and the system is tested with the help of a representative. This step ensures the integrity of the circuit and adequate diaphragm contraction. The radio receiver and silastic coils are placed in the subcutaneous pocket and retested. Care must be taken to leave enough slack in the wiring so that the phrenic nerve is not under traction. A 20-Fr chest tube is place through the caudal-most incision where it will not interfere with the wire, and the lung is inflated under direct vision. Wounds are closed in the usual fashion, and occlusive dressings are applied. The patient then requires repositioning, and the procedure is repeated on the opposite side. It is customary to obtain a chest X-ray at the conclusion of the procedure. If there is no evidence of pneumothorax, the chest tubes may be removed while the patient is still under anesthesia. The patient is left intubated and placed in the intensive care unit. The total operative time is typically 3–4 h, and patients require aggressive pulmonary hygiene and physiotherapy to help prevent pneumonia. Patients are generally discharged 24–48 h later.

Cervical Technique

This technique was originally described by Glenn et al. [7] in 1976 and has undergone minor modifications to suit the modern-day needs of the implants. This is the preferred technique due to ease of patient positioning, implant placement, and shorter recovery time as compared with the thoracoscopic approach. The patient is placed supine on the operating table and intubated with a single-lumen endotracheal tube. A small roll is placed under the shoulders to accentuate the upper chest and lower neck. Gentle traction can be applied to the shoulders bilaterally via tape to maintain them caudally. Care is taken to ensure that the patient's head is not rotated to either the right or left side. Antibiotics are administered, and a sterile surgical field is prepared, including the entire neck down to the nipples bilaterally. The sternocleidomastoid (SCM) muscles are palpated bilaterally. Approximately 5 cm above the clavicle, a horizontal incision is marked. The area is infiltrated with 0.5% bupivacaine. A 2- to 3-cm horizontal incision is carried out over the lateral border of the SCM. The SCM is easily identified under the platysma muscle. Care is taken to mobilize the lateral border of the SCM, working both inferiorly and superiorly to the level of the incision. Once the SCM is freed, it is mobilized medially. It may be gently retracted medially by an assistant with a blunt handheld retractor. The body of the anterior scalene will be found on the posterior side of the SCM. The phrenic nerve will either be immediately identifiable or the surgeon may first need to mobilize the internal

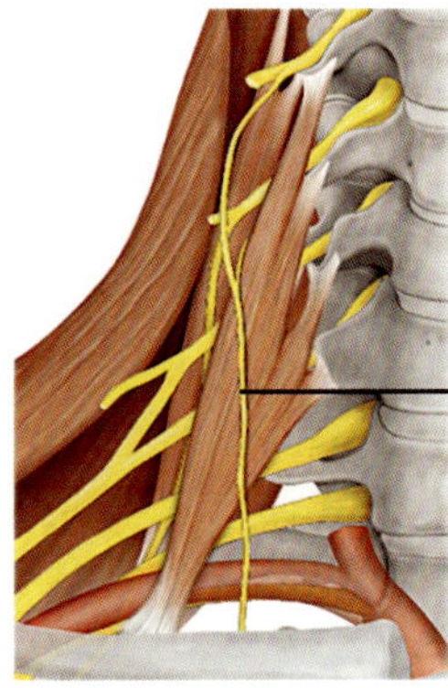

Fig. 5. Anatomic depiction of the phrenic nerve. The phrenic nerve lies directly anterior to the anterior scalene muscle as it courses inferiorly and slightly medially between the levels of the midbody of C5 and the midbody of C7. Approaching the nerve at this location is advantageous because vascular structures remain inferior to the surgical field and the nerve has received all of its contributions from the C3–C5 nerve roots.

jugular vein medially. Typically, this is not necessary if the incision is 5 cm above the clavicle. The phrenic nerve will be approximately 0.5 cm in diameter at this location, directly overlying the anterior scalene muscle (fig. 5). Occasionally, an accessory phrenic nerve may be observed, but its caliber is smaller. If there is any question about its location, the accessory phrenic nerve can be traced superiorly to the lateral border of the anterior scalene muscle where it clearly emerges from the anterior ramus of C5. It also lies laterally to the phrenic nerve. This nerve does not need to be incorporated into the pacing lead. Attention is then turned toward fashioning the subcutaneous pocket. Halfway between the clavicle and the nipple, 0.5% bupivacaine is injected and an approximately 3-cm incision is made. A small subcutaneous pocket is created, and a tonsil clamp is used to tunnel from the pocket to the cervical incision site, superficial to the clavicle. The male end of the wire is gently grasped on the silastic tubing, and the tonsil clamp is brought back through to the subcutaneous pocket. The male end is then connected to the radio receiver, and heavy suture is used to tie the two together. The phrenic nerve is then laid over the groove in the platinum lead, and a 4-0 nonabsorbable suture is used to secure the lead in place around the nerve (fig. 6). The lead should be anchored to the nearby anterior scalene muscle or SCM, such that the lead does not cause a kink in the nerve when laid flat without tension. The system is tested with the help of a representative, and the diaphragm will contract with good force at low impedance if the circuit is intact. The radio receiver and extra wire are then placed in the subcutaneous pocket and retested to ensure functionality prior to closing the incisions in layers (fig. 7). The procedure is then repeated on the opposite side of the patient without need to re-prep the skin or reposition (fig. 8). The total surgical time is approximately 1 h. At the authors' institution, most of the patients do not live in the immediate vicinity and are typically discharged from the hospital the next morning. There is no medical contraindication to discharge on the same day as the procedure.

Fig. 6. Leads attached to the phrenic nerve via the cervical approach. The SCM seen at the top of the picture is gently displaced medially by a cerebellar retractor. The twin-lead version of the Avery Mark IV Breathing Pacemaker System™ is being implanted. The superior lead has been attached to the phrenic nerve and is held closed by a Weck clip. The phrenic nerve is seen distally before the second lead is secured to the nerve. The anterior scalene, which lies deep to the phrenic nerve, is not shown.

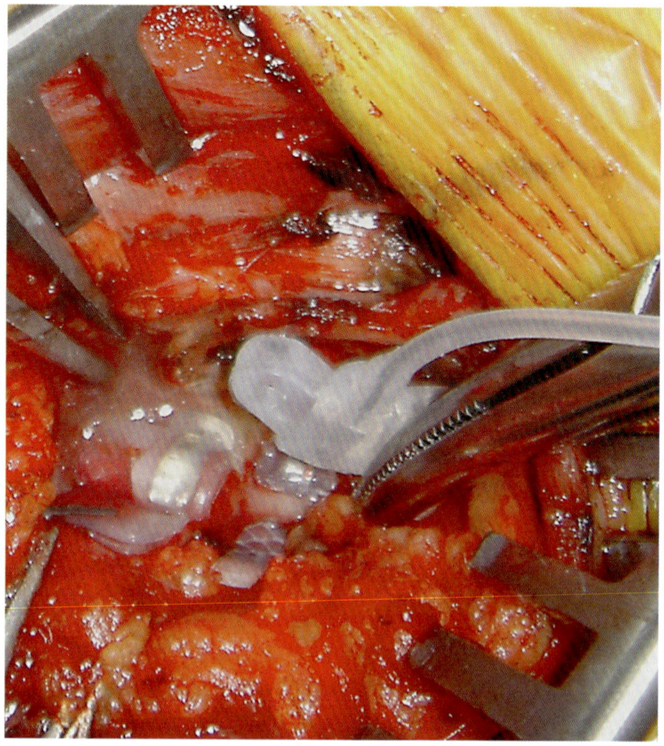

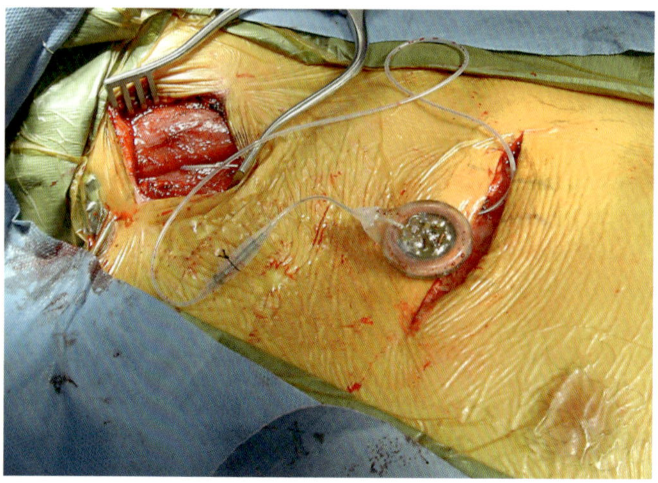

7

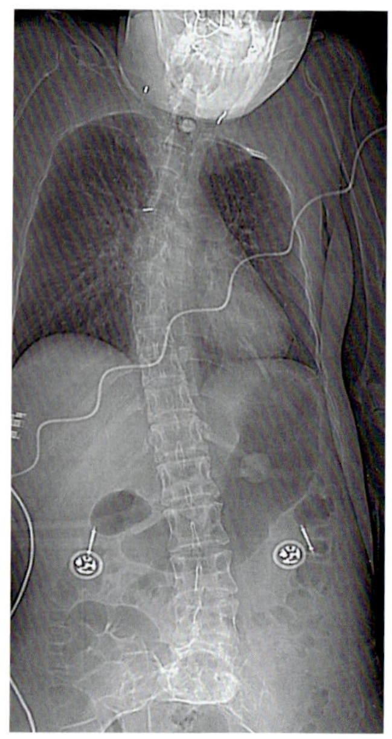

8

(*For legends see next page.*)

Follow-Up Care

Return to clinic appointments are typically 2 weeks from the date of surgery when the wound is assessed for integrity. While some surgeons prefer to delay pacing for 6 weeks to allow fibrotic scar formation around the lead when placed thoracoscopically, this is not necessary after using the cervical approach.

When diaphragm pacing and conditioning is initiated, patients are admitted to a rehabilitation unit or hospital for 2–3 days. The amplitude, rate, and time of phrenic nerve stimulation are adjusted to achieve the desired tidal volume and ventilation determined by noninvasive measures such as pulse oximetry and end-tidal PCO_2. Initially, most patients are able to tolerate 1–2 h of pacing per day. This is somewhat dependent on the physiology of the patients and their medical condition. The phase of endurance training will then take place on an outpatient basis. Pacing is increased 1 h each week until the pacing goal is reached. Pacing is replaced with mechanical ventilation at the first sign of fatigue because patients can decompensate quickly. The initiation of pacing and conditioning/endurance training is typically managed by a pulmonary care, physical medicine and rehabilitation, or neurorehabilitation physician.

Complications

Typical complications of anesthesia, infection, and bleeding are possible. Procedure-specific complications include possible injury to the phrenic nerve and surrounding vascular structures. The battery life of the radio receiver can be 5 years or more with the current state of technology. Patients can expect to need a revision at that time. Shaul et al. [8] presented a total of 9 patients, including one who had pneumonia and one who had a liver laceration. Glenn et al. [9] retrospectively collected a multicenter complication profile that essentially represented a meta-analysis of several centers; therefore, the statistical data are limited. Despite this, they found a 4.5% rate of infection and a 5–15% rate of pacing failure that was attributed to iatrogenic nerve injury.

Fig. 7. Cervical implant placement. This is a right-sided intraoperative image after the lead has been placed and the distal wiring has been tunneled and connected to the radio receiver. Note that the wire emerges from the lateral aspect of the SCM and is tunneled superficially to the clavicle where the male end of the connector is secured to the radio receiver with a silk tie. Excess wiring is then coiled in the subcutaneous pocket behind the radio receiver, and the wounds are closed in layers.

Fig. 8. X-ray showing placement of bilateral phrenic nerve stimulation system. This scout image from a computed tomography scan shows leads from both a right thoracoscopic and bilateral cervical approach in a patient that had phrenic nerve stimulation performed over 20 years ago. The radio receivers were placed over the abdomen at that time, and the pacers were verified as functional 20 years after placement.

Outcomes

In well-selected patients, phrenic nerve pacing provides an opportunity for partial or complete freedom from mechanical ventilation. Current outcome data are difficult to amalgamate because the number of patients that fit current indications for phrenic nerve stimulation is small. Data are scattered across multiple centers and are typically collected in a retrospective manner without matched controls. Nevertheless, the multicenter study conducted by Glenn et al. [9] from 1966 through 1988 showed that 84% of patients had gained significant respiratory support from their stimulator. The majority of these patients were able to pace for at least 12 h a day. A total of 16% experienced failure. Over 45% of the patients in the study were able to pace for 24 h per day. More recent data from 1998 indicate that 18 of 22 patients were able to pace continuously for 24 h. The remaining 4 patients paced during sleep [10].

An analysis of unpublished data conducted by the authors addresses quality of life outcomes in patients who have received the Avery Mark IV Breathing Pacemaker System™. These data contain 127 patients worldwide, the vast majority of whom had their implant placed for congenital central hypoventilation syndrome or SCI. Only 25–30% of these patients were able to pace for 24 h per day as compared to the preceding numbers. In contrast, over 90% of patients were using their pacers, which is a higher rate than reported elsewhere. Moreover, 96% of all patients stated that their pacer improved their quality of life, and 84% of patients said their pacemaker had a positive impact on their school/work and social life. Over 50% of quadriplegic patients also believed that their phrenic nerve pacers improved their ability to swallow, speak, and smell compared to mechanical and other means of positive pressure ventilation. When surgical indications are less stringently applied, these outcomes are not as favorable. The outcomes data show that phrenic nerve stimulation is safe, effective, and can positively impact numerous metrics in properly selected patients.

Future Directions

The field of neuromodulation is rapidly evolving as technology improves and physicians and industry partners learn more about the physiologic properties of peripheral nerves and derangements that occur because of injury, infection, metabolic insults, and other pathologies. Surgeons are continuously applying new neuromodulation techniques. A major limitation is the clinical indication for SCI patients at C3 and above. The most common location for SCI is at C4–C6. Krieger et al. [11] and Krieger and Krieger [12] have reported reanimation of the diaphragm after intercostal to phrenic nerve anastomosis for patients with SCI below C3 [11, 12]. More recently, a technique modification leading to direct diaphragmatic muscular pacing has been applied to patients with amyotrophic lateral sclerosis and poliomyelitis. Patients with amyotrophic lateral sclerosis are able to delay ventilator dependency for an average of 2 years if pacing is utilized [13, 14]. These techniques, if proved fruitful, will provide new indications for the procedure and may allow more patients to live independently of mechanical ventilation.

References

1 Hufeland CW: De usu vis electricae in asphyxia experimentis illustrato. Inaugural dissertation, Göttingen, 1873.

2 Duchenne G-B: De l'électrisation localisée et de son application à la pathologie et à la thérapeutique par courants induits et par courants galvaniques interrompus et continus. 3ème éd. Paris, Baillière, 1872.

3 Judson JP, Glenn WW: Radio-frequency electrophrenic respiration. Long-term application to a patient with primary hypoventilation. JAMA 1968;203: 1033–1037.

4 History of phrenic nerve pacing. Avery Biomedical Devices. http://www.averybiomedical.com/additional-resources/history-of-pacing (accessed on December 26, 2014).

5 Sarnoff SJ, Sarnoff LC, Whittenberger JL: Electrophrenic respiration. VII. The motor point of the phrenic nerve in relation to external stimulation. Surg Gynecol Obstet 1951;93:190–196.

6 Versteegh MI, Braun J, Voigt PG, Bosman DB, Stolk J, Rabe KF, Dion RA: Diaphragm plication in adult patients with diaphragm paralysis leads to long-term improvement of pulmonary function and level of dyspnea. Eur J Cardiothorac Surg 2007;32:449–456.

7 Glenn WW, Holcomb WG, Shaw RK, Hogan JF, Holschuh KR: Long-term ventilator support for diaphragm pacing in quadriplegia. Ann Surg 1976;183: 566–577.

8 Shaul DB, Danielson PD, McComb JG, Keens TG: Thoracoscopic placement of phrenic nerve electrodes for diaphragmatic pacing in children. J Pediatric Surg 2002;37:974–978.

9 Glenn WW, Brouillette RT, Dentz B, Fodstad H, Hunt CE, Keens TG, Marsh HM, Pande S, Piepgras DG, Vanderlinden RG: Fundamental considerations in pacing of the diaphragm for chronic ventilator insufficiency: a multi-center study. Pacing Clin Eletrophysiol 1988;11:2121–2127.

10 Garrido-Garcia H, Mazaira Alvarez J, Martín Escribano P, Romero Ganuza J, La Banda F, Gambarrutta C, Garcia ME, Labarta C, Arroyo O, Sebastián de la Cruz F, Gutierrez R, García Moreno J: Treatment of chronic ventilator failure using diaphragmatic pacemaker. Spinal Cord 1998;36:310–314.

11 Krieger A, Gropper M, Adler R: Electrophrenic respiration after intercostals to phrenic anastomosis in a patient with anterior spinal artery syndrome: technical case report. Neurosurgery 1994;35:760–764.

12 Krieger L, Krieger A: The intercostals to phrenic nerve transfer: an effective means of reanimating the diaphragm in patients with high cervical spine injury. Plast Reconstr Surg 2000;103:1255–1261.

13 Onders R, Carlin A, Elmo M, Sivashakaran S, Katirji B, Schilz R: Amyotrophic lateral sclerosis: the Midwestern surgical experience with the diaphragm pacing stimulation system shows that general anesthesia can be safely performed. Am J Surg 2009;197:386–390.

14 Onders R, Elmo M, Khansarinia S, Bowman B, Yee J, Road J, Bass B, Dunkin B, Ingvarsson PE, Oddsdóttir M: Complete worldwide operative experience in laparoscopic diaphragm pacing: results and differences in spinal cord injured patients and amyotrophic lateral sclerosis patients. Surg Endosc 2009;23:1433–1440.

Prof. Daniel H. Kim, MD, FAANS, FACS, Director of Spinal Neurosurgery/Reconstructive Peripheral Nerve Surgery
Memorial Hermann Health System, Department of Neurosurgery
University of Texas Health Science Center at Houston
6400 Fannin St., Ste. 2150
Houston, TX 77030 (USA)
E-Mail daniel.h.kim@uth.tmc.edu

Slavin KV (ed): Stimulation of the Peripheral Nervous System. The Neuromodulation Frontier.
Prog Neurol Surg. Basel, Karger, 2016, vol 29, pp 76–82 (DOI: 10.1159/000434658)

Trigeminal Ganglion Stimulation

Jean-Pierre Van Buyten

Multidisciplinary Pain Center, AZ Nikolaas, Sint-Niklaas, and Clinique du Parc Léopold (CHIREC Hospitals), Brussels, Belgium

Abstract

Facial pain in the distribution of the trigeminal nerve, commonly identified as trigeminal neuralgia, should not be confused with trigeminal neuropathic pain. The latter is caused by an accidental and nonintentional nerve lesion. When the first-line pharmacological treatment fails to provide satisfactory pain relief, surgical treatment, such as microvascular decompression and neurodestructive interventions (radiofrequency or cryotherapy), is not indicated. The logical choice of technique becomes neuromodulation, but it may be challenging to perform in the facial area. Although the initial results of trigeminal ganglion stimulation were promising, they often were of short duration because of lead migration and inadequate stimulation coverage in the trigeminal nerve distribution. To ensure accurate placement and proper anchoring, a custom-made electrode was developed and produced, and its stereotactic implantation is guided by electromagnetic navigation. This technique has been used at our center for several years; the published results show at least 30% of pain relief in 75% of the patients and considerable reduction in medication use.

The term 'craniofacial pain' describes a variety of conditions that tend to respond to different approaches when it comes to pharmacological and interventional therapy. The success of any chosen treatment mainly depends on an accurate diagnosis. A recent review of the differential diagnosis and management of facial pain [1] states that the accuracy of diagnosis of facial pain depends on the consulted physician; based on this, the recommendation to treat chronic facial pain by a multidisciplinary team was made. In the past, any pain occurring in the distribution region of the trigeminal nerve often led to the diagnosis of trigeminal neuralgia, whereas in some cases the diagnosis

Table 1. Burchiel's classification of facial pain syndromes (adapted from Burchiel [3])

Diagnosis	History/pattern	Causes
Spontaneous onset		
TN type I	>50% paroxysmal pain	Neurovascular compression of trigeminal nerve or unknown
TN type II	<50% paroxysmal pain	Neurovascular compression of trigeminal nerve or unknown
Symptomatic TN	TN due to multiple sclerosis, tumors, etc.	Demyelination
Atypical facial pain	Somatoform pain disorder	
Peripheral trigeminal injury		
TNP	Incidental nonintentional injury	ENT/oral surgery, facial trauma, stroke, etc.
Trigeminal deafferentation pain	Trigeminal injury from peripheral ablation	RF rhizotomy, glycerol rhizolysis, GKR, balloon compression, etc.
Postinfection		
Postherpetic neuralgia	Herpes zoster outbreak	Shingles involving trigeminal distribution

ENT = Ear, nose, and throat; GKR = Gamma-Knife radiosurgery; RF = radiofrequency; TN = trigeminal neuralgia.

of trigeminal neuropathic pain (TNP) would have been more accurate. Subsequently, various therapies including high doses of carbamazepine, tricyclic antidepressants, opioids, surgical treatment with microvascular decompression procedures, and neurodestructive procedures of the trigeminal nerve were proposed. Although the last approach is preferred for the treatment of classic trigeminal neuralgia, in treatment of pharmacologically refractory TNP, success of neurodestructive interventions can hardly be expected. Sweet's [2] large-scale study showed that these neurodestructive procedures did not have any beneficial effect and instead aggravated pain symptoms in 73% of the patients. These findings suggested that an alternative treatment method is required. Appropriate treatment selection should be based on a correct subdiagnosis of the facial pain.

Two classification methods are useful for the diagnosis of craniofacial pain. The commonly used classification schema proposed by Burchiel [3] is based on the patient's symptoms and history (table 1). The second classification is the International Classification of Headache Disorders (ICHD), which may also help in establishing a proper diagnosis [4].

Neuromodulation Techniques for Facial Pain and Headache

The use of neuromodulation techniques for the management of intractable facial pain and headache was a direct spin-off of the gate control theory [5]. The first trials with low-intensity stimulation of peripheral nerves via implanted electrodes were performed by Wall and Sweet [6] using electrical stimulation applied to trigeminal branches on themselves. The improvement in anatomic knowledge and development of appropriate procedural equipment has resulted in neuromodulation becoming an integral part of the current treatment algorithm of facial pain and headache syndromes.

Neuromodulation of the Gasserian Ganglion

Shelden et al. [7] first attempted electrical stimulation of the trigeminal nerve in 1962. Meyerson and Håkanson [8] sutured a bipolar plate electrode to the dura overlying the gasserian ganglion using an open craniotomy technique. This technique involved high risks mainly because of the required approach and was soon abandoned. A major weakness in this approach was the fact that the stimulation parameters could not be tested prior to the permanent implantation. In 1978 and 1984, Steude [9] and Meglio [10] described the first percutaneous technique for gasserian ganglion stimulation. In a large implant series, Steude [11, 12] concluded that 86% of patients with TNP, and 100% of patients with trigeminal deafferentation pain had relief from gasserian ganglion stimulation. In Toronto, Tasker and colleagues reported similar results [13].

Although complications were rare, the most common problem was electrode dislocation due to the unique anatomy of the foramen ovale [14, 15]. Thus, several shapes and sizes of electrodes were used to try to overcome this problem, including a 'sigma' electrode, 'quinta' trigeminal anchored electrode, and a sacral nerve root stimulation electrode (Model 3889; Medtronic Neurological, Minneapolis, Minn., USA). The size of the electrodes seems to affect the incidence of displacements and the rate of discomforting dysesthesia. In the experience of Mehrkens and Steude [14], a 0.7-mm electrode (SP, Medtronic) became displaced in 10% of cases but did not produce dysesthesias, whereas a 0.9-mm electrode (Model 3483 SNS, Medtronic) had no dislocations but resulted in dysesthesias in 18% of the patients. The 'anchor electrode' (Quinta, Model 3981, Medtronic) was 1.2 mm in diameter and was associated with dysesthesias in 30% of cases and became dislodged in about 30% of cases [14]. The general impression was that larger electrodes seem to be less prone to displacements, but have a higher chance of eliciting dysesthesia [14]. To reduce the incidence of dislocation and improve the precision of the electrode placement, a custom-made Tripolar Bent Tined TGS Lead (Model 09053, Medtronic Neurological; fig. 1) was introduced along with a technique that involves real-time 3D tip-tracked electromagnetic guidance [16].

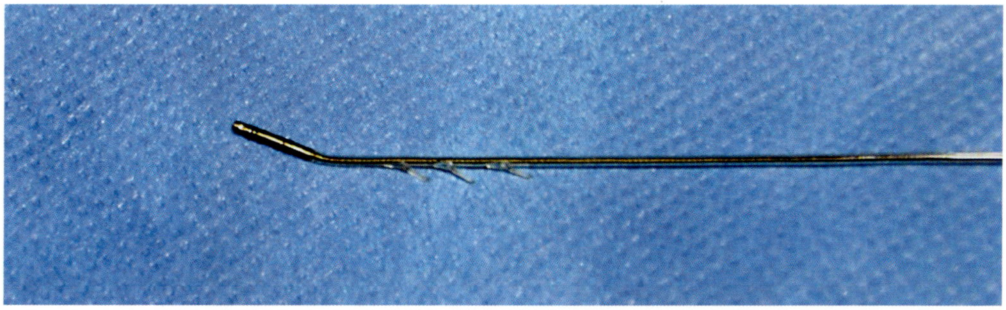

Fig. 1. Custom-made Tripolar Bent Tined TGS Lead (Model 09053, Medtronic Neurological). Modified from Van Buyten et al. [17].

Technique of Gasserian Ganglion Stimulation

The procedure is performed in two stages. The first is a trial lasting at least 4 weeks with an externalized electrode. On the day prior to implant, a 3D computed tomography (CT) scan of the head is acquired and used to guide needle placement into the foramen ovale using the O-arm®-coupled electromagnetic neuronavigational system (Medtronic). In the operating room the patient is placed in the supine position on a radiolucent table. With proper monitoring, sedation is given using propofol (Diprivan®; AstraZeneca, Wilmington, Del., USA). The O-arm® is placed around the head of the patient, allowing continuous high-definition fluoroscopy. To place the lead, an intraoperative CT scan is acquired, and a 3D reconstruction is used to calculate the path to the gasserian ganglion through the foramen ovale. Based on the 3D images, entry and target points are set and a virtual track is proposed in axonal, coronal, and sagittal planes (fig. 2). A local anesthetic is then injected at the entry point. A small incision is made lateral to the labial commissure, and a 15-gauge needle is inserted. In our center, all incisions are made by a plastic surgeon to obtain the most aesthetic result after wound healing.

The needle is then guided by 3D real-time electromagnetic tip tracking into the foramen ovale [16]. Under continuous fluoroscopic control, the electrode is inserted until its tip reaches the clivus. At that moment the patient is awakened, and a test-stimulation performed until paresthesia is evoked in the area of neuropathic pain. The needle is withdrawn under continuous fluoroscopic control to assure that the electrode remains in the correct position, and a nonabsorbable braided 4-0 suture (Mersilene; Ethicon, Somerville, N.J., USA) is placed on the electrode at the entry site. No anchor is used. The patient is then re-sedated and the electrode tunneled subcutaneously between the maxilla and mandibular region. A second suture is then placed in a preauricular position. We chose this position to prevent traction on the lead by movement of the neck and jaw (fig. 3). Finally, in case of a positive trial, an internal pulse generator (Itrel 3 or similar device, Medtronic) is placed in

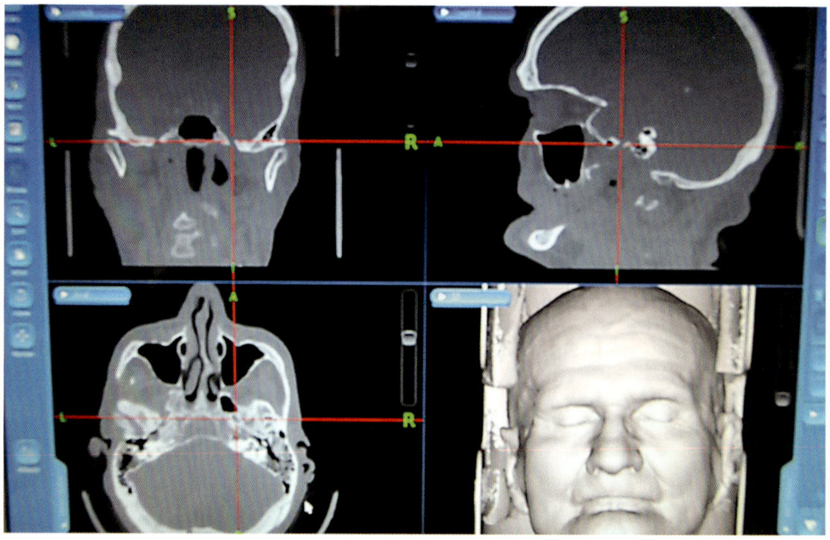

Fig. 2. View of the screen of the navigation station with coronal, axial, and sagittal views of the foramen ovale.

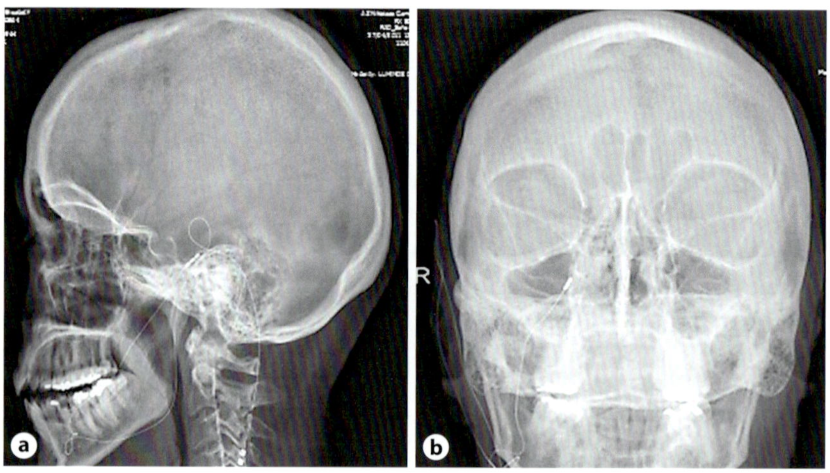

Fig. 3. Lateral (**a**) and anteroposterior (**b**) fluoroscopic images of the electrode. Modified from Van Buyten et al. [17].

the infraclavicular fossa. Skull-base X-ray and CT scan confirmation films are then obtained.

The special electrode design is more flexible after removal of the stylet, reducing traction or irritation with movement of the head and face. The electrode diameter of 1.2 mm was chosen for better stability – despite earlier concerns, it did not elicit dysesthesias in our series. Because of the negative experience with various anchoring devices that have not reduced the risk of dislodgement (and could create facial area irritation), Mersilene sutures are used to fix the electrode subcutaneously at the mandibular and preauricular region.

Results of Gasserian Ganglion Stimulation

The most comfortable frequency of stimulation has proven to be 50 Hz. Pulse width is initially programmed at 450 μs. The amplitude of the stimulus varies between 0.2 and 2.5 V. Higher amplitudes tend to activate the masseter muscle or the periorbital muscles, giving rise to visible contractions of the jaw and blurred vision. Since low voltages are used for stimulation, battery longevity is expected to be high. In a series of 8 patients, 6 patients experienced at least 30% pain relief [17]. Medication intake was significantly reduced and 4 patients stopped opioid treatment completely. Two patients had minor dislocation that required revision. No major complications were observed.

Conclusions

Trigeminal neuropathy may be extremely painful and refractory to conservative management. Neurostimulation of the gasserian ganglion has been documented to provide lasting pain relief. The problem of electrode dislocation has largely been solved by the use of a custom-made electrode and suturing the electrode subcutaneously. Electromagnetic guidance allows precise electrode placement and avoids unexpected injury of the adjacent anatomical structures.

References

1 Zakrzewska JM: Differential diagnosis of facial pain and guidelines for management. Br J Anaesth 2013; 111:95–104.

2 Sweet WH: Percutaneous methods for the treatment of trigeminal neuralgia and other faciocephalic pain; comparison with microvascular decompression. Semin Neurol 1988;8:272–279.

3 Burchiel KJ: A new classification for facial pain. Neurosurgery 2003;53:1164–1167.

4 Headache Classification Subcommittee of the International Headache Society. The International Classification of Headache Disorders: 2nd ed. Cephalalgia 2004;24:9–160.

5 Melzack R, Wall PD: Pain mechanisms: a new theory. Science 1965;150:971–979.

6 Wall PD, Sweet WH: Temporary abolition of pain in man. Science 1967;155:108–109.

7 Shelden CH, Pudenz RH, Doyle J: Electrical control of facial pain. Am J Surg 1967;114:209–212.

8 Meyerson BA, Håkanson S: Suppression of pain in trigeminal neuropathy by electric stimulation of the gasserian ganglion. Neurosurgery 1986;18:59–66.

9 Steude U: Percutaneous electro stimulation of the trigeminal nerve in patients with atypical trigeminal neuralgia. Neurochirurgia (Stuttg) 1978;21:66–69.

10 Meglio M: Percutaneous implantable chronic electrode for radiofrequency stimulation of the gasserian ganglion: a perspective in the management of trigeminal pain. Acta Neurochir Suppl 1984;33:521–525.

11 Steude U: Chronic trigeminal nerve stimulation for the relief of persistent pain; in Gildenberg P, Tasker R (eds): Textbook of Stereotactic and Functional Neurosurgery. New York, McGraw-Hill, 1998, pp 1557–1564.
12 Steude U: Percutaneous electrical stimulation of the gasserian ganglion in patients with atypical trigeminal neuralgia. A new technique for percutaneous test stimulation and permanent implantation of a stimulation device; in Erdmann W, Oyama T, Pernak MJ (eds): The Pain Clinic 1. Utrecht, VNU Science Press, 1985, pp 239–246.
13 Taub E, Munz M, Tasker RR: Chronic electrical stimulation of the gasserian ganglion for the relief of pain in a series of 34 patients. J Neurosurg 1997;86: 197–202.
14 Mehrkens JH, Steude U: Chronic electrostimulation of the trigeminal ganglion in trigeminal neuropathy: current state and future prospects. Acta Neurochir Suppl 2007;97:91–97.
15 Osenbach R. Neurostimulation for the treatment of intractable facial pain. Pain Med 2006;7:S126–S136.
16 Van Buyten JP, Smet I, Van de Kelft E: Electromagnetic navigation technology for more precise electrode placement in the foramen ovale: a technical report. Neuromodulation 2009;12:244–249.
17 Van Buyten JP, Hens C: Chronic stimulation of the gasserian ganglion in patients with trigeminal neuropathy: a case series. J Neurosurg Rev 2011;1:73–77.

Dr. Jean-Pierre Van Buyten
Multidisciplinary Pain Center
AZ Nikolaas
Moerlandstraat, 1, BE–9100 Sint-Niklaas (Belgium)
E-Mail vanbuyten@skynet.be

Slavin KV (ed): Stimulation of the Peripheral Nervous System. The Neuromodulation Frontier.
Prog Neurol Surg. Basel, Karger, 2016, vol 29, pp 83–93 (DOI: 10.1159/000434659)

Carotid Sinus/Nerve Stimulation for Treatment of Resistant Hypertension and Heart Failure

Dali Yin · Konstantin V. Slavin
Department of Neurosurgery, University of Illinois at Chicago, Chicago, Ill., USA

Abstract
Hypertension and cardiovascular disease are leading causes of morbidity and mortality worldwide. The prevalence of resistant hypertension remains high and is expected to increase. Moreover, there are limitations to therapeutic interventions aimed at treating resistant hypertension and heart failure despite the wide availability of therapeutic agents and dietary and lifestyle modification. Device-based therapy by baroreflex activation via carotid sinus/nerve stimulation is currently undergoing investigation, and promising findings from clinical trials have been published. Baroreflex activation therapy may represent a new approach for treatment of these conditions by reducing sympathetic drive and increasing parasympathetic activity. Here we describe a new technology which is designed to deliver carotid sinus stimulation to electrically activate the carotid baroreceptors and baroreflex, thereby reducing blood pressure and improving cardiac function. The theory, surgical techniques, and clinical trials of carotid sinus stimulation are highlighted.

Resistant Hypertension

The prevalence of hypertension in the United States is estimated to be 33.6%, affecting more than 76 million adults with an estimated cost over USD 76.6 billion in 2010 [1]. Hypertension is a significant risk factor for stroke, heart failure (HF), myocardial infarction, and renal failure [2]. Moreover, 20–30% of hypertensive patients have treatment-resistant hypertension [3–5], and this rate is expected to increase in the future. Resistant hypertension is diagnosed when patients cannot decrease blood pressure (BP) to <140/90 mm Hg for the general population and <130/80 mm Hg for patients with diabetes mellitus, coronary artery disease, or chronic kidney disease in spite of treatment with three antihypertensive agents of different classes, including a diuretic [6]. Resistant hypertension is frequently associated with stroke, chronic kidney disease, heart disease, diabetes, and obesity [6, 7]. In such patients, new treatment approaches are needed to control BP and reduce hypertension-induced morbidities [2, 6, 8–12]. Studies have shown that the mechanisms of causing resistant hypertension are related to overflowing sympathetic activity and impaired baroreflex regulation [13–17].

Sympathetic Activity and Baroreflex Mechanism

The carotid sinus contains numerous baroreceptors that are sensitive to pressure changes in the arterial blood. Hering's nerve, which is a branch of the glossopharyngeal nerve, innervates the carotid sinus baroreceptors (fig. 1). An increase in BP leads to activation of the baroreceptors that are sensitive to stretch in the carotid sinus and aortic arch [18, 19]. Therefore, the firing rates increase in the afferent signals in the carotid body via the glossopharyngeal nerve and aortic bodies via vagus nerves to the solitary tract nucleus in the medulla oblongata [2, 18]. The brain interprets increased signals as an elevated BP and attempts to counteract it by transmitting signals to various end organs through a decrease in sympathetic drive and an increase in parasympathetic tone [2, 19]. The carotid baroreflex plays an important role in the control of both short-term and long-term regulation of BP to prevent excessive increases and drops, and to influence the structural and functional changes in both the heart and kidneys [2, 11].

Lohmeier et al. [13–16] have extensively investigated the mechanism of action of baroreflex activation on BP reduction in both normotensive and hypertensive animals. It has been shown that electrical baroreflex stimulation decreases BP through reduction of sympathetic activity as demonstrated by a decrease in plasma norepinephrine levels and preventing activation of the renin-angiotensin-aldosterone system. Patients with damage to baroreflex afferent or efferent nerve fibers present with baroreflex impairment and autonomic dysfunction, respectively [8, 20, 21]. Compensatory changes in the function of the sympathetic nervous system are an important component of primary hypertension and HF [6]. Decreased parasympathetic tone and increased sympathetic activity increase peripheral vascular resistance, reduce renal blood flow, and enhance sodium retention, thus contributing to adverse cardiac and vascular changes in terms of both structure and shape [6, 22]. The poor prognosis in different disease states including hypertension and HF is related to the sympathetic activation [8, 23]. It has also been reported that the degree of renal dysfunction in patients with different severities of kidney disease correlates well with the level of sympathetic activity [24, 25].

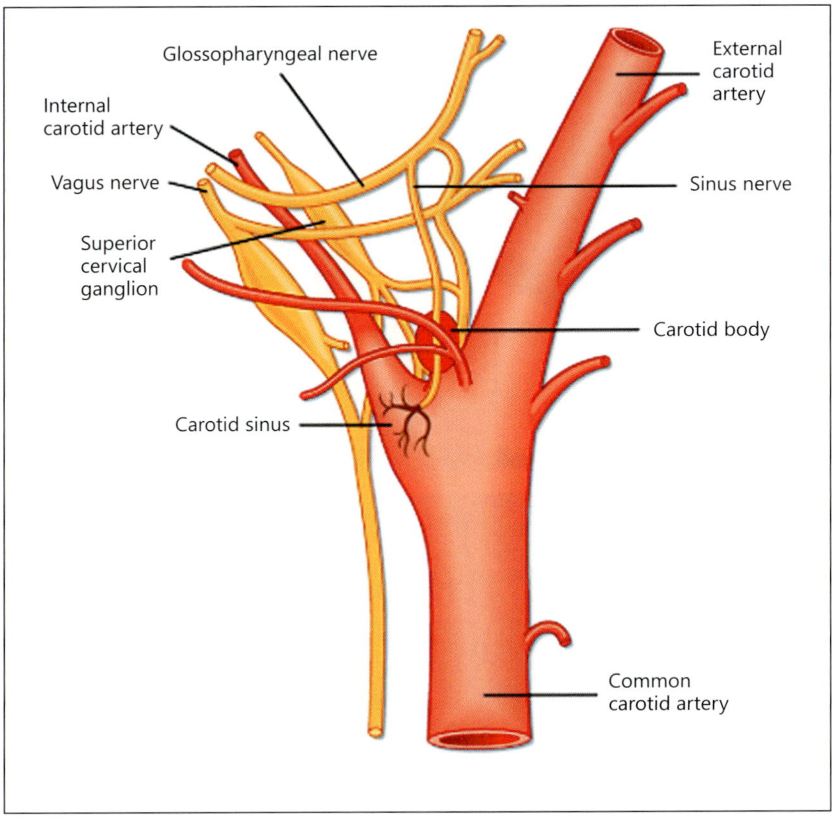

Fig. 1. Anatomy of the carotid sinus and sinus nerve (Koeppen and Stanton [41], with permission from Elsevier). The sinus nerve of Hering innervates the carotid sinus baroreceptors, which is a branch of the glossopharyngeal nerve.

Electrical Carotid Sinus/Nerve Stimulation

The rationale for carotid sinus stimulation is based on the evidence that the brain is able to sense the electrical stimulus as BP increases. As described in the body's natural baroreflex system, the impulses from stimulation are transmitted to the brainstem, which functions to modulate sympathetic and vagal outflows. Then, baroreflex efferent structures are regulated to counteract the discerned increase in BP through reducing sympathetic drive and increasing parasympathetic tone, which lead to a decrease in BP [8, 9].

Electrical stimulators directly activating afferent baroreflex nerves (baroreceptors) were evaluated in the treatment of refractory hypertension and angina in the late 1950s, but failed due to technical issues [26–28]. A dedicated surgical device, Implantable Barostim System (Barostim Rheos and Barostim *neo*™, CVRx Inc., Minneapolis, Minn., USA), for the treatment of resistant hypertension has been developed to deliver baroreflex activation therapy (BAT) via carotid sinus stimulation [2, 6, 8–10, 12,

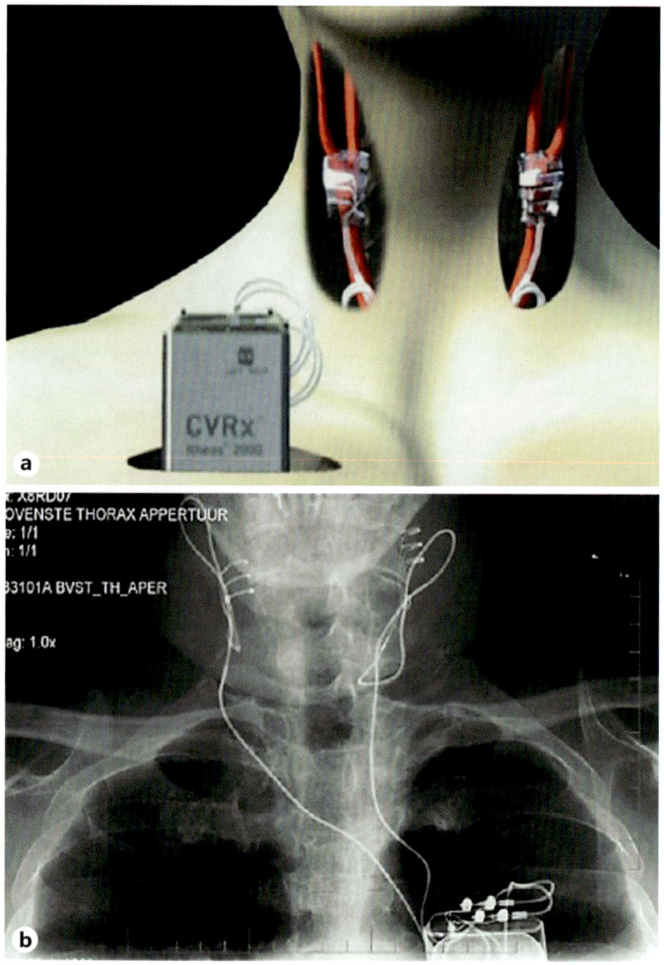

Fig. 2. a Bilateral implant of carotid sinus leads and subclavicular placement of the IPG of the Rheos device (courtesy of CVRx Inc., reproduced with permission). **b** Postoperative radiograph showing position of the carotid sinus leads and IPG (Tordoir et al. [9], with permission from Elsevier).

29]. This novel system uses perivascular electrodes to provide chronic baroreflex activation, and also addresses the challenges of the earlier devices [9, 30]. BAT is a unique approach to treat hypertension and HF, in which electrical stimulation of baroreceptors in the carotid sinus induces reduction in sympathetic drive to the heart, vasculature, and kidneys, as well as an increase in parasympathetic activity [29]. The stimulation system consists of three components: (1) bilateral carotid sinus leads, (2) an implantable pulse generator (IPG), and (3) a programmer system (fig. 2) [2, 31, 32]. There are two different types of carotid sinus leads, with the smaller electrode capable of covering the free wall of the carotid sinus and the larger one recommended for use in bigger arteries or larger anatomic variants of the carotid sinus [2]. The dimensions of IPG are 90 mm (height) × 48 mm (width) × 12 mm (thickness), and the weight is 95 g. The IPG delivers stimulation to the baroreceptor in the vessel walls of carotid sinuses of between 1 and 7.5 V of activation energy. The computer-based programmer system enables noninvasive communication with and control of the IPG via radiofrequency coupling [2]. The patient can also temporarily turn off the IPG. The first-generation carotid sinus stimulator, Rheos system, applies electrical impulses bilaterally using an electrode that is wrapped around the carotid sinus.

A second-generation system, the Barostim *neo* system, is comprised of an IPG and a lead (fig. 3), and is controlled with a laptop computer-based programming system via radiofrequency telemetry [33]. The pulse generator is implanted unilaterally in the chest wall ipsilateral to the stimulated carotid sinus. The electrode portion of the lead consists of a single platinum-iridium disc coated with iridium oxide attached concentrically to a circular insulated backer [33]. This system is CE marked for the treatment of hypertension and is undergoing clinical evaluation in the United States.

Surgical Implantation

The implant of a carotid sinus stimulation system is frequently performed under general anesthesia. The Rheos system depends on a bilateral implantation of the electrodes on both the left and right carotid sinus, and is no longer used. The newly introduced Barostim *neo* device only requires unilateral placement for carotid sinus stimulation, simplifying the surgical procedure without decreasing its effectiveness.

The surgical implantation technique for the Rheos system has been described previously [9, 10]. Here we focus on the surgical procedure for placement of the Barostim *neo* device. In brief, the patient is placed in the supine position. The right side of the patient's neck and upper part of the chest are prepped and draped in standard sterile fashion. After application of a local anesthetic, a straight incision is made below the right clavicle. The soft tissues are dissected and a pocket is created above the fascia and below the skin in order to accommodate the IPG. The second incision is made on the right side of the neck over the carotid bifurcation. After the carotid sheath is opened, the common carotid artery, internal jugular vein, and vagus nerve are identified. The carotid artery bifurcation is dissected, and carotid sinus mapping is then performed until the location where it provides the optimal hemodynamic response is found with reduction of systolic BP by at least 10–20 mm Hg and heart rate by 5–10 beats/min. The stimulation parameters are 3 V and 100 Hz for impulses and 480 μs for pulse width. Once a desirable area is identified, the electrode is sutured in place. It is important to mention that the surgical technique of placing the electrode on the carotid sinus does not pose a high risk of damaging the carotid sinus nerve. The subcutaneous tunneling procedure is performed, allowing the lead to be connected to the IPG. Unilateral implantation reduces the complexity and duration of the implant procedures [6], thereby reducing the possibility of nerve injury and other procedure-related safety issues. Figure 3b provides an illustration of the implant sites of the carotid sinus leads and IPG. After surgery, a special programmer device is used to interrogate the implanted system. The parameters of stimulation are programmed before hospital discharge and 1 month after the implantation.

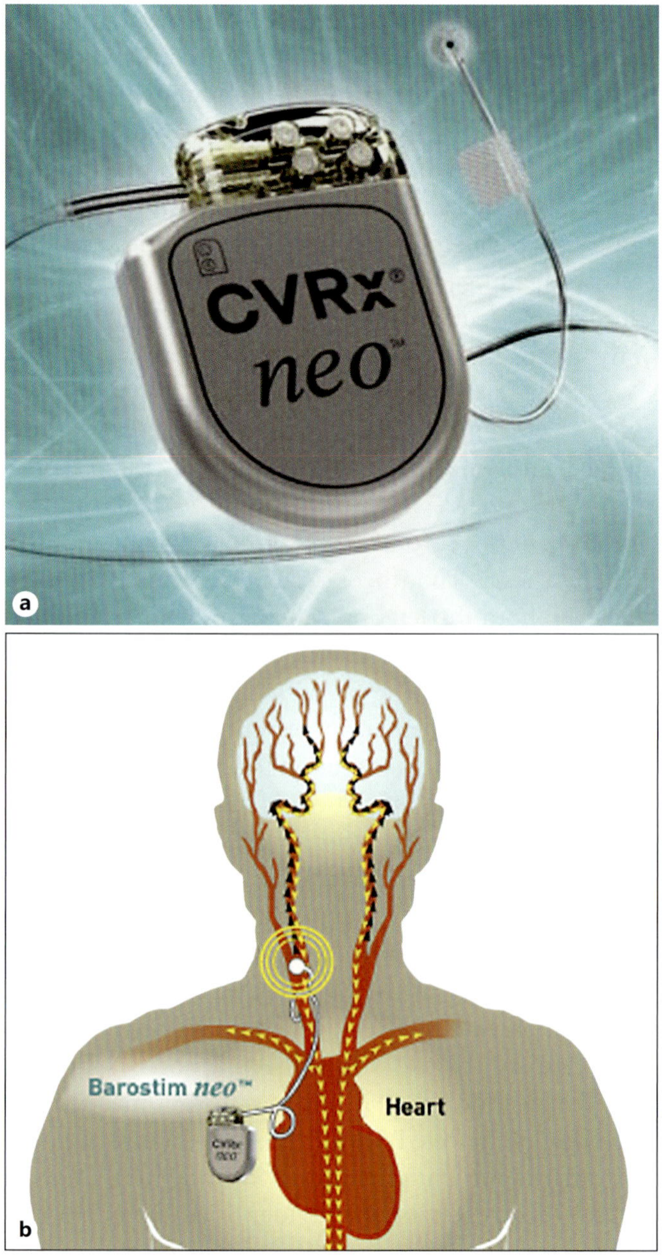

Fig. 3. a Barostim *neo* device with unilateral carotid sinus lead and IPG (courtesy of CVRx Inc., reproduced with permission). **b** The device activates baroreceptors in the wall of the carotid sinus, which stimulate the afferent and efferent pathways of the autonomic nervous system (courtesy of CVRx Inc., reproduced with permission). The brain responds by modulating efferent pathways, which relaxes the blood vessels and slows the heart rate. The increase in parasympathetic tone and decrease in sympathetic drive result in the restoration of sympathetic-vagal balance, which reduces BP and improves cardiac structure and function.

Carotid Sinus Stimulation in Animal Models

Animal studies have provided the basis for the initial investigations of carotid sinus stimulation on patients. The hypothesis that electrical carotid sinus stimulation could lower BP was first demonstrated in not only normotensive conscious [13], but also obese dogs [15]. Carotid sinus stimulation resulted in a substantial reduction in plasma norepinephrine, suggesting that the depressor response may be related to a long-standing sympathetic inhibition [13–16]. It has also been shown that carotid sinus stimulation is particularly promising in the treatment of sympathetically driven arterial hypertension [13–16]. The experiments in animals gave us important insight into the mechanisms of mediating the depressor response to electrical carotid sinus stimulation. Moreover, these studies indicated that satisfactory treatment could also depend on the underlying pathophysiology of the hypertension [8]. Due to page limitations, we do not present here detailed results of the animal studies.

Carotid Sinus Stimulation in Patients with Resistant Hypertension

The effect of carotid sinus stimulation was first investigated in an acute setting. Schmidli et al. [34] in 2007 showed that short-term electrical carotid baroreceptor stimulation lowered BP. The data from Tordoir et al. [9] indicate the Rheos device can be used to control high BP with a low risk of adverse events. Moreover, the multicenter phase II Rheos feasibility trial showed that this implantable device for carotid sinus stimulation can be placed safely and result in a significant acute reduction in BP [10]. These findings support clinical development of BAT as a new approach to treat resistant hypertension. Furthermore, the results obtained in the United States parallel those obtained in Europe, reinforcing earlier experimental studies [2].

Following these acute studies, the effect of chronic carotid sinus stimulation on lowering BP and its safety in patients with resistant hypertension was evaluated [8]. The European Device-Based Therapy in Hypertension Trial (DEBuT-HT) showed that carotid sinus stimulation decreased systolic and diastolic BP by 21 and 12 mm Hg, respectively, below the baseline measurement after 3 months of treatment. In 17 patients with 2 years of follow-up, BP was decreased by 33 and 22 mm Hg below the baseline measurement [8, 35]. In this study, patients were able to decrease the average number of antihypertensive medications from 5.0 at baseline to 3.4 at 4 years after stimulation. The data also demonstrate that the BP reduction with the Rheos system is sustained, and suggest that an implantable device can replace medication treatment as a chronic therapeutic option in patients with resistant hypertension [2].

The Rheos Pivotal Trial evaluated the effect of BAT on 265 patients with resistant hypertension in an FDA-approved double-blind, randomized, prospective, multicenter, placebo-controlled phase III clinical trial [6]. The study showed that BAT significantly benefits the patients in terms of endpoints of sustained efficacy, BAT safety, and device safety. At 12 months, reductions in systolic BP (up to 35 mm Hg) were observed in all subjects as compared with BP before implantation. Additionally, over 50% of patients were able to achieve a systolic BP of ≤140 mm Hg with BAT. Furthermore, BAT-induced BP reduction was maintained over long-term follow-up of 22–53 months [29].

The safety of the Implantable Baroreflex Hypertension Therapy device and procedure from the DEBuT-HT study was reported in 2010 [2, 30]. No carotid stenosis or orthostatic hypotension was found in this study. The safety results from the Rheos Pivotal Trial showed the procedural complications include nerve damage (9%), surgical complications (5%), respiratory complications (2%), and wound complications (2%) [2]. There were only very few serious adverse events related to the device during the long-term follow-up [36]. Taken together, BAT via carotid sinus stimulation has been demonstrated to be safe and efficacious, and is the only treatment option for resistant hypertension [6, 33].

Recently, the second-generation system for BAT, Barostim *neo* system with unilateral implantation of electrodes was evaluated in a clinical trial [33], and the data showed that it provided a better safety profile and similar efficacy as the Barostim Rheos system. The most impressive finding in this study is that the minimally invasive system for BAT led to substantial systolic BP reductions of 26 mm Hg on average at 6 months, in which a similar therapeutic effect was obtained as compared to the 21-mm Hg decrease in the DEBuT trial at 3 months [30] and 26-mm Hg reduction in the Rheos Pivotal Trial at 6 months [6]. Furthermore, 43% of the resistant hypertensive patients achieved systolic BP <140 mm Hg by 6 months of therapy [33]. An international study of the Barostim *neo* device in hypertension has already completed patient enrollment (n = 40).

Carotid Sinus Stimulation in Patients with Heart Failure

HF continues to be a major public health problem in terms of patient morbidity and mortality, as well as cost to the healthcare system, impacting more than 5 million Americans [37–39]. The pathophysiology of HF is mediated by autonomic dysfunction, including sympathetic activation and diminished baroreflex sensitivity, which correlate well with mortality risk of HF [40]. Cardiac sympathetic drive contributes to development of hypertrophy of left ventricle, and increases myocardial automaticity, which can promote ventricular tachyarrhythmias and sudden death [37]. Evidence of the adverse prognostic role of sympathetic activation in patients with HF provides a concept behind management of adrenergic influences [40]. Therefore, carotid sinus stimulation may have the potential to benefit HF patients. A recent report has shown that chronic BAT via carotid sinus stimulation markedly and persistently reduced sympathetic drive of patients with class III HF (New York Heart Association Functional Classification) while increasing baroreflex sensitivity and improving ejection fraction, functional capacity, clinical status, and quality of life [40]. Further studies with BAT for treatment of HF are ongoing.

Conclusions and Future Direction

BAT via carotid sinus stimulation may represent a novel therapeutic strategy for treatment of resistant hypertension and HF. The efficacy of BAT has been evaluated in clinical trials, and the findings have shown that it may provide long-term BP control and improvement of cardiac function by reducing sympathetic drive and increasing parasympathetic tone. In addition, the implantable carotid sinus stimulation system provides unique opportunities for research on physiology of baroreflex in human. A new system for carotid sinus stimulation that involves a unilateral implant procedure has been developed (see above) and further evaluation is currently underway in Europe. At the same time, the design of the device can be further optimized with development of a smaller, lighter, longer-lasting IPG and addition of a closed-loop stimulation design that enables it to find the best set of parameters for each patient automatically and avoid side effects that are caused by overstimulation. With the advancement of technology and promising clinical data, the implantable BAT system may get regulatory approval as an alternative treatment for patients with resistant hypertension and HF in the future.

References

1 Writing Group Members, Lloyd-Jones D, Adams RJ, Brown TM, Carnethon M, Dai S, De Simone G, Ferguson TB, Ford E, Furie K, Gillespie C, Go A, Greenlund K, Haase N, Hailpern S, Ho PM, Howard V, Kissela B, Kittner S, Lackland D, Lisabeth L, Marelli A, McDermott MM, Meigs J, Mozaffarian D, Mussolino M, Nichol G, Roger VL, Rosamond W, Sacco R, Sorlie P, Roger VL, Thom T, Wasserthiel-Smoller S, Wong ND, Wylie-Rosett J; American Heart Association Statistics Committee and Stroke Statistics Subcommittee: Heart disease and stroke statistics – 2010 update: a report from the American Heart Association. Circulation 2010;121:e46–e215.

2 Ng MM, Sica DA, Frishman WH: Rheos: an implantable carotid sinus stimulation device for the nonpharmacologic treatment of resistant hypertension. Cardiol Rev 2011;19:52–57.

3 Calhoun DA, Jones D, Textor S, Goff DC, Murphy TP, Toto RD, White A, Cushman WC, White W, Sica D, Ferdinand K, Giles TD, Falkner B, Carey RM; American Heart Association Professional Education Committee: Resistant hypertension: diagnosis, evaluation, and treatment: a scientific statement from the American Heart Association Professional Education Committee of the Council for High Blood Pressure Research. Circulation 2008;117:e510–e526.

4 Acelajado MC, Calhoun DA: Resistant hypertension, secondary hypertension, and hypertensive crises: diagnostic evaluation and treatment. Cardiol Clin 2010;28:639–654.

5 Sarafidis PA, Bakris GL: Resistant hypertension: an overview of evaluation and treatment. J Am Coll Cardiol 2008;52:1749–1757.

6 Bisognano JD, Bakris G, Nadim MK, Sanchez L, Kroon AA, Schafer J, de Leeuw PW, Sica DA: Baroreflex activation therapy lowers blood pressure in patients with resistant hypertension: results from the double-blind, randomized, placebo-controlled Rheos Pivotal Trial. J Am Coll Cardiol 2011;58:765–773.

7 Cuspidi C, Macca G, Sampieri L, Michev I, Salerno M, Fusi V, Sebvergnini B, Meani S, Magrini F, Zanchetti A: High prevalence of cardiac and extracardiac target organ damage in refractory hypertension. J Hypertens 2001;19:2063–2070.

8 Jordan J, Heusser K, Brinkmann J, Tank J: Electrical carotid sinus stimulation in treatment resistant arterial hypertension. Auton Neurosci 2012;172:31–36.

9 Tordoir JH, Scheffers I, Schmidli J, Savolainen H, Liebeskind U, Hansky B, Herold U, Irwin E, Kroon AA, de Leeuw P, Peters TK, Kieval R, Cody R: An implantable carotid sinus baroreflex activating system: surgical technique and short-term outcome from a multi-center feasibility trial for the treatment of resistant hypertension. Eur J Vasc Endovasc Surg 2007;33:414–421.

10 Illig KA, Levy M, Sanchez L, Trachiotis GD, Shanley C, Irwin E, Pertile T, Kieval R, Cody R: An implantable carotid sinus stimulator for drug-resistant hypertension: surgical technique and short-term outcome from the multicenter phase II Rheos feasibility trial. J Vasc Surg 2006;44:1213–1218.

11 Taylor JG, Bisognano JD: Baroreflex stimulation in antihypertensive treatment. Curr Hypertens Rep 2010;12:176–181.

12 Navaneethan SD, Lohmeier TE, Bisognano JD: Baroreflex stimulation: a novel treatment option for resistant hypertension. J Am Soc Hypertens 2009;3:69–74.
13 Lohmeier TE, Irwin ED, Rossing MA, Serdar DJ, Kieval RS: Prolonged activation of the baroreflex produces sustained hypotension. Hypertension 2004;43: 306–311.
14 Lohmeier TE, Dwyer TM, Hildebrandt DA, Irwin ED, Rossing MA, Serdar DJ, Kieval RS: Influence of prolonged baroreflex activation on arterial pressure in angiotensin hypertension. Hypertension 2005;46: 1194–1200.
15 Lohmeier TE, Dwyer TM, Irwin ED, Rossing MA, Kieval RS: Prolonged activation of the baroreflex abolishes obesity-induced hypertension. Hypertension 2007;49:1307–1314.
16 Lohmeier TE, Hildebrandt DA, Dwyer TM, Barrett AM, Irwin ED, Rossing MA, Kieval RS: Renal denervation does not abolish sustained baroreflex-mediated reductions in arterial pressure. Hypertension 2007;49:373–379.
17 Heusser K, Tank J, Engeli S, Diedrich A, Menne J, Eckert S, Peters T, Sweep FC, Haller H, Pichlmaier AM, Luft FC, Jordan J: Carotid baroreceptor stimulation, sympathetic activity, baroreflex function, and blood pressure in hypertensive patients. Hypertension 2010;55:619–626.
18 Chapleau MW: Arterial baroreflexes; in Izzo JL Jr, Sica DA, Black HR (eds): Hypertension Primer, ed 4. Dallas, American Heart Association, 2008, pp 120–123.
19 Zar T, Peixoto AJ: Paroxysmal hypertension due to baroreflex failure. Kidney Int 2008;74:126–131.
20 Ketch T, Biaggioni I, Robertson R, Robertson D: Four faces of baroreflex failure: hypertensive crisis, volatile hypertension, orthostatic tachycardia, and malignant vagotonia. Circulation 2002;105:2518–2523.
21 Heusser K, Tank J, Luft FC, Jordan J: Baroreflex failure. Hypertension 2005;45:834–839.
22 Grassi G: Sympathetic neural activity in hypertension and related diseases. Am J Hypertens 2010;23: 1052–1060.
23 Grassi G, Cattaneo BM, Seravalle G, Lanfranchi A, Mancia G: Baroreflex control of sympathetic nerve activity in essential and secondary hypertension. Hypertension 1998;31:68–72.
24 Hausberg M, Mark AL, Winniford MD, Brown RE, Somers VK: Sympathetic and vascular effects of short-term passive smoke exposure in healthy nonsmokers. Circulation 1997;96:282–287.
25 Zilch O, Vos PF, Oey PL, Cramer MJ, Ligtenberg G, Koomans HA, Blankenstijn PJ: Sympathetic hyperactivity in haemodialysis patients is reduced by short daily haemodialysis. J Hypertens 2007;25:1285–1289.
26 Parsonnet V, Rothfeld EL, Raman KV, Myers GH: Electrical stimulation of the carotid sinus nerve. Surg Clin North Am 1969;49:589–596.
27 Rothfeld EL, Parsonnet V, Raman KV, Zucker IR, Tiu R: The effect of carotid sinus nerve stimulation on cardiovascular dynamics in man. Angiology 1969;20:213–218.
28 Peters TK, Koralewski HE, Zerbst E: The principle of electrical carotid sinus nerve stimulation: a nerve pacemaker system for angina pectoris and hypertension therapy. Ann Biomed Eng 1980;8: 445–458.
29 Bakris GL, Nadim MK, Haller H, Lovett EG, Schafer JE, Bisognano JD: Baroreflex activation therapy provides durable benefit in patients with resistant hypertension: results of long-term follow-up in the Rheos Pivotal Trial. J Am Soc Hypertens 2012;6: 152–158.
30 Scheffers IJ, Kroon AA, Schmidli J, Jordan J, Tordoir JJ, Mohaupt MG, Luft FC, Haller H, Menne J, Engeli S, Ceral J, Eckert S, Erglis A, Narkiewicz K, PhilippT, de Leeuw PW: Novel baroreflex activation therapy in resistant hypertension: results of a European multi-center feasibility study. J Am Coll Cardiol 2010;56:1254–1258.
31 Sica DA, Lohmeier TE: Baroreflex activation for the treatment of hypertension: principles and practice. Expert Rev Med Devices 2006;3:595–601.
32 Scheffers IJ, Kroon AA, Tordoir JH, de Leeuw PW: Rheos Baroreflex Hypertension Therapy System to treat resistant hypertension. Expert Rev Med Devices 2008;5:33–39.
33 Hoppe UC, Brandt MC, Wachter R, Beige J, Rump LC, Kroon AA, Cates AW, Lovett EG, Haller H: Minimally invasive system for baroreflex activation therapy chronically lowers blood pressure with pacemaker-like safety profile: results from the Barostim *neo* trial. J Am Soc Hypertens 2012;6:270–276.
34 Schmidli J, Savolainen H, Eckstein F, Irwin E, Peters TK, Martin R, Kieval R, Cody R, Carrel T: Acute device-based blood pressure reduction: electrical activation of the carotid baroreflex in patients undergoing elective carotid surgery. Vascular 2007;15: 63–69.
35 Mohaupt MG, Schmidli J, Luft FC: Management of uncontrollable hypertension with a carotid sinus stimulation device. Hypertension 2007;50:825–828.

36 Bakris G, Bisognano J, Nadim M, Sanchez L, Sica D, Schafer J: Potential of implantable carotid sinus stimulator for drug-resistant hypertension. Proceedings of the 23rd Scientific Meeting of the International Society of Hypertension, Vancouver, 2010, p 151.
37 Georgakopoulos D, Little WC, Abraham WT, Weaver FA, Zile MR: Chronic baroreflex activation: a potential therapeutic approach to heart failure with preserved ejection fraction. J Card Fail 2011;17:167–178.
38 Croft JB, Giles WH, Pollard RA, Keenan NL, Casper ML, Anda RF: Heart failure survival among older adults in the United States: a poor prognosis for an emerging epidemic in the Medicare population. Arch Intern Med 1999;159:505–510.
39 Stewart S, MacIntyre K, Capewell S, McMurray JJ: Heart failure and the aging population: an increasing burden in the 21st century? Heart 2003;89:49–53.
40 Gronda E, Seravalle G, Brambilla G, Costantino G, Casini A, Alsheraei A, Lovett EG, Mancia G, Grassi G: Chronic baroreflex activation effects on sympathetic nerve traffic, baroreflex function, and cardiac haemodynamics in heart failure: a proof-of-concept study. Eur J Heart Fail 2014;16:977–983.
41 Koeppen BM, Stanton BA: Beme and Levy Physiology, ed 6. Amsterdam, Elsevier, 2010.

Dali Yin, MD
Department of Neurosurgery, University of Illinois at Chicago
912 South Wood Street, M/C 799, Rm. 451N
Chicago, IL 60612 (USA)
E-Mail daliyin@uic.edu

Slavin KV (ed): Stimulation of the Peripheral Nervous System. The Neuromodulation Frontier.
Prog Neurol Surg. Basel, Karger, 2016, vol 29, pp 94–105 (DOI: 10.1159/000434660)

Hypoglossal Nerve Stimulation for Obstructive Sleep Apnea

Gimbada B. Mwenge[a, d] · Philippe Rombaux[b, d] · Benoit Lengele[c] · Daniel Rodenstein[a, d]

Departments of [a]Pneumology, [b]ENT and [c]Plastic Surgery, and [d]Center for Sleep Medicine, Cliniques Universitaires Saint-Luc, Université Catholique de Louvain, Brussels, Belgium

Abstract

Obstructive sleep apnea (OSA) is a very frequent affliction that affects about 1–5% of the adult population in its severe form. Continuous positive airway pressure (CPAP) is the most commonly used treatment and is highly effective, but its use is limited by low long-term adherence rates and overall poor acceptance among the patients. Therefore, there is a need for developing alternative approaches to OSA treatment, including a more 'natural' concept of maintaining an open airway through neuromodulation. Here we review the concept, scientific rationale, and technical details of hypoglossal nerve stimulation. We also review results of published clinical studies with several hypoglossal stimulation devices that are being investigated today. Hypoglossal nerve stimulation appears to be a very promising treatment for patients with moderate-to-severe OSA. If its efficacy is confirmed, it will probably be complementary with CPAP therapy and initially aimed at patients unable or unwilling to use CPAP. Once it becomes a standard therapy, its advantages might prove sufficient to challenge CPAP as the first-line therapy.

The Tongue

The human tongue is a curious structure. It is a critical functional structure (no more and no less than other vital structures such as the lungs or heart). The newborn could not survive if he could not suck milk from the mother's nipple and then swallow the milk. The tongue is essential for both activities. Your tongue is essential to chew, suck, drink, eat, swallow, talk, sing, whistle, play wind instruments, lap, and even kiss if both of you wish. You can project your tongue (in fact only part of it) out of your body, twist it, turn it, bend it, and retract it; in fact, you can give it almost any shape you can think of. All this is the result of muscular activity of at least 8 pairs of muscles [1, 2], most of which, including all the intrinsic muscles and the genioglossus muscle (believed to be the main protractor muscle), are controlled on each side by a single nerve, the hypoglossal nerve or XIIth cranial nerve. This is mainly a pure motor nerve, with only a small minority of sensory fibers.

The tongue can perform all these movements and achieve all these spatial positions because it is a hydrostat [3]. This is a three-dimensional structure with a high water (or water-like) content, making it incompressible, meaning that its volume cannot be modified by an applied force. However, such a structure can maintain its volume unchanged, whereas its shape can be modified. Imagine a cylinder with a given diameter (in cross section) and a given length. This cylinder can maintain a fixed volume while decreasing its diameter and increasing its length. This is exactly what you do when you pull your tongue out of your body. In the tongue, as in all hydrostats, it is the particular spatial arrangement of the muscle fibers that gives it its freedom of movement and almost infinite changing shape [4].

The tongue has 4 pairs of intrinsic muscles, i.e. muscular bundles that are entirely contained within the tongue and do not connect the tongue to adjacent structures [1]. There are longitudinal muscles, one on top and one at the bottom, a transverse muscle, and a vertical muscle, all four on each hemitongue. The fibers are intermerged and mix with fibers from 4 pairs of extrinsic muscles. The latter connect the tongue to adjacent structures, most of which are mobile, with only one being a fixed attachment in the base of the skull (the styloid apophysis, on the back and above the tongue). The tongue is attached on the front to the back side of the mandible, a very mobile bone; to the hyoid bone on the back and down, this being the most unarticulated bone in the body, and to the skull base and the soft palate on the back and above, a double muscular curtain hanging downwards from the styloid process of the temporal bone (styloglossus muscle) and behind the hard palate (palatoglossus muscle). It is the intermerged characteristic of the muscular bands that contract at the same time that gives the tongue its exquisite mobility. Fibers that elongate the bottom of the tongue may contract simultaneously with fibers retracting the top part of the tongue while transverse fibers in the right hemitongue contract and the ones in the left hemitongue relax; one can think of any such combination resulting in almost any kind of deformation of the shape of the tongue.

From the grossly anatomical point of view, the tongue has three main parts. One is contained within the mouth, is mostly horizontal (when you are sitting or standing), and fills the oral cavity when the mouth is closed. The second part is behind the former, is mostly vertical (again, except if you are lying down on your back and everything needs a 90° turn), and forms the frontal part of the throat, the part of the body that anatomists designate as the pharynx (more precisely the oro- and hypopharynx). The third part is submerged below the floor of the mouth. Figure 1 shows this schematic view of tongue anatomy.

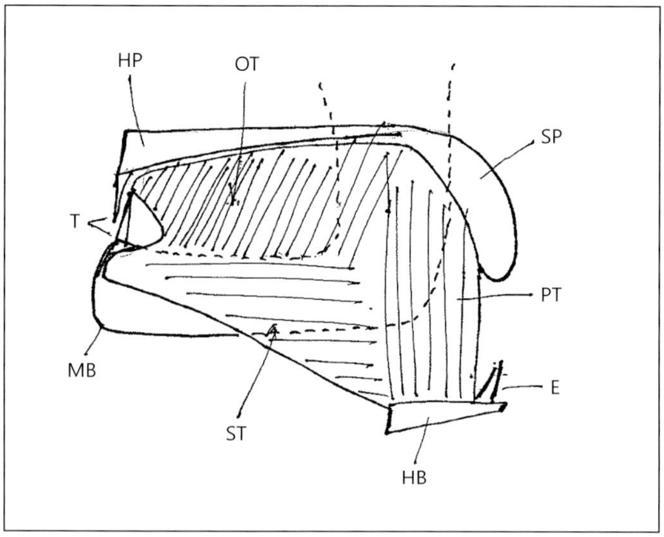

Fig. 1. Schematic representation of tongue anatomy, seen from the side. E = Epiglottis; HB = hyoid bone; HP = hard palate; MB = mandible bone; OT (slanting lines) = oral portion of the tongue; PT (vertical lines) = pharyngeal portion of the tongue; SP = soft palate; ST (horizontal lines) = submerged tongue, below the floor of the mouth; T = teeth.

Breathing

Humans need oxygen to fuel their myriad of cells, most of which are far from the atmosphere and cannot just extract oxygen from ambient air. Cells produce carbon dioxide when they work, and this needs to be disposed of as it is built to avoid accumulation. The body has a single organ where oxygen from the atmosphere is captured and carbon dioxide is disposed of – the lungs. There are two lungs, contained in (and protected by) the thoracic cavity. From the lungs, oxygen is distributed to the rest of the body by the blood, pumped by the heart into the clean vascular channels (the arterial system). The same blood transports back the carbon dioxide to the lungs through the waste vascular system (the veins).

To connect the lungs to the atmosphere so that oxygen-rich and carbon dioxide-poor ambient air can replenish the oxygen-depleted and carbon dioxide-enriched lung gas, a complex system of air channels, called bronchi, are distributed throughout the lungs. There is one main bronchus for each lung that divides in progressively smaller and smaller tubes that reach the lung periphery and finally the alveoli, which are tiny balloons where the air and blood exchange gases. The two main bronchi unite to form the air pipe, called the trachea, which ends in the larynx (the Adam's apple is part of the larynx). This includes the vocal cords. It is their vibrations when air flows through them that produce the sounds that, after some acoustic transformation, characterize our voice. The larynx connects to the throat or pharynx, which finally connects with two horizontal galleries: the mouth and the nasal passages. The pharynx is thus part of the breathing circuit, and is also part of the digestive circuit allowing food to run downwards to the esophagus, stomach, and beyond.

The air column has a continuous alternating to-and-fro tidal movement – first down into the lungs, then up out into the atmosphere. This is produced by an aspirating negative pressure pump that lowers the pressure inside the thorax below atmospheric pressure while it expands, sucking ambient air into the lungs, then stopping its action and allowing the accumulated elastic pressure to go back to atmospheric pressure, chasing the alveolar gas out into the atmosphere. The negative pressure pump is formed by the respiratory muscles, the diaphragm, and all accessory muscles.

Thus, breathing requires the development of negative pressure within the airways (including the pharynx) for inspiration, then the return to atmospheric pressure for expiration.

Sleep

Humans sleep for several hours every day. Sleep is a temporary and self-subsiding partial disconnection from the external environment, but also from the bodily environment. Sleep is essentially a brain activity, but since the brain is the master of everything, sleep affects the entire body. While sleep affects breathing through several effects, probably the most conspicuous is the sharp increase in the resistance of the airways to flow, which explains the decrease in the volume of each breath, the tidal volume. The resistance increases essentially within the pharynx. The pharynx, whose anterior wall is partly formed by the tongue, is an entirely muscular tube, lacking structural support. Its 'rigidity' is given by the resting tonus of the muscles forming its walls. This rigidity is necessary to sustain the negative inspiratory pressure that will tend to suck in the walls if they are floppy. And this is exactly what sleep does to pharyngeal walls: it decreases muscle tone everywhere, also in the pharynx, making the pharyngeal walls less rigid and therefore more prone to partially collapse during inspiration. Thus, the pharyngeal cross-sectional diameter decreases, the resistance to airflow increases and tidal volume decreases. If for any reason the pharynx is already narrow, then the collapse may be so impressive that airflow is almost abolished or stopped altogether. If the pharynx remains closed for more than 10 s, with breathing interrupted, oxygen will start to fall in the blood since pulmonary gas will be depleted from oxygen that will not be replenished. This is called apnea in sleep.

The Sleep Apnea Disease

There are human beings that have many apneas when they sleep. Apneas only appear during sleep; these people have no problem breathing while awake. But during sleep, complete or incomplete apneas are always present. They may last for 20 or 30 s each and present every minute, amounting to as many as 50 or 60 apneas per hour slept. This is not trivial as it affects health in a serious way. This sleep apnea syndrome as it is called, leads to arterial hypertension, myocardial infarction, stroke, unrefreshing sleep, excessive of sleepiness, decreased concentration, and ultimately reduced survival [5, 6]. It is very frequent, affecting about 1% of adult population with what is considered severe disease (more than 30 breathing interruptions per hour). And all that happens behind the sleeping tongue.

Sleep Apnea Treatment

There is an efficient treatment for OSA used by many patients throughout the world. It consists of preventing pharyngeal collapse by pushing apart the walls of the pharynx during sleep. This is achieved through an increase in the pressure of the air column in the upper airways above atmospheric pressure. A turbine is connected through wide bore tubing to a mask placed upon the nose and maintained in place with elastic traps passed around the head. The pressure in the system is raised a small amount above ambient pressure (something around 10 cm of water, or 1% of ambient pressure), which is enough to keep the walls of the pharynx apart and push the tongue forward and the lateral walls away. The device, called continuous positive airway pressure (CPAP) has to be used all night and every night in order to obtain compete relief from the disease as well as longstanding protection against the serious effects of the disease on health, including improvement in survival [5, 6].

Unfortunately, the high flows necessary to obtain the positive airway pressure impose a very high workload on the nasal mucosa, which has to heat and humidify the air current. In many patients, this leads to a breakdown of the mucosal capacity, with consequent mucosal congestion, complete nasal obstruction, aqueous rhinitis, sneezing attacks, and complete arrest of the efficiency of CPAP. In addition, many patients have nasal polyps that render the nasal passages narrow to start with. On top of this, many patients feel psychologically constrained by the need to use the external device all night every night, experience claustrophobia, or encounter serious rejection of the treatment by their bed partner. Others experience skin problems (irritation, wounds, scars). These many reasons explain why 30–50% of patients with severe sleep apnea start CPAP treatment but are unable to remain under treatment and finally abandon it altogether in the first year of therapy [7, 8]. Therefore, they remain untreated and subject to the symptoms and health risks of the disease. The search for an alternative therapy is as old as CPAP itself, and great hopes are placed on neurostimulation.

Hypoglossal Nerve Stimulation

Since the role of upper airway muscles is prominent in OSA, the potential beneficial effects of upper airway, specifically tongue, muscle, and nerve stimulation, have been studied very early on. Animal studies performed in cats, rats, rabbits, and dogs demonstrated that stimulation of the hypoglossal nerve or of the branches innervating the genioglossus muscle, stimulation of the genioglossus (considered as the main protractor) muscle together with retractor muscles, or direct stimulation of the genioglossus muscle all lead to the same result: enlargement of the pharyngeal lumen [9]. Human trials were also performed shortly after the introduction of CPAP treatment, using either stimulation of the hypoglossal nerve or the genioglossus muscle transdermally with intramuscular needle electrodes or with specially designed implanted nerve electrodes [10]. These trials produced varied results. In some experiments patients were awakened by stimulation, in other experiments favorable results (increases in nasal flow, resolution of apneas, decreases in critical closing pressure) were obtained without perturbing sleep. Reproducibility between patients was poor and it was difficult to predict the response to stimulation from anthropometric or physiologic data.

After an acute study in 5 volunteer patients with OSA submitted to hypoglossal nerve stimulation (HGNS) suggested feasible and potentially useful effects, a first clinical trial was initiated with a unilateral implantable system consisting of a cuffed hypoglossal nerve electrode positioned on the medial branch of the hypoglossal nerve innervating the genioglossus muscle and an implanted stimulator placed subcutaneously in the upper thorax. The Inspire I system from Medtronic (Minneapolis, Minn., USA) included a separate pressure sensor to detect intrathoracic inspiratory pressure that was fixed in a hole drilled on the manubrium sternale [11]. Stimulation was applied only during inspiration. Stimulation parameters were adjusted with a transcutaneous programming device. The system was activated at bedtime by the patient with a remote control unit. Out of the 8 implanted patients, beneficial results were obtained in 7, with significant reductions in the apnea-hypopnea index (AHI) and lesser drops in oxygen saturation. Stimulation did not provoke pain or arousal from sleep, the characteristics of which tended to improve, and tolerance appeared excellent throughout the 6 months of the study [11]. In the long term, most devices stopped functioning because of technical defects [10].

This first promising clinical trial was followed by a decade without any apparent further development. However, as it would later become evident, the concept continued stimulating the imagination of researchers and entrepreneurs. Indeed, the prevalence of OSA and the economic value of CPAP make any new remedy for the disease a desirable investment possibility.

By the end of the first decade of the 21st century, three new clinical trials were underway, sponsored by three different and independent firms: Apnex (St. Paul, Minn., USA), Inspire (Maple Grove, Minn., USA), and ImThera Medical (San Diego, Calif., USA) (table 1). All three were performed in volunteer patients with OSA who had tried CPAP therapy but refused to use it long term, were noncompliant, or refused to have a CPAP trial altogether.

Apnex and Inspire followed the same principles set forward by the Medtronic trial: unilateral inspiratory stimulation of the medial branch of the hypoglossal nerve from an implanted stimulator placed subcutaneously in the upper thorax in order to cause

Table 1. Summary of the published pilot studies

	n	Mean BMI	Type of stimulation	Study duration	AHI[a]	ODI[a]	MAI[a]	ESS[a]	Complications	Comments
Apnex	21	32.7	Insp.	6 months	43.1/19.5	16.8/9.1	43.8/23.5	12.1/8.1	2 patients explanted; plastic guards on lower teeth to protect from tongue abrasion	definition of obstructive hypopneas?
Inspire 1[b]	22 14 6	 30.7 27.8	Insp.	6 months	 51.1/56.1 26.1/7.7	 36.7/45.0 14.5/6.7	 NA NA	11/7.6 for all subjects ending the study (n = 28)	1 infection, explanted	2 patients excluded (lost for follow-up and infection); final results (n = 20)
Inspire 2	9	28.9	Insp.	6 months	38.9/10	32.1/9.5	NA	see above	1 patient explanted for failed stimulation	1 patient failed stimulation; final results (n = 8)
Inspire STAR Trial	126	28.4	Insp.	12 months + 7 days	32/15.3	28.9/13.9	28.9/14.8	11.6/7	2 device revisions, frequent tongue abrasions	randomized therapy – withdrawal trial at 12 months (n = 46)
ImThera	14	31	Cont.	12 months	45.2/21.0	29.2/15.3	36.8/24.9	10.8/7.9	1 patient not Implanted, 2 transient tongue paresis	final results (n = 13) multicontact electrode

Insp. = Inspiratory; Cont. = continuous; ESS = Epworth Sleepiness Scale (note that for the Inspire data, the results are combined for Inspire 1 and Inspire 2); MAI = microarousal index; ODI = oxygen desaturation index. [a] Values are means; baseline/final results. [b] There were initially 22 patients, but 2 dropped out; 14 patients showed no change in the AHI and 6 showed a >50% reduction.

a contraction of the genioglossus muscle. Inspiration was identified with a separate sensor, a double impedance sensor positioned over the lower ribs of both hemithoraces in the case of the Apnex device, and an effort sensor placed between the intercostal muscles in the fourth intercostal space with the Inspire II device.

The first published report was from Apnex Medical [12]. The HGNS clinical trial was performed in Australia. Of 37 screened subjects, 21 were implanted (14 males) and followed up for 6 months. The inclusion criteria called for disease severity between 20 and 100 apnea-hypopnea events per hour of sleep, but with at least 80% of events being hypopneas. BMI had to be <40 and age between 21 and 70 years. Efficacy was assessed through changes in the AHI and in questionnaires on sleep quality and daytime sleepiness. The results showed a >50% reduction in the AHI at 3 and 6 months stimulation, an improvement in sleep-related questionnaires, and in some indices of sleep quality (percentage of deep and paradoxical sleep and sleep efficiency). This study was followed by a larger scale phase 2–3 clinical trial, which apparently failed to produce the expected results – the AHI fell from 45 to 25 as a mean, slightly less than the expected 50% decrease – leading to a stop in the development of the device and closure of Apnex.

The Inspire II trial was published shortly thereafter [13]. It was a 6-month-long two-part study, the first with wide inclusion and exclusion criteria and the second with narrower criteria based on the findings of the first part, including pharyngeal appearance during a drug-induced sleep endoscopy procedure. Initially, the patients had to have a BMI <35 and AHI >25 events per hour. From the 20 patients implanted in the first part of the study, 14 showed no change in the AHI, one of the two selected outcomes, whereas 6 patients showed a >50% reduction in AHI and a final index after 6 months of stimulation lower than 20 events per hour. These patients were younger and their BMI was lower than the patients who failed to improve on stimulation. The narrower part 2 criteria were a BMI <32, AHI between 20 and 50 events per hour, and a nonconcentric collapse on drug-induced sleep endoscopy at the level of the soft palate. Nine patients responding to these criteria were implanted in part 2, 8 were assessed at 6 months and 7 showed the expected outcome results.

The Inspire II trial was followed by a larger multicentric 1-year phase 2–3 trial (STAR trial). The study was completed in March 2014 [14, 15]. It included 126 patients refusing or unable to stand CPAP therapy, with BMI <32, AHI between 20 and 50 events per hour, absence of complete concentric collapse at the palatal level on drug-induced sleep endoscopy, and absence of significant central apneas or positional disease (apneas being numerous in dorsal decubitus but absent or minimal in other positions). The AHI decreased after 1 year from 32 to 15 events per hour as a mean and from 29 to 9 events per hour as a median. Sixty-six percent of the participants achieved a final AHI 50% lower than their initial value and with absolute values below 20 events per hour. Twenty-three responder patients were studied again 2 weeks after stopping stimulation and compared to 23 other responder patients continuing stimulation. In the first group, values worsened to levels similar to baseline ones, whereas in the second group the improvements at 1 year were maintained. After publication of these results, the FDA granted approval for the Inspire device.

ImThera Medical developed a device with different principles. Stimulation was delivered during both inspiration and expiration, like a tonic rather than a phasic stimulation, making use of separate sensors to identify inspiration unnecessary. In addition, the cuffed electrode had an array of six contacts positioned around the main trunk of the hypoglossal nerve, targeting all muscles in the hemilateral tongue. Finally,

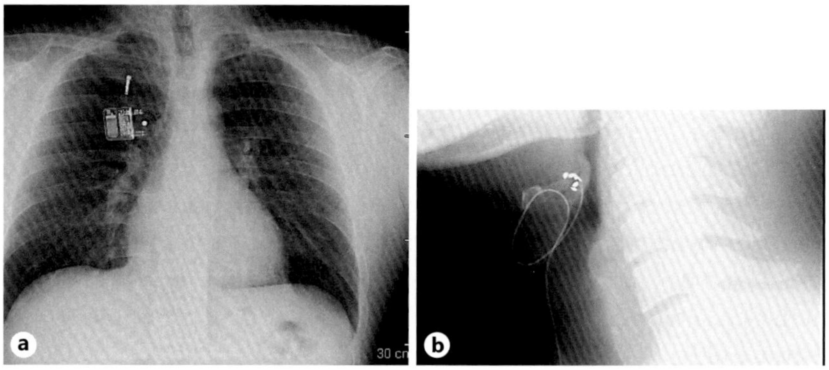

Fig. 2. Imthera Medical device. **a** Chest radiograph showing the position of the IPG over the right hemithorax with the connector leading to the ascending lead. **b** Detail of lateral radiograph of the neck depicting the electrode contacts around the main trunk of the hypoglossal nerve and a safety strain relief loop preventing excessive traction on the lead.

the implanted stimulator was smaller, but had to be recharged daily with the help of a remote controller and charger coil positioned above the implant with a pair of magnets (fig. 2). The initial clinical study [16] was a 1-year study performed in 14 patients (1 female). Thirteen of them were successfully implanted; one patient was not implanted due to technical defects of the implant. Inclusion criteria were age 25–70 years, BMI 25–40, AHI >20 events per hour, Mallampati score 1–3 (scoring system used to determine the potential level of difficulty and risk in intubating a patient undergoing surgery based on visual inspection of the oral cavity), and palatine tonsils grades 0–2. Patients were 50.3 years old on average and had a mean BMI of 30.5. At the 1-year follow-up, the AHI had decreased by more than 50% (from 45.2 to 21), with 10 patients showing final results below 30 events per hour; however, 3 patients did not reach this point. The oxygen desaturation index and sleep fragmentation indices showed similar improvements (from 29.2 to 15.3 and from 36.8 to 24.9 events per hour, respectively). In addition, in the patients who improved on stimulation, the effect lasted at least for the first night without stimulation, a remnant effect that CPAP does not demonstrate [17]. This suggests a possible disease-modifying effect. Following this initial trial, a larger phase 2–3 trial is underway. Table 1 summarizes the main characteristics of these first studies.

Comparisons between Continuous Positive Airway Pressure and Hypoglossal Stimulation

According to the results available to date, unilateral hypoglossal stimulation can alleviate OSA to the point of decreasing the disease load to safe levels (i.e. levels that do not lead to long-term cardiovascular morbidity and mortality) expressed as the number of apneas and hypopneas, number and depth of oxygen saturation drops, and degree of sleep fragmentation, as well as improving symptoms. The reported improvements with CPAP are more impressive, with complete or almost complete disappearance of sleep-related disordered breathing events, complete normalization of oxygen saturation, and normalization of sleep characteristics and length. CPAP therapy appears to suppress the cardiovascular morbidity and mortality due to sleep apnea [5, 18] – something hypoglossal stimulation has not proven yet.

A main difference between the two types of therapy relies on their effect on the pathophysiology of sleep apnea. The disease is assumed to result from the loss in muscle tongue of pharyngeal (mainly tongue) muscles. HGNS aims to restore the muscle tone necessary to avoid pharyngeal lumen collapse. In essence, it is a physiologically sound correction of the mechanism causing the disease. It is 'natural'. By contrast, CPAP grants the permeability of the pharyngeal airway by pushing away the pharyngeal walls, resulting in a decrease, if not abolition, of any residual muscle tonus. In essence it is a very efficient antiphysiologic remedy to the disease. It is 'unnatural'. This might account for the absence of remnant effect of CPAP, whereas hypoglossal stimulation might produce a persistent improvement even if not applied for a night.

The tolerance to treatment is variable for CPAP. Many patients accept the therapy well, sleep with their device all nights for a great part of the night or for the whole night, and go on using the device for years. However, many patients are completely unable to stand the mask and machine, and very rapidly abandon CPAP after the start of therapy even if the polysomnographic control demonstrates the efficacy of the treatment. In these patients, the advantages of hypoglossal stimulation (unobtrusive, silent, 'natural') become evident. In all the published trials on neurostimulation, patients had tried and failed to consistently use CPAP, or had refused even to try it. With HGNS, tolerance appears less problematic than with CPAP, but in all trials there is a minority of patients who do not achieve the desired endpoint (usually referred to as nonresponders).

An obvious difference between hypoglossal stimulation and CPAP is the need for surgery in the former. Contrary to previous surgical attempts to treat OSA, surgery is not the treatment of OSA when considering hypoglossal stimulation, but is a necessary unavoidable first step. Therefore, safety has to be maximal and complications of surgery should be regarded as major drawbacks to this approach. Up to now, no serious injury and no deaths have been reported, but 3 patients had to be explanted due to infections in the first two trials described above.

Another difference worth considering concerns the titration process whereby the treatment 'dose' is determined for an individual patient. With CPAP, titration consists of determining the minimal pressure that abolishes apneas and hypopneas and stabilizes both sleep and oxygen saturation without waking the patient. This is done either manually, when the operator slowly increases the pressure and observes the polysomnographic tracings until the desired normalization is achieved, or with so-called 'intelligent machines (autoPAPs)' that perform the process according to some proprietary algorithm. Titrating CPAP generally takes less than 1 h, and the physiologic effects are immediate. Once a given pressure has shown its efficacy, it seldom needs adaptations unless there are substantial changes in BMI. Titration of a neurostimulation device is entirely different both in the process itself and in the timing of titration. Titration does not start until 1 month after surgical implantation, and may require several weeks until the desired result is obtained. Currently, it seems unrealistic to expect to achieve a final definition of the stimulation settings in a single night. In addition, neurostimulation offers a greater variety of separate elements that can be applied: stimulation intensity, frequency, duration, and (in the case of ImThera's device) number and position of active or inactive contacts. Thus, titration is more complex and takes more time.

Finally, in what will probably become an essential issue for comparing the two treatments, provided that hypoglossal stimulation confirms the promising results obtained so far, is the price of the devices. This should be viewed in the context of a cost-utility analysis, and not just as a price comparison.

Conclusions

HGNS appears to be a very promising treatment for patients with moderate-to-severe OSA. If its efficacy is confirmed and the titration process made simpler, it will probably become an alternative to CPAP and initially aimed at patients unable or unwilling to use CPAP. Once it becomes a standard therapy, its advantages might prove sufficient to challenge CPAP as the first-line therapy.

References

1 Sanders I, Mu L: A three-dimensional atlas of human tongue muscles. Anat Rec (Hoboken) 2013;296: 1102–1114.
2 Mu L, Sanders I: Human tongue neuroanatomy: nerve supply and motor endplates. Clin Anat 2010; 23:777–791.
3 Gilbert RJ, Napadow VJ, Gaige TA, Weden VJ: Anatomical basis of lingual hydrostatic deformation. J Exp Biol 2007;210:4069–4082.
4 Balley EF, Huang YH, Fregosi RF: Anatomic consequences of intrinsic tongue muscle activation. J Appl Physiol 2006;101:1377–1385.
5 Sullivan CE, Issa FG, Berthon-Jones M, Eves L: Reversal of obstructive sleep apnoea by continuous positive airway pressure applied through the nares. Lancet 1981;1:862–865.
6 Marin JM, Carrizo SJ, Vicente E, Agusti AG: Long-term cardiovascular outcomes in men with obstructive sleep apnoea-hypopnoea with or without treatment with continuous positive airway pressure: an observational study. Lancet 2005;365:1046–1053.
7 Sucena M, Liistro G, Aubert G, Rodenstein DO, Pieters T: Continuous positive airway treatment for sleep apnoea: compliance increases with time in continuing users. Eur Respir J 2006;27:761–766.
8 Smith I, Nadig V, Lasserson TJ: Educational, supportive and behavioural interventions to improve usage of continuous positive airway pressure machines for adults with obstructive sleep apnoea. Cochrane Database Syst Rev 2009;15:CD007736.
9 Fairbanks DW, Fairbanks DN: Neurostimulation for obstructive sleep apnea: Investigations. Ear Nose Throat J 1993;72:52–57.

10 Kezirian EJ, Boudewyns A, Eisele DW, Schwartz AR, Smith PL, Van de Heyning PH, De Backer WA: Electrical stimulation of the hypoglossal nerve in the treatment of obstructive sleep apnea. Sleep Med Rev 2010;14:299–305.

11 Schwartz AR, Bennett ML, Smith PL, De Backer W, Hedner J, Boudewyns A, Van de Heyning P, Ejnell H, Hochban W, Knaack L, Podszus T, Penzel T, Peter JH, Goding GS, Erickson DJ, Testerman R, Ottenhoff F, Eisele DW: Therapeutic electrical stimulation of the hypoglossal nerve in obstructive sleep apnea. Arch Otolaryngol Head Neck Surg 2001;127: 1216–1223.

12 Eastwood PR, Barnes M, Walsh JH, Maddison KJ, Hee G, Schwartz AR, Smith PL, Malhotra A, McEvoy RD, Wheatley JR, O'Donoghue FJ, Rochford PD, Churchward T, Campbell MC, Palme CE, Robinson S, Goding GS, Eckert DJ, Jordan AS, Catcheside PG, Tyler L, Antic NA, Worsnop CJ, Kezirian EJ, Hillman DR: Treating obstructive sleep apnea with hypoglossal nerve stimulation. Sleep 2011;34:1479–1486.

13 Van de Heyning PH, Badr MS, Baskin JZ, Cramet Bornemann MA, De Backer WA, Dotan Y, Hohenhorst W, Knaack L, Lin HS, Maurer JT, Netzer A, Odland RM, Oliven A, Strohl KP, Vanderveken OM, Verbraecken J, Woodson BT: Implanted upper airway stimulation device for obstructive sleep apnea. Laryngoscope 2012;122:1626–1633.

14 Strollo PJ Jr, Soose RJ, Maurer JT, de Vries N, Cornelius J, Froymovich O, Hanson RD, Padhya TA, Steward DL, Gillespie MB, Woodson BT, Van de Heyning PH, Goetting MG, Vanderveken OM, Feldman N, Knaack L, Strohl KP; STAR Trial Group: Upper-airway stimulation for obstructive sleep apnea. N Engl J Med 2014;370:139–149.

15 Woodson BT, Gillespie MB, Soose RJ, Maurer JT, de Vries N, Steward DL, Baskin JZ, Padhya TA, Lin HS, Mickelson S, Badr SM, Strohl KP, Strollo PJ Jr; STAR Trial Investigators: Randomized controlled withdrawal study of upper airway stimulation on OSA: short- and long-term effect. Otolaryngol Head Neck Surg 2014;151:880–887.

16 Mwenge GB, Rombaux P, Dury M, Lengelé B, Rodenstein D: Targeted hypoglossal neurostimulation for obstructive sleep apnea. A 1-year pilot study. Eur Respir J 2013;41:360–367.

17 Rodenstein D, Rombaux P, Lengele B, Dury M, Mwenge GB: Residual effect of THN hypoglossal stimulation in obstructive sleep apnea: a disease-modifying therapy. Am J Respir Crit Care Med 2013; 187:1276–1278.

18 Young T, Finn L, Peppard PE, Szklo-Coxe M, Austin D, Nieto FJ, Stubbs R, Hla KM: Sleep disordered breathing and mortality: eighteen-year follow-up of the Wisconsin sleep cohort. Sleep 2008;31:1071–1078.

Daniel Rodenstein, MD, PhD
Department of Pneumology and Center for Sleep Medicine
Cliniques Universitaires Saint-Luc, Université Catholique de Louvain
Av. Hippocrate 10, BE–1200 Brussels (Belgium)
E-Mail daniel.rodenstein@uclouvain.be

Slavin KV (ed): Stimulation of the Peripheral Nervous System. The Neuromodulation Frontier.
Prog Neurol Surg. Basel, Karger, 2016, vol 29, pp 106–116 (DOI: 10.1159/000434661)

Sphenopalatine Ganglion Stimulation in Neurovascular Headaches

Jean Schoenen

Headache Research Unit, Department of Neurology, CHR Citadelle, Liège University, Liège, Belgium

Abstract

The interest for the sphenopalatine ganglion (SPG) in neurovascular headaches dates back to 1908 when Sluder presented his work on the role of the SPG in 'nasal headaches', which are now part of the trigeminal autonomic cephalalgias and cluster headache (ICHD-III-beta). Since then various interventions with blocking or lesional properties have targeted the SPG (transnasal injection of lidocaine and other agents, alcohol or steroid injections, radiofrequency lesions, or even ganglionectomy); success rates vary, but benefit is usually transient. Here we briefly review some anatomo-physiological characteristics of the SPG and hypotheses about its pathophysiological role in neurovascular headaches before describing recent therapeutic results obtained with electrical stimulation of the SPG. Based on results of a prospective randomized controlled study, SPG stimulation appears to be an effective treatment option for patients with chronic cluster headaches; efficacy data indicate that acute electrical stimulation of the SPG provides significant attack pain relief and in many cases pain freedom compared to sham stimulation. Moreover, in some patients SPG stimulation has been associated with a significant and clinically meaningful reduction in cluster headache attack frequency; this preventive effect of SPG stimulation warrants further investigation. For migraine attacks, the outcome of a proof-of-concept study using a temporary electrode implanted in the pterygopalatine fossa was less encouraging; however, an ongoing multicenter trial is evaluating the efficacy of long-term SPG stimulation against sham stimulation for acute and preventive treatment in patients with frequent migraine.

Interest in the sphenopalatine ganglion (SPG) in neurovascular headaches dates back to 1908 when Sluder [1] presented his work on the 'role of the sphenopalatine (or Meckel's) ganglion in nasal headaches', which are now part of the trigeminal autonomic cephalalgias and cluster headache (CH) (ICHD-III-beta) [2]. Since then various interventions with blocking or lesional properties have targeted the SPG such as transnasal injection of lidocaine and other agents [3, 4], alcohol or steroid injections

[5], radiofrequency lesions [6–8], or even ganglionectomy [9]. Success rates vary, but benefit is usually transient [10].

We will briefly review some anatomophysiological characteristics of the SPG and hypotheses about its pathophysiological role in neurovascular headaches before describing recent therapeutic results obtained with electrical stimulation of the SPG.

Anatomophysiology of the Sphenopalatine Ganglion

The SPG is the largest extracranial parasympathetic ganglion located in the pterygopalatine fossa, where it is closely associated with sensory and sympathetic fibers (see review by Khan et al. [11]). Its parasympathetic fibers originate in the superior salivary nucleus (SSN) of the pons and supply extra- and intracerebral arteries, the lacrimal gland, nasal mucosa, and conjunctiva. Sympathetic fibers come from the pericarotid plexus and pass through the SPG to innervate the lacrimal gland and nasal and palatine mucosa. Only a few fibers from the sphenopalatine branches of the maxillary nerve enter the SPG, forming the sensory root. They innervate areas such as the posterior nasopharynx via the lesser palatine nerve.

Physiologically, low-frequency electrical stimulations of the SPG (10–20 Hz) in animal studies produce dilatation of intra- and extracranial arteries, increased cerebral blood flow and plasma protein extravasation in dura mater.

The trigeminoparasympathetic reflex consists of a brainstem connection between trigeminal afferents and parasympathetic efferents of the facial nerve that synapse in the SPG. The reflex was broadly demonstrated in animal and human studies, showing that trigeminal ganglion stimulation leads to intra- and extracranial vasodilatation, increased regional cerebral blood flow and increased facial temperature, a response that is abolished by lesioning the facial nerve. Thus, when the trigeminal-parasympathetic reflex is activated, the postganglionic parasympathetic fibers from the SPG release neurotransmitters and vasodilators that activate sensory trigeminal fibers causing further activation of the trigeminal pain pathway, which in turn causes further parasympathetic outflow [12, 13] (fig. 1).

Pathogenic Role of the Sphenopalatine Ganglion in Neurovascular Headaches

There is no doubt that the cranial autonomic symptoms that characterize CH attacks are predominantly due to activation of the parasympathetic system, and thus the SPG. It is postulated that upon nociceptive activation of nociceptors belonging to the ophthalmic nerve during a CH attack, the trigeminoparasympathetic reflex is activated. Fibers from the trigeminocervical complex project to the superior salivatory nucleus and activate facial parasympathetic efferents. As parasympathetic activation leads to vasodilation of meningeal arteries, a vicious circle further increasing trigeminal

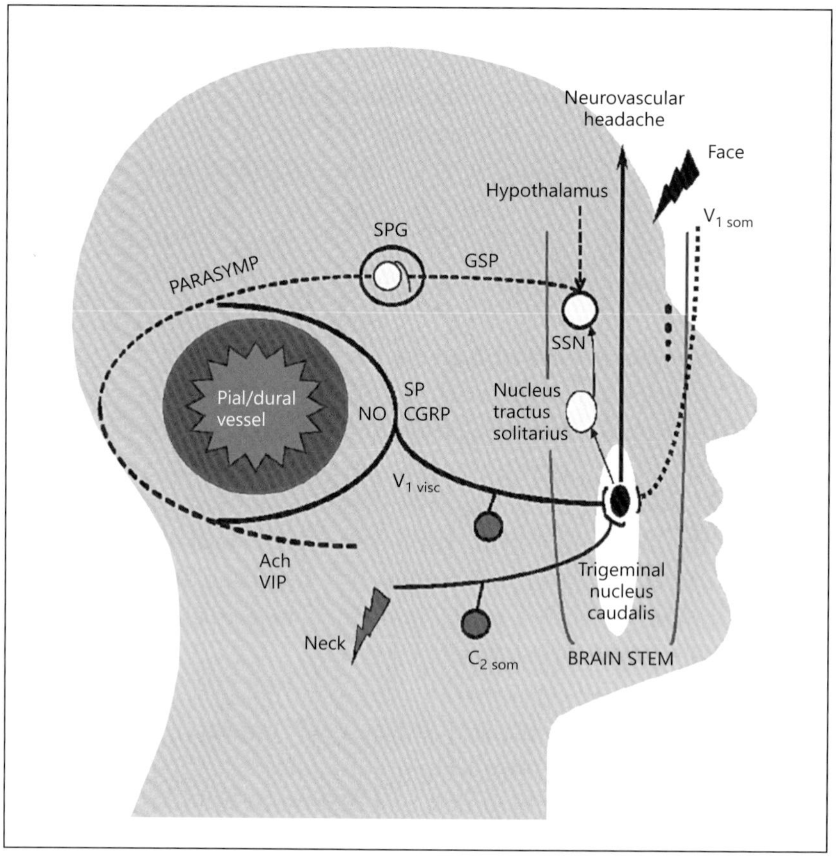

Fig. 1. Schematic outline of the trigeminoparasympathetic circuit. Trigeminovascular afferents (dark lines) belonging to the visceral part of the ophthalmic nerve innervate the meninges and relay in the spinal trigeminal nucleus, from where the SSN can be activated via nucleus tractus solitarius. The parasympathetic fibers (gray dashed lines) innervate meningeal vessels, lacrimal glands, and nasal mucosa via the SPG, producing cranial autonomic symptoms on the side of the headache. The SSN can activate trigeminovascular nociceptors in the spinal trigeminal nucleus and can be activated by descending afferents, e.g. from the hypothalamus.

activation has been proposed [14]. This hypothesis is supported by a recent study showing that low-frequency stimulation of the SPG is able to induce attacks in CH patients [15]. Interestingly, low-frequency stimulation of the SSN in cats leads to firing of trigeminovascular neurons in the trigeminocervical complex, which is inhibited by oxygen inhalation, an established treatment for CH attacks [16].

Cranial autonomic symptoms may also occur during migraine attacks, although they are usually less prominent than in CH. As mentioned, SPG activation produces meningeal vasodilatation and plasma protein extravasation, both of which may be involved in migraine pathogenesis [11]. Burstein and Jakubowski [17] have proposed that common migraine triggers, such as stress, may activate brain areas that project to the SSN. The SSN would then stimulate the release of vasoactive intestinal peptide, nitric oxide, and acetylcholine from meningeal terminals of SPG neurons. The resulting dilatation of intracranial blood vessel and local release of inflammatory molecules would activate meningeal nociceptors, and thus produce the migraine headache. The results of a randomized controlled trial (RCT) showing that during a migraine attack intranasal lidocaine 4% is able to relieve the headache in 35.8% of patients [18] could be considered as support for the 'parasympathetic' theory of migraine pathogenesis. However, there is no proof that lidocaine acts on the headache only via the SPG, and not by influencing sensory afferents. All things considered, the experimental evidence that the trigeminoparasympathetic circuit is pathogenically relevant is much weaker in migraine than in CH.

The SPG is thought to play a role in other pain syndromes besides headaches like trigeminal and sphenopalatine neuralgia, atypical facial pain, muscle pain, vasomotor rhinitis, eye disorders, and herpes infection. Clinical trials have shown that SPG blockade can be helpful in these pain disorders [19].

Sphenopalatine Ganglion Neurostimulation: Available Data

The data showing that blocking or lesioning the SPG may be helpful in neurovascular headaches and that low-frequency stimulation of the SPG in animals induces changes that may be associated with migraine and CH attacks led to the concept that high-frequency stimulation might on the contrary have an inhibitory effect that would be beneficial for acute treatment [11].

Cluster Headache

It is commonly accepted that subcutaneous injections of the 5-HT1B/D agonist sumatriptan are at present the most effective treatment for CH attacks. In the sole available RCT [20], pain relief and pain freedom at 15 min was obtained in 74 and 46% of patients, respectively. Sumatriptan, however, is contraindicated in patients with cardiovascular disease, and many CH patients are heavy smokers and thus at risk for cardiovascular disease. The next most effective acute therapy after sumatriptan is oxygen inhalation, which has a 78% success rate [21]. Various preventive treatments are available for CH such as steroids, verapamil, lithium, topiramate, methysergide, and valproate, but their use may be limited by intolerance or contraindications [22]. Moreover, 10–20% of patients develop the chronic form of CH without remissions and many of them become resistant to preventive drugs. In such patients, invasive neurostimulation methods were studied and found useful in 60–70% of the patients. Deep hypothalamic stimulation is effective but risky. Occipital nerve stimulation is as effective, but also associated with a rather high incidence of adverse effects, e.g. lead migration, infection, and battery depletion (for a review, see Magis and Schoenen [23]).

Therefore, there is room in CH for safer acute treatments and for more effective and better tolerable preventive therapies.

In 2010, a proof-of-concept study on the response of CH patients to acute electrical stimulation of the SPG was published by Ansarinia et al. [24]. In 6 patients in whom attacks occurred spontaneously or were induced in the hospital, stimulation of the SPG with a removable stimulating electrode introduced in the pterygopalatine fossa abolished pain in 11 of 18 attacks (61%) and reduced pain by ≥50% in 3 more attacks. Based on these data, Autonomic Technologies Inc. (ATI; Redwood, Calif., USA) developed an implantable SPG microstimulator and sponsored a prospective, randomized, blinded, multicenter study (Pathway CH-I) to test its efficacy and safety in drug-resistant chronic CH patients [25].

Protocol

The ATI SPG Neurostimulator is implanted under general anesthesia using a minimally invasive, transoral, gingival buccal technique such that the stimulating electrodes on the integral lead are positioned within the pterygopalatine fossa close to the SPG and the body – on the lateral-posterior maxilla medial to the zygoma and anchored to the zygomatic process of the maxilla (fig. 2). The position of the SPG Neurostimulator is verified with an X-ray immediately after implantation, and, if needed, at later time points. Thirty-two chronic CH patients with unilateral attacks in 6 European clinical sites participated in the Pathway CH-I study. After postimplantation healing and titration periods, 4 patients had dropped out and 28 with a mean weekly attack frequency of 17.4 were randomized 1:1:1 to effective, subthreshold, or sham stimulation during an 8-week or 30-attack experimental period. Parameters of effective stimuli were adjusted to provoke paresthesias in the root of the nose or a treatment during an attack (mean intensity: 1.6 mA; mean frequency: 120.4 Hz; mean pulse width: 389.7 µs) and subperception stimuli were at 85% of the lowest effective amplitude. Patients were instructed to apply the remote controller on the face to treat ipsilateral CH attacks that were at least of moderate pain intensity (categorical pain scale: 0 = none; 1 = mild; 2 = moderate; 3 = severe; 4 = very severe) and to stimulate for 15 min, whereafter they were allowed to use acute medications if needed. Pain scores were recorded using a custom electronic headache diary included in the ATI Remote Controller prior to each use and 15, 30, 60, and 90 min after the start of stimulation. The primary efficacy endpoint was pain relief, i.e. a change from 2, 3, or 4 on the categorical pain scale to 0 or 1 at 15 min after the start of stimulation. Secondary endpoints were pain freedom at 15 min, pain relief and freedom at 30, 60, and 90 min, as well as disability changes assessed by the Headache Impact Test (HIT-6) and quality of life changes assessed with the Short-Form Health Survey (SF-36v2). Safety was assessed by tabulating all device- or procedure-related serious adverse events from the implantation procedure to the end of the experimental period.

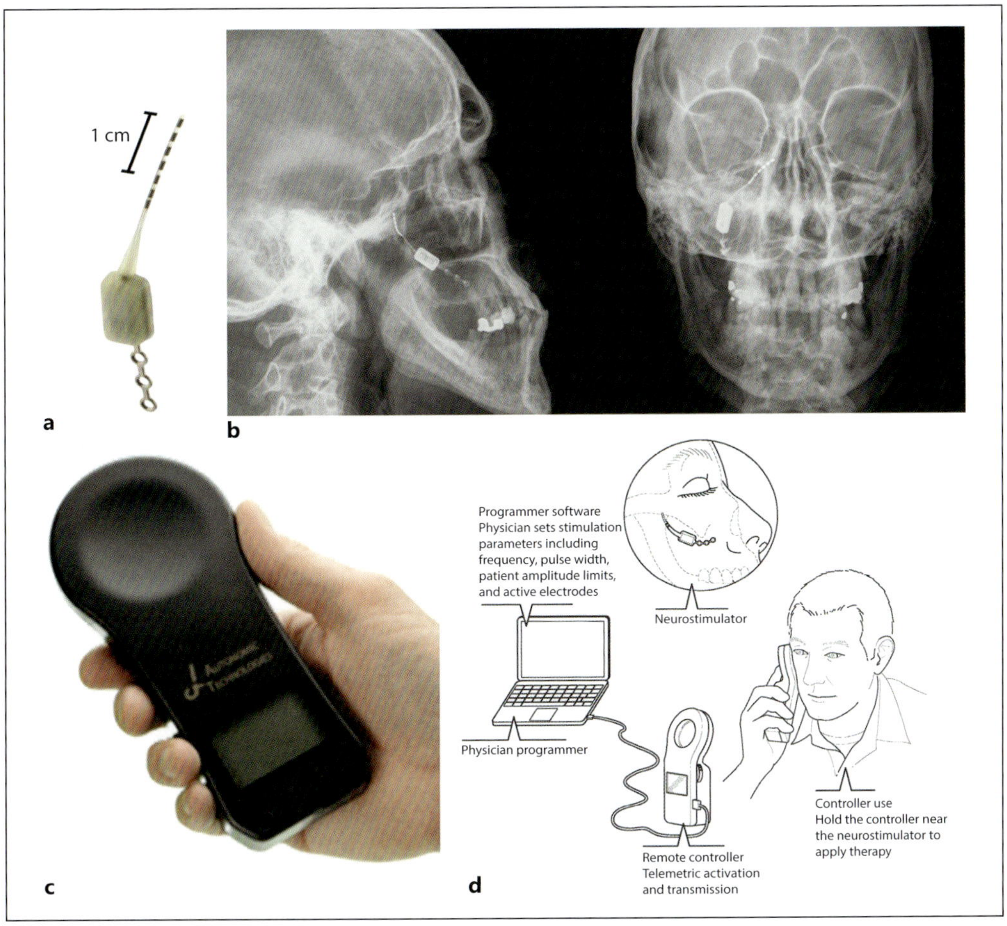

Fig. 2. The ATI Neurostimulator Pulsante™ (**a**, available in four lengths) is a miniaturized device with an integral lead containing six electrodes that is implanted in the pterygopalatine fossa through the gums of the upper maxilla. **b** Lateral and anteroposterior X-rays showing the neurostimulator body anchored to the zygomatic process of the maxilla and the lead with its tip next to the anatomical location of the sphenopalatine ganglion. The handheld ATI Remote Controller (**c**) is positioned by the patient on the jaw to activate the implanted neurostimulator; it also allows the physician to program the stimulation parameters (**d**) (images courtesy of Autonomic Technologies Inc.).

Efficacy Data

During the course of study, the SPG stimulation decreased attack frequency in a number of patients so that out of the 28 evaluable patients only 14 treated enough attacks to be analyzed for acute response. Pain relief at 15 min was achieved in 67.1% of attacks treated by these 14 patients with full stimulation, compared to 7.4% after sham stimulation and 7.3% after subthreshold stimulation. Pain freedom was obtained in 34.1 and 1.5%, respectively. Among the 14 patients, 9 (64%) were considered acute responders since they had pain relief at 15 min in at least 50% of the full stimulation-treated attacks. Overall, 9 out of the 28 patients in the experimental period (32%) reported pain relief of 50% or more at 15-min stimulation.

Twelve out of the randomized 28 patients (43%) were frequency responders with an average 88% reduction of weekly attack frequency. In total, 19 patients out of 28 (68%) experienced an acute response, a frequency response, or both: n = 7 (25%), n = 10 (36%), and n = 2 (7%), respectively. SPG stimulation resulted in a statistically and clinically significant reduction in headache disability.

On completion of the Pathway CH-I trial, patients had the opportunity to enroll in an open long-term follow-up. Among 14 patients who reached 18 months postimplantation, SPG stimulation (average duration 8.6 min) was effective in 84% of the 2,166 analyzable attacks. Efficacy was highest (93%) in attacks of moderate severity, which were also the most frequent attacks treated with SPG stimulation (72%), and lowest in very severe attacks (29%).

Safety Data

As other maxillofacial surgeries, implantation of the ATI Neurostimulator induces standard perioperative adverse effects like local pain, swelling, hematoma, seroma, and sensory disturbances. Among the 32 operated patients in the Pathway CH-I trial, there were 5 device- or procedure-related serious adverse events: 3 misplacements needing a revision procedure, and 2 postimplantation migrations of the electrode needing explantation. Sensory disturbance in the distribution of the maxillary nerve occurred in 81% of the patients with loss of sensation being the most common (21 of 32 events in 19 of 32 patients). Sensory deficit resolved after an average of 97 days (range: 31–259), but in 6 patients, though being mild or moderate, it had not resolved at the time of the report, and in one patient with an electrode migration who had to be explanted because of neuropathic pain, a mild sensory deficit persisted 1 year after the procedure. During and after the Pathway CH-I trial, advancements in surgical instruments and additional surgical experience have decreased surgical time by 25%, the number of adverse events by 23%, and the rate of explants or revisions by 83%.

Mechanism of Action

As mentioned above, in a double-blind randomized crossover study, low-frequency (5 Hz) stimulation applied to the 6 CH patients implanted with the ATI Neurostimulator triggered an attack in 3 of them. These attacks were effectively treated with high-frequency (120 Hz) stimulation [15].

The prominent autonomic symptoms associated with CH attacks result from increased cranial parasympathetic outflow that is thought to activate trigeminal afferents via the trigeminovascular system [12]. High-frequency electrical stimulation of the SPG may block the parasympathetic efferents, thereby turning off the efferent arm of the trigeminal-autonomic reflex, which is thought to be due to depletion of stored neurotransmitter(s). From a pathophysiological perspective, the positive results of the Pathway CH-I trial confirm that the cranial parasympathetic system plays a crucial role in the occurrence as well as recurrence of CH attacks.

Electrical stimulation in the region of the SPG also acts on the neighboring sensory fibers of the maxillary nerve, producing paresthesias in the nasopharynx, soft palate, nasal cavity, and palatal gingiva. In the Pathway CH-I study, these paresthesias guided the programming of stimulation parameters. Whether the activation of sensory fibers of the maxillary nerve contributes to the therapeutic effect is unlikely, but remains to be explored.

The mechanisms of action may be different between the acute and preventive effects of SPG stimulation, which is suggested by the absence of a correlation between the two effects in many Pathway CH-I patients. Assuming that it can be confirmed in an adequate RCT, the preventive effect might be associated with modulation of centers involved in descending pain control, similar to that found in chronic CH patients after occipital nerve stimulation [26].

Migraine

For the treatment of migraine attacks, analgesics, NSAIDs, and triptans are currently available. Triptans are the most effective, although the pain-free rate hardly exceeds 30% after 2 h. Triptans may also have unpleasant side effects and they are contraindicated in patients with cardiovascular disease. Moreover, the overuse of analgesics and triptans is the most prevalent chronifying factor of migraine [27]. Preventive therapies in migraine have at best a 50% responder rate of 50–60%, and the most efficient preventive drugs like the anticonvulsants topiramate and valproate are not tolerated by many patients. In addition, patients suffering from chronic migraine become notoriously resistant to preventive therapies [28]. Therefore, there is room for more efficacious and better tolerated treatments. In the last decade, several neuromodulation methods have been explored, including electrical stimulation of peripheral nervous structures [23]. Transcutaneous supraorbital nerve stimulation with a new device was found to be superior to placebo in an RCT of episodic migraineurs, but the 50% responder rate was just below 40% [29].

As mentioned above, there is some evidence for interictal autonomic dysfunctions in migraine, and cranial autonomic symptoms can accompany the attack [11]. It remains to be shown, however, whether these autonomic symptoms are epiphenomena due to the trigeminovascular activation or if they also contribute to the headache and central sensitization, as suggested by some trials [27].

A proof-of-concept study on the potential utility of SPG stimulation in migraine was conducted similarly to that performed in CH [30]. As for CH, the authors implanted a removable stimulation needle lead in the pterygopalatine fossa in 11 patients with medically refractory migraine: 9 with medication overuse headache and 2 with episodic migraine. The interventions were performed in an outpatient procedure room. Patients had spontaneous or induced migraine headaches and were, in a cross-over protocol, either effectively or sham stimulated at the peak of their headache and associated migrainous features, i.e. several hours after pain onset. Patients had 1–3 peaks of headache stimulated for a mean of 3 min with a mean amplitude of 1.2 V, mean frequency of 57 Hz, and mean pulse width of 394 μs.

SPG stimulation produced complete abolition of pain within 3 min in 5 out of 15 headache peaks treated in 2 patients (33.3%). In 3 of 15 attacks, <50% headache relief was achieved. One patient had headache relief with SPG stimulation, but also with sham stimulation. No adverse effects occurred during this study.

These results paved the way for the ongoing Pathway MIG-I trial, where the efficacy of effective stimulation with the ATI SPG Neurostimulator is being evaluated against sham stimulation for acute and preventive treatment in patients with frequent migraine. No data are available yet.

Conclusions

There is evidence that the SPG plays a role in the pathophysiology of neurovascular headaches. Based on available studies, the evidence looks much more convincing in CH than in migraine. In both headache types, however, there is a need for more efficient and better tolerable treatments, particularly in the most severely affected patients.

In experimental animals, low-frequency stimulation of the SPG produces vascular and meningeal changes that are thought to be associated with migraine and CH. A contrario, stimulation at high frequency is thought to inhibit parasympathetic output by exhausting transmitter synthesis and release. Based on this rationale, proof-of-concept studies have been performed with SPG stimulation by removable needle electrodes implanted in the pterygopalatine fossa during CH or migraine attacks, abolishing the pain in 61 and 33% of attacks, respectively.

The hitherto only sham-controlled RCT of SPG stimulation was performed in chronic CH with the implantable ATI Neurostimulator. In 14 out of 28 evaluable patients, effective SPG stimulation for 15 min produced significant pain relief in 61% of attacks, compared to 7% for ineffective stimulation. Incidentally, this study suggested that repeated SPG stimulation was also able to decrease attack frequency. Overall, 25% of the patients had an acute response, 36% had a frequency response, and 7% experienced both. The Pathway CH-I trial clearly shows that SPG stimulation with the implantable ATI Neurostimulator is able to abort CH attacks. The possible preventive effect needs to be verified in a proper RCT. The acute effect must be weighed against the adverse effects of the surgical intervention that are comprised of perioperative local symptoms and in particular long-lasting sensory disturbances due to injury of branches of the maxillary nerve.

The patients enrolled in the Pathway CH-I trial were severely disabled chronic CH patients. These patients became resistant to the available preventive drugs, but their attacks usually still responded fully and rapidly (within 5–10 min) to injectable sumatriptan and sometimes to oxygen inhalation. Therefore, they are above all in need of a better preventive treatment. SPG stimulation was most effective in attacks of moderate severity and thus treated early. In severe attacks, e.g. which awake patients during night, SPG stimulation was much less effective than injectable sumatriptan. One major advantage of SPG stimulation, however, is that it can be repeated several times over a 24-hour period in patients with multiple attacks and can be used by patients with cardiovascular contraindications for injectable sumatriptan.

Contrary to SPG stimulation, occipital nerve stimulation has a convincing preventive effect in refractory chronic CH patients as it is seldom useful during an attack. Therefore, the two neuromodulation methods are not comparable at this stage, and could be complementary. Assuming that the preventive effect of SPG stimulation can be proven in CH, the effect size and, more importantly, the benefit/adverse effect ratio have to be compared with those of occipital nerve stimulation.

During migraine attacks, the outcome of the proof-of-concept study using a removable electrode implanted in the pterygopalatine fossa was less encouraging than in CH attacks since only 1 out of 3 attacks was interrupted. Nonetheless, an RCT of the effect of SPG stimulation with the ATI Neurostimulator (Pathway MIG-I) has been launched in frequent migraine. Besides a possible action on the attack, most patients and their treating practitioners would welcome a stimulation-induced reduction of attack frequency.

References

1 Sluder G: The role of the sphenopalatine (or Meckel's) ganglion in nasal headaches. NY Med J 1908;87: 989–990.
2 Headache Classification Committee of the International Headache Society (IHS). ICHD-III-beta: The International Classification of Headache Disorders, 3rd edition (beta version). Cephalalgia 2013;33:629–808.
3 Devoghel JC: Cluster headache and sphenopalatine block. Acta Anaesthesiol Belg 1981;32:101–107.
4 Felisati G, Arnone F, Lozza P, Leone M, Curone M, Bussone G: Sphenopalatine endoscopic ganglion block: a revision of a traditional technique for cluster headache. Laryngoscope 2006;116:1447–1450.
5 Pipolo C, Bussone G, Leone M, Lozza P, Felisati G: Sphenopalatine endoscopic ganglion block in cluster headache: a reevaluation of the procedure after 5 years. Neurol Sci 2010;31(suppl 1):S197–S199.
6 Sanders M, Zuurmond WW: Efficacy of sphenopalatine ganglion blockade in 66 patients suffering from cluster headache: a 12- to 70-month follow-up evaluation. J Neurosurg 1997;87:876–880.
7 Narouze S, Kapural L, Casanova J, Mekhail N: Sphenopalatine ganglion radiofrequency ablation for the management of chronic cluster headache. Headache 2009;49:571–577.
8 Chua NH, Vissers KC, Wilder-Smith OH: Quantitative sensory testing may predict response to sphenopalatine ganglion pulsed radiofrequency treatment in cluster headaches: a case series. Pain Pract 2011; 11:439–445.
9 Meyer JS, Binns PM, Ericsson AD, Vulpe M: Sphenopalatine ganglionectomy for cluster headache. Arch Otolaryngol 1970;92:475–484.
10 Levin M: Nerve blocks in the treatment of headache. Neurotherapeutics 2010;7:197–203.
11 Khan S, Schoenen J, Ashina M: Sphenopalatine ganglion neuromodulation in migraine: what is the rationale? Cephalalgia 2014;34:382–391.

12 May A, Goadsby PJ: The trigeminovascular system in humans: pathophysiologic implications for primary headache syndromes of the neural influences on the cerebral circulation. J Cereb Blood Flow Metab 1999;19:115–127.
13 Goadsby PJ: Pathophysiology of cluster headache: a trigeminal autonomic cephalgia. Lancet Neurol 2002;1:251–257.
14 Jürgens TP, Schoenen J, Rostgaard J, Hillerup S, Láinez MJ, Assaf AT, May A, Jensen RH: Stimulation of the sphenopalatine ganglion in intractable cluster headache: expert consensus on patient selection and standards of care. Cephalalgia 2014;34:1100–1110.
15 Schytz HW, Barløse M, Guo S, Selb J, Caparso A, Jensen R, Ashina M: Experimental activation of the sphenopalatine ganglion provokes cluster-like attacks in humans. Cephalalgia 2013;33:831–841.
16 Akerman S, Holland PR, Lasalandra MP, Goadsby PJ: Oxygen inhibits neuronal activation in the trigeminocervical complex after stimulation of trigeminal autonomic reflex, but not during direct dural activation of trigeminal afferents. Headache 2009;49: 1131–1143.
17 Burstein R, Jakubowski M: Unitary hypothesis for multiple triggers of the pain and strain of migraine. J Comp Neurol 2005;493:9–14.
18 Maizels M, Geiger AM: Intranasal lidocaine for migraine: a randomized trial and open-label follow-up. Headache 1999;39:543–551.
19 Piagkou M, Demesticha T, Troupis T, Vlasis K, Skandalakis P, Makri A, Mazarakis A, Lappas D, Piagkos G, Johnson EO: The pterygopalatine ganglion and its role in various pain syndromes: from anatomy to clinical practice. Pain Pract 2012;12:399–412.
20 The Sumatriptan Cluster Headache Study Group: Treatment of acute cluster headache with sumatriptan. N Engl J Med 1991;325:322–326.
21 Cohen AS, Burns B, Goadsby PJ: High-flow oxygen for treatment of cluster headache: a randomized trial. JAMA 2009;302:2451–2457.
22 Evers S, Afra J, Frese A, Goadsby PJ, Linde M, May A, Sandor PS: Cluster headache and other trigemino-autonomic cephalgias; in Gilhus NE, Barnes MP, Brainin M (eds): European Handbook of Neurological Management, ed 2. Oxford, Wiley-Blackwell, 2011, vol 1, pp 179–190.
23 Magis D, Schoenen J: Advances and challenges in neurostimulation for headaches. Lancet Neurol 2012;11:708–719.
24 Ansarinia M, Rezai A, Tepper SJ, Steiner CP, Stump J, Stanton-Hicks M, Machado A, Narouze S: Electrical stimulation of sphenopalatine ganglion for acute treatment of cluster headaches. Headache 2010;50: 1164–1174.
25 Schoenen J, Jensen RH, Lantéri-Minet M, Láinez MJ, Gaul C, Goodman AM, Caparso A, May A: Stimulation of the sphenopalatine ganglion (SPG) for cluster headache treatment. Pathway CH-1: a randomized, sham-controlled study. Cephalalgia 2013;33:816–830.
26 Magis D, Bruno MA, Fumal A, Gérardy PY, Hustinx R, Laurey S, Schoenen J: Central modulation in cluster headache patients treated with occipital nerve stimulation: an FDG-PET study. BMC Neurol 2011; 11:25.
27 Coppola G, Schoenen J: Management of acute and chronic migraine. Curr Opin Support Palliat Care 2012;6:177–182.
28 Silberstein SD, Latsko M, Schoenen J: Preventive antimigraine drugs; in Fernández-de-las-Peñas C, Chaitow L, Schoenen J (eds): Contemporary Issues in Physical Therapy and Rehabilitation Medicine. Multidisciplinary Management of Migraine. Burlington, Jones & Bartlett Learning, 2013, pp. 91–102.
29 Schoenen J, Vandersmissen B, Jeangette S, Herroelen L, Vandenheede M, Gérard P, Magis D: Migraine prevention with a supraorbital transcutaneous stimulator: a randomized controlled trial. Neurology 2013;80:697–704.
30 Tepper SJ, Rezai A, Narouze S, Steiner C, Mohajer P, Ansarinia M: Acute treatment of intractable migraine with sphenopalatine ganglion electrical stimulation. Headache 2009;49:983–989.

Prof. Jean Schoenen
Headache Research Unit, Department of Neurology
CHR Citadelle, Liège University
Blvd du XII de Ligne, BE–4000 Liège (Belgium)
E-Mail jschoenen@ulg.ac.be

Slavin KV (ed): Stimulation of the Peripheral Nervous System. The Neuromodulation Frontier.
Prog Neurol Surg. Basel, Karger, 2016, vol 29, pp 117–126 (DOI: 10.1159/000434662)

Occipital Nerve Stimulation for Migraine: Update from Recent Multicenter Trials

Todd J. Schwedt · A. Laine Green · David W. Dodick

Department of Neurology, Mayo Clinic Arizona, Phoenix, Ariz., USA

Abstract

Occipital nerve stimulation (ONS) continues to be investigated for the treatment of refractory chronic migraine. Results from case series and from prospective, sham-controlled clinical trials remain inconclusive regarding the efficacy of ONS for migraine treatment. Safety and implantation techniques require improvements since rates of lead migration, infection, and persistent stimulator-related pain continue to be high. Existing data justify further ONS trials with carefully chosen primary outcome(s), adequate statistical power, and improved surgical techniques.

Occipital nerve stimulation (ONS) has been investigated for the treatment of chronic migraine patients who are refractory to more conventional therapy. 'Chronic migraine' is the diagnosis when a patient has headaches on at least 15 days per month including at least 8 days per month on which symptoms meet diagnostic criteria for migraine. The International Classification of Headache Disorders-3 beta diagnostic criteria for chronic migraine are illustrated in table 1 [1]. Chronic migraine affects approximately 2% of the general population [2]. Most commonly, chronic migraine develops in a patient who has had a slow progression in headache frequency over years, thus transforming from episodic migraine (fewer than 15 headache days/month) to chronic migraine. Approximately 3–14% of people with episodic migraine transform to chronic migraine each year [3, 4].

Chronic migraine exerts substantial negative effects on the individual sufferer and results in significant societal costs. Chronic migraineurs average 22 headache days per month, although a subset of chronic migraineurs have continuous headache pain [5]. Compared to episodic migraine, chronic migraine is associated with headaches of

Table 1. International Classification of Headache Disorders-3 beta: diagnostic criteria for chronic migraine

A. Headache (tension-type-like and/or migraine-like) on ≥15 days per month for >3 months and fulfilling criteria B and C
B. Occurring in a patient who has had ≥5 attacks of migraine without aura and/or migraine with aura
C. On ≥8 days per month for >3 months, fulfilling any of the following:
   a. Migraine without aura diagnostic criteria
   b. Migraine with aura diagnostic criteria
   c. Believed by the patient to be migraine at onset and relieved by a triptan or ergot derivative
D. Not better accounted for by another headache diagnosis

longer duration and more severe intensity [6]. People with chronic migraine have elevated rates of comorbid psychiatric disorders, other pain disorders, altered sleep, and fatigue [7–10]. As would be expected, chronic migraine is associated with greater disability than episodic migraine, resulting in more days of work or school missed (8.2% of people with chronic migraine miss ≥5 days/3 months vs. 2.2% with episodic migraine), more days of reduced productivity at work/school (33.8% of people with chronic migraine have significantly reduced productivity on ≥5 days/3 months vs. 12.3% with episodic migraine), more missed days of work around the house (57.4% of chronic migraine sufferers miss ≥5 days/3 months vs. 24.3% with episodic migraine), and more family and social activities missed (36.9% of chronic migraineurs miss ≥5 days/3 months vs. 9.5% with episodic migraine) [11]. Very severe migraine-related disability is reported by over 60% of people with chronic migraine and about 90% have at least moderate migraine-related disability [6, 12, 13]. Societal costs from chronic migraine are enormous. According to the Global Burden of Disease 2010 study, migraine is responsible for about 1% of all disability-adjusted life years [14]. Direct costs from chronic migraine are estimated to be close to USD 3,500–4,150 per person per year [6, 15].

Treatment of chronic migraine focuses on prophylactic measures aimed at reducing the frequency and severity of migraine headaches and associated symptoms. Prophylactic measures often include lifestyle modifications, migraine trigger avoidance, physical therapy, behavioral therapy, and optimized pharmacologic therapy. Similar to the procedure for treating episodic migraine, medication selection for chronic migraine prophylaxis is often influenced by individual physician experience and/or a trial-and-error process, with many chronic migraineurs being unresponsive (or having effects wane over time) to selected therapies. Although it is generally assumed that medications effective for episodic migraine are also effective for chronic migraine, pharmacologic prevention of chronic migraine has been inadequately studied. The highest level of evidence (randomized controlled trials) for chronic migraine prophylaxis exists for topiramate and onabotulinumtoxin A, the latter being FDA approved for chronic migraine prophylaxis.

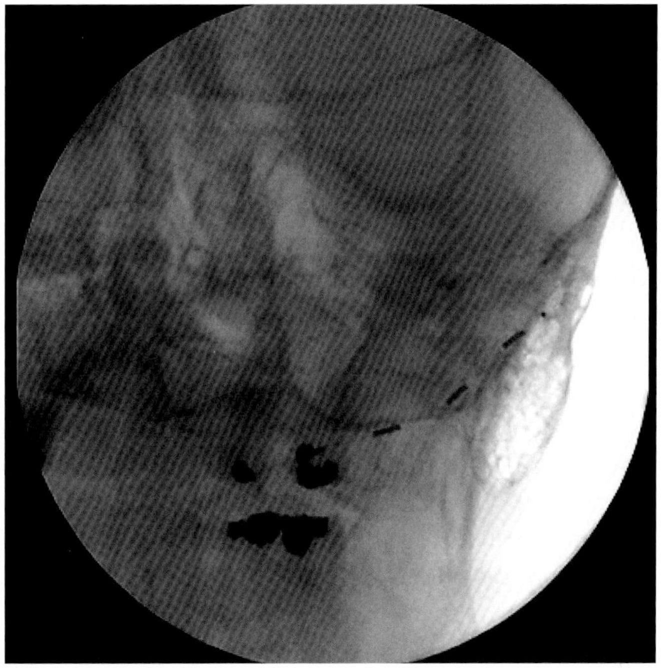

Fig. 1. ONS lead insertion: unilateral ONS lead.

Despite the use of best available practices for chronic migraine prevention, a proportion of patients will not respond and are thus considered refractory to conventional therapy. Estimates of refractory migraine prevalence in the general population are lacking. Approximately 5% of patients seen in a headache clinic have refractory migraine [16]. Although the definition of 'refractory' can be debated, recommendations have been published [17–20]. The American Headache Society has proposed the following criteria for refractory chronic migraine: (1) headaches cause significant interference with function or quality of life despite modification of triggers, lifestyle factors, and adequate trials of medications with established efficacy, and (2) patient failed adequate trials of preventive medications, alone or in combination, from at least 2 of 4 drug classes including beta-blockers, anticonvulsants, tricyclics, and calcium-channel blockers, and (3) patient failed adequate trials of abortive medications, including both a triptan and dihydroergotamine intranasal or injectable formulation and either nonsteroidal anti-inflammatory drugs or combination analgesics, unless contraindicated. For this group of refractory chronic migraineurs, there is interest in interventional therapies. One such therapy is ONS (fig. 1).

Although the mechanism(s) by which ONS might effectively treat migraine is not completely known, ONS likely exerts its effect via peripheral and central mechanisms. Stimulation-induced activation of large sensory afferents likely results in suppression of nociceptive traffic in the smaller pain fibers [21]. This may represent a diffuse noxious inhibitory control-like response. Furthermore, ONS may alter nociceptive pain processing in the migraine brain. A PET study of 8 chronic migraine patients who were successfully treated with ONS showed regional cerebral blood flow changes that correlated with pain scores in several regions of the migraine 'pain matrix', including the dorsal rostral pons, anterior cingulate cortex, and cuneus [22].

Case Series of Occipital Nerve Stimulation for Chronic Migraine

There have been several published, open-label, uncontrolled case series of ONS treatment for chronic migraine. Although the level of evidence resulting from these case series is low, these early studies served as a basis to justify and design prospective sham-controlled trials.

The largest case series included 25 chronic migraine patients who had migraine for a median of 10 years and failed to respond to an average of 7 migraine medications prior to ONS [23]. Ten patients decided to use their stimulator continuously while 15 patients stimulated intermittently. At a mean follow-up of 18 months, headache frequency was reduced from 76/90 days pre-ONS to 38/90 days with ONS ($p < 0.001$), 88% of the patients had at least a 50% reduction in headache frequency or severity, and there were substantial reductions in the use of migraine-abortive medications and migraine-related disability. Adverse events included lead migration in 9 patients and infection in 1 patient.

A second ONS series included 10 patients with chronic migraine [24]. The number of years with migraine ranged from 2 to 25 years. All patients had substantial relief from occipital nerve blockade before the decision was made to treat with ONS. Patients had an 'on the table trial' of ONS followed by immediate battery internalization. At 1 month, 9 patients reported >90% pain relief and 1 reported 75–90% pain relief. At 6 months, 7/9 patients continued to have >90% relief and 2 had 75–90% relief (1 patient was lost to follow-up). Complications included infection in 2 patients.

An ONS study of 15 patients with refractory headaches included 8 patients with chronic migraine and pain that involved the C2 distribution [25]. At an average follow-up of 17.8 months, headache frequency was reduced to 60/90 days from 90/90 days ($p = 0.04$), headache severity was reduced to 4.5 (on a scale of 1–10) from 6.75 ($p = 0.009$), and there were substantial reductions in headache-related disability and depression. Adverse events included lead migration in 3 patients, need for implanted pulse generator revision in 1 patient, neck stiffness in 1 patient, and persistent incision-site pain in 1 patient.

In a series of 8 patients, ONS resulted in an excellent response in 4 (complete suppression or rare breakthrough headaches), very good response in 2 (complete suppression most of the time with breakthrough headaches on ~10 days/month), and good response in 2 (continued constant headaches but with severity reduced by 50–75%) [22]. All patients had significant reduction or discontinuation of headache medications. Adverse events included lead migration in 3 patients and abdominal hematoma related to the implanted pulse generator in 1 patient.

One-year migraine-related disability outcomes were collected from 3 patients with refractory chronic migraine treated with ONS [26]. Two patients had >90% reduction in disability and 1 patient had between 25 and 49% reduction in disability.

Two large centers that specialize in neuromodulation examined, retrospectively, their experiences with ONS over a 6-year period (2007–2012) [27]. Twenty-five patients had an ONS implanted but only 23 were analyzed. Seventeen patients had ONS for chronic migraine. Other diagnoses included occipital neuralgia (n = 3), idiopathic intracranial hypertension (n = 1), cluster headache (n = 1), and cervicogenic headache (n = 1). With respect to the migraine subjects, 53% had a ≥50% reduction in the number of headaches and/or pain intensity. The average follow-up was 40 ± 27 months. Five patients had migraine pain that originated in the trigeminal distribution while 11 patients had pain that originated in the occipital area. Eighty percent of the trigeminal pain distribution patients had sustained pain relief, while 45% of the occipital pain distribution patients had significant relief over time. The most frequent complications were related to lead issues and overall 43% of the subjects had at least one surgical revision. There were three infections. Eight patients eventually had their ONS removed (4 = ineffective, 2 = infection and ineffective, 1 = granuloma and skin erosion, 1 = psychological reasons).

Combined occipital and supraorbital nerve stimulation has also been employed for treatment of refractory chronic migraine [28, 29]. In a study of 8 refractory chronic migraine patients, 7 had at least 50% improvement in pain during a 5-day percutaneous combined supraorbital and ONS trial, and thus received permanent implants [28]. After a median follow-up duration of 15 months (range: 1–35), all 7 patients reported substantial benefits from stimulation. Six patients reported at least 90% improvement in their headaches and 1 patient reported 60% improvement. Five patients were able to discontinue medications and the other 2 had marked reductions in medication intake. Disability was reduced, with all patients returning to 'fully functional lifestyles'. Complications included infection in 1 patient, lead migration in 1 patient, and 1 patient had an allergic reaction to the titanium in the pulse generator.

In a separate study of combined supraorbital and ONS, 3 out of 3 patients with refractory chronic migraine derived >50% benefit from percutaneous trial stimulation over 24–72 h and thus had permanent implantation [29]. One patient had permanent implantation of occipital leads only and 2 had combined occipital and supraorbital leads. After a mean follow-up of 4 months (range: 4–6), all 3 reported substantial benefits with >50% reductions in headache. One patient required surgical revision due to lead migration.

Prospective Randomized Crossover Study

One study has evaluated ONS in a prospective randomized crossover study [30]. In this study, eligible subjects had a diagnosis of chronic migraine with or without medication overuse headache and had to have failed 2 prophylactic treatments (efficacy or intolerable to side effects) and not be taking prophylactic medication at the start of the study. Those that had a reduction (≥50%) in the number or severity of attacks following a temporary percutaneous stimulation trial (15–30 days) underwent placement of an internal pulse generator. They were randomized (1:1) to two different groups: stimulator 'on' or 'off'. Those in the stimulator 'off' arm could switch their stimulator on if the frequency or severity of their headaches increased by 30%. After 4 weeks, the patients crossed over (except for those who had already switched from the stimulator 'off' arm to the stimulator 'on' arm). Follow-up was to occur at 3, 6, and 12 months. Amongst the 34 enrolled patients, the average frequency of headaches was 5.8 ± 1.6 days per week. One patient withdrew after the consent procedure and one withdrew after a stimulator infection. Thirty-two patients completed the study with an average follow-up of 45 ± 23 days. Sixty-six percent had a ≥50% reduction in the number and severity of headaches, 22% had a ≥50% reduction in the severity of headaches, and 9% had a ≥50% reduction in the number of headaches. Three percent of the patients did not achieve any of these outcomes. Even though a number of patients required their stimulators to be turned on, when allocated to the 'off' group, there was no difference in the 'off' times between the groups. Both groups had improvement in disability scores and quality of life scores based on the MIDAS and SF-36 questionnaires, respectively. Triptan and nonsteroidal anti-inflammatory drug use dropped significantly from 20 and 25 doses per month to 3 and 2 doses per month at the 1-year follow-up. Five adverse events were recorded: 2 implantation site infections and 3 lead migrations. The main study limitations were that is was a small single-center trial and the lack of a control group.

Randomized Sham-Controlled Clinical Trials of Occipital Nerve Stimulation for Chronic Migraine

Two randomized sham-controlled trials of ONS for treatment of refractory chronic migraine have been completed [31, 32].

The smaller of the two clinical trials was designed with the intention of collecting further data regarding safety and efficacy of ONS for chronic migraine [31]. There was no a priori selected primary outcome and the study was not powered to draw conclusions regarding efficacy and safety. The study included 77 subjects who had migraine for an average of 22 years with chronic migraine for 10 years. On average, subjects had 23 days per month with headache and were refractory to migraine prophylactic medications from at least 2 different classes. Subjects all had headache pain within the occipital nerve territory and all subjects had transient relief of pain following occipital nerve blockade. Patients overusing abortive migraine medications were excluded. Migraine prophylactic medications were allowed as long as there were no changes in the medications or doses within 4 weeks of enrollment. Subjects were randomized in a 2:1:1 ratio either to adjustable stimulation (i.e. active treatment), preset-stimulation for 1 min daily (i.e. sham stimulation), or continued medical management. Stimulator implantation was preceded by paresthesia testing, and only those subjects who felt paresthesias within the regions of their head pain had the stimulator implanted.

Numerous measures of efficacy were examined after 3 months of stimulation; for most of these, active ONS was numerically superior (although not meeting statistical significance in many cases) to sham stimulation and continued medical management. Patients in the adjustable stimulation group had a reduction in headache days from 22.4 to 15.7 days per month. Active stimulation was significantly superior for a few disability and quality of life outcomes when independently analyzed (not multiple comparison corrected). Complications within the first 3 months (of stimulation) included lead migration in 24% of subjects and infection in 14%.

In the larger of the two multicenter clinical trials, 157 refractory chronic migraine subjects were randomized (2:1) to active stimulation or sham stimulation [32]. Patients had experienced migraine for about 23 years, with an average of approximately 22 days with headache per month, and had severe migraine-related disability. Only patients who had a successful stimulation trial (≥50% reduction in pain or adequate paresthesia coverage in the painful areas) received implantation of the permanent system and were included in the analysis.

The primary outcome of this study was the proportion of subjects in each group who were 'responders', defined as ≥50% reduction in average pain intensity with no increase in average headache duration at 12 weeks. There were no differences in the proportion of responders in the active stimulation group (17.1%) versus the sham stimulation group (13.5%). However, active stimulation was superior to sham stimulation for several secondary outcomes including the proportion of patients achieving 10, 20, and 30% reduction in pain intensity; 10, 20 and 30% reductions in headache frequency; reductions in migraine-related disability, and the proportion of subjects self-rating their headache pain relief as 'good' or 'excellent'. There were 107 adverse events reported (73 in the active stimulation group, 34 in the sham stimulation group). The most common adverse events included persistent pain and/or numbness at the implanted pulse generator/lead site (21.5% of all adverse events), lead migration (18.7%), infection (6.5%), and unintended stimulation effects (6.5%) [32].

Long-term results of this cohort of 157 migraine patients who were followed for an additional 40 weeks in an open-label fashion indicate that there was a significant reduction in number of headache days [6.7 ± 8.4 days in the intent-to-treat group ($n = 157$), $p < 0.001$, and 7.7 ± 8.7 days in those patients actually meeting criteria for intractable chronic migraine ($n = 125$), $p < 0.001$] [33]. Both disability scores and pain and distress measures improved in both groups. The percentage of patients who achieved a reduction of 30 and 50% in headache days and/or headache intensity was 59.5 and 47.8%, respectively. There were a total of 183 device-/procedure-related adverse events during the study, of which 85 (40.7%) required surgical intervention and 18 (8.6%) required hospitalization.

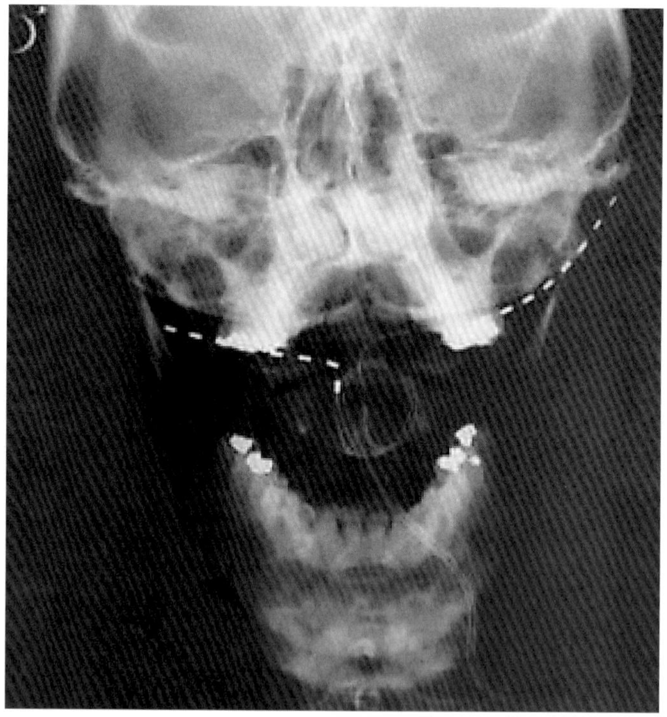

Fig. 2. Occipital nerve stimulator lead migration: bilateral ONS leads with a stress relief loop in the mid-cervical region; the right ONS lead is inferiorly displaced.

Conclusions

ONS may be a reasonable therapy for some patients with refractory chronic migraine. Case series and prospective clinical trials have shown small-to-modest benefits of ONS over sham stimulation, albeit with relatively high rates of adverse events. The only prospective clinical trial adequately powered and designed to test a primary outcome for efficacy failed to show superiority of ONS over sham stimulation for the primary outcome. However, secondary analyses suggest some benefit from ONS.

Given the substantial pain and disability that refractory chronic migraine causes, the undeniable need for effective treatments for this patient group, the biologic plausibility of ONS for migraine treatment, and the existing study results, further investigations of ONS for the treatment of refractory chronic migraine are needed. Future studies need to use carefully chosen primary outcome and secondary outcome measures (s) and include enough subjects so that they are adequately powered. They also need to reduce the potential placebo effect in the preimplantation stimulation trials. These future studies should continue to investigate patient characteristics (e.g. headache location) that may predict ONS treatment response, optimal stimulation parameters, modified surgical techniques that lead to lower rates of adverse events (fig. 2), and the potential benefits of combined occipital and supraorbital stimulation. They should also follow patients for extended intervals in order to collect data on long-term safety and efficacy.

References

1 Headache Classification Committee of the International Headache Society (IHS): The International Classification of Headache Disorders, 3rd edition (beta version). Cephalalgia 2013;33:629–808.

2 Castillo J, Muñoz P, Guitera V, Pascual J: Kaplan Award 1998. Epidemiology of chronic daily headache in the general population. Headache 1999;39:190–196.

3 Scher AI, Stewart WF, Liberman J, Lipton RB: Prevalence of frequent headache in a population sample. Headache 1998;38:497–506.

4 Katsarava Z, Schneeweiss S, Kurth T, Kroener U, Fritsche G, Eikermann A, Diener HC, Limmroth V: Incidence and predictors for chronicity of headache in patients with episodic migraine. Neurology 2004;62:788–790.

5 Bigal ME, Rapoport AM, Lipton RB, Tepper SJ, Sheftell FD: Assessment of migraine disability using the migraine disability assessment (MIDAS) questionnaire: a comparison of chronic migraine with episodic migraine. Headache 2003;43:336–342.

6 Stokes M, Becker WJ, Lipton RB, Sullivan SD, Wilcox TK, Wells L, Manack A, Proskorovsky I, Gladstone J, Buse DC, Varon SF, Goadsby PJ, Blumenfeld AM: Cost of health care among patients with chronic and episodic migraine in Canada and the USA: results from the International Burden of Migraine Study (IBMS). Headache 2011;51:1058–1077.

7 Juang KD, Wang SJ, Fuh JL, Lu SR, Su TP: Comorbidity of depressive and anxiety disorders in chronic daily headache and its subtypes. Headache 2000;40:818–823.

8 Peres MF, Zukerman E, Young WB, Silberstein SD: Fatigue in chronic migraine patients. Cephalalgia 2002;22:720–724.

9 Peres MF, Young WB, Kaup AO, Zukerman E, Silberstein SD: Fibromyalgia is common in patients with transformed migraine. Neurology 2001;57:1326–1328.

10 Kelman L, Rains JC: Headache and sleep: examination of sleep patterns and complaints in a large clinical sample of migraineurs. Headache 2005;45:904.

11 Bigal ME, Serrano D, Reed M, Lipton RB: Chronic migraine in the population: burden, diagnosis, and satisfaction with treatment. Neurology 2008;71:559–566.

12 Blumenfeld AM, Varon SF, Wilcox TK, Buse DC, Kawata AK, Manack A, Goadsby PJ, Lipton RB: Disability, HRQoL and resource use among chronic and episodic migraineurs: results from the International Burden of Migraine Study (IBMS). Cephalalgia 2011;31:301–315.

13 Buse DC, Manack AN, Fanning KM, Serrano D, Reed ML, Turkel CT, Lipton RB: Chronic migraine prevalence, disability, and sociodemographic factors: results from the American Migraine Prevalence and Prevention Study. Headache 2012;52:1456–1470.

14 Murray CJ, Vos T, Lozano R, Naghavi M, Flaxman AD, et al: Disability-adjusted life years (DALYs) for 291 diseases and injuries in 21 regions, 1990–2010: a systematic analysis for the Global Burden of Disease Study 2010. Lancet 2012;380:2197–2223.

15 Lantéri-Minet M, Duru G, Mudge M, Cottrell S: Quality of life impairment, disability and economic burden associated with chronic daily headache, focusing on chronic migraine with or without medication overuse: a systematic review. Cephalalgia 2011;31:837–850.

16 Irimia P, Palma JA, Fernandez-Torron R, Martinez-Vila E: Refractory migraine in a headache clinic population. BMC Neurol 2011;11:94.

17 Schulman EA, Peterlin BL, Lake AE 3rd, Lipton RB, Hanlon A, Siegel S, Levin M, Goadsby PJ, Markley HG: Defining refractory migraine: results of the RHSIS survey of American Headache Society members. Headache 2009;49:509–518.

18 D'Amico D, Leone M, Grazzi L, Bussone G: When should 'chronic migraine' patients be considered 'refractory' to pharmacological prophylaxis? Neurol Sci 2008;29(suppl 1):S55–S58.

19 Schulman EA, Lake AE 3rd, Goadsby PJ, Peterlin BL, Siegel SE, Markley HG, Lipton RB: Defining refractory migraine and refractory chronic migraine: proposed criteria from the Refractory Headache Special Interest Section of the American Headache Society. Headache 2008;48:778–782.

20 Bussone G: Clinicial considerations on chronic migraine, pharmacoresistance and refractoriness. Neurol Sci 2010;31(suppl 1):S83–S85.

21 Melzack R, Wall PD: Pain mechanisms: a new theory. Science 1965;150:971–979.

22 Matharu MS, Bartsch T, Ward N, Frackowiak RSJ, Weiner R, Goadsby PJ: Central neuromodulation in chronic migraine patients with suboccipital stimulators: a PET study. Brain 2004;127:220–230.

23 Popeney C, Aló K: Peripheral neurostimulation for the treatment of chronic, disabling transformed migraine. Headache 2003;43:369–375.

24 Oh MY, Ortega J, Bellotte JB, Whiting DM, Aló K: Peripheral nerve stimulation for the treatment of occipital neuralgia and transformed migraine using a C1-2-3 subcutaneous paddle style electrode: a technical report. Neuromodulation 2004;7:103–112.

25 Schwedt TJ, Dodick DW, Hentz J, Trentman TL, Zimmerman RS: Occipital nerve stimulation for chronic headache – long-term safety and efficacy. Cephalalgia 2007;27:153–157.
26 Trentman TL, Rosenfeld DM, Vargas BB, Schwedt TJ, Zimmerman RS, Dodick DW: Greater occipital nerve stimulation via the Bion microstimulator: implantation technique and stimulation parameters clinical trial: NCT00205894. Pain Physician 2009;12: 621–628.
27 Palmisani S, Al-Kaisy A, Arcioni R, Smith T, Negro A, Lambru G, Bandikatla V, Carson E, Martelletti P: A six year retrospective review of occipital nerve stimulation practice – controversies and challenges of an emerging technique for treating refractory headache syndromes. J Headache Pain 2013;14:67–76.
28 Reed KL, Black SB, Banta CJ, Will K: Combined occipital and supraorbital neurostimulation for the treatment of chronic migraine headache: initial experience. Cephalalgia 2010;30:260–271.
29 Royster EI, Crumbley K: Initial experience with implanted peripheral nerve stimulation for the treatment of refractory cephalgia. Ochsner J 2011;11: 147–150.
30 Serra R, Marchioretto R: Occipital nerve stimulation for chronic migraine: a randomized trial. Pain Physician 2012;15:245–253.
31 Saper JR, Dodick DW, Silberstein SD, McCarville S, Sun M, Goadsby PJ; ONSTIM Investigators: Occipital nerve stimulation for the treatment of intractable chronic migraine: ONSTIM feasibility study. Cephalalgia 2011;31:271–285.
32 Silberstein SD, Dodick DW, Saper J, Huh B, Slavin KV, Sharan A, Reed K, Narouze S, Mogilner A, Goldstein J, Trentman T, Vaisma J, Ordia J, Weber P, Deer T, Levy R, Diaz RL, Washburn SN, Mekhail N: Safety and efficacy of peripheral nerve stimulation of the occipital nerves for the management of chronic migraine: results from a randomized, multicenter, double-blinded, controlled study. Cephalalgia 2012; 32:1165–1179.
33 Dodick DW, Silberstein SD, Reed KL, Deer TR, Slavin KV, Huh B, Sharan AD, Narouze S, Mogilner AY, Trentman TL, Ordia J, Vaisman J, Goldstein J, Mekhail N: Safety and efficacy of peripheral nerve stimulation of the occipital nerves for the management of chronic migraine: long-term results from a randomized, multicenter, double-blinded, controlled study. Cephalalgia 2015;35:344–358.

Todd J. Schwedt, MD
Department of Neurology
Mayo Clinic Arizona
5777 East Mayo Boulevard
Phoenix, AZ 85054 (USA)
E-Mail schwedt.todd@mayo.edu

Slavin KV (ed): Stimulation of the Peripheral Nervous System. The Neuromodulation Frontier.
Prog Neurol Surg. Basel, Karger, 2016, vol 29, pp 127–138 (DOI: 10.1159/000434666)

Peripheral Nerve Stimulation for Back Pain

Paul Verrills[a] • Marc Russo[b, c]

[a]Metro Pain Group, Melbourne, Vic., and [b]Hunter Pain Clinic, and [c]Australian Pain Research Center, Newcastle, N.S.W., Australia

Abstract

Peripheral nerve stimulation (PNS) generally refers to stimulation of a named nerve via direct placement of a lead next to the nerve either via a percutaneous or open approach; in peripheral nerve field stimulation (PNFS), leads are subcutaneously placed to stimulate the region of affected nerves, cutaneous afferents, or the dermatomal distribution of the nerves which converge back to the spinal cord. Recently, there has been a renewed interest in using the PNS approach for many otherwise refractory pain conditions; however, PNFS appears to be more effective for the management of low back pain and therefore more attractive. Here we discuss procedural details of PNFS trial and implant, and provide scientific and clinical rationale for placing PNFS electrodes at a certain depth under the skin. We also summarize results of published studies on use of PNFS in the management of low back pain and list the criteria that are used for proper patient selection. Our experience and the published studies provide evidence that PNFS is a safe and well-tolerated pain control option for intractable pain conditions, including chronic low back pain. Notably, achieving efficacious pain relief relies on correct patient selection and the optimal placement of the leads, ensuring, in particular, a lead depth of 10–12 mm from the surface to maximize the target sensation (mediated by fast-adapting Aβ fibers) of PNFS, which is believed to be most effective for the pain relief.

Electrical neuromodulation generally involves the selective application of a programmable pulse waveform through a series of electrodes, within a lead, to stimulate afferent nerve fibers and subsequently reduce the perception of pain.

Historically, spinal cord stimulation (SCS) has primarily been used for widespread leg, buttock, and (to some extent) back pain, particularly following failed back surgery [1–6]. Traditionally, however, SCS has not adequately covered and relieved axial back pain. This has led to individuals experimenting with the placement of subcutaneous leads within areas of significant pain. Peripheral nerve stimulation (PNS) generally refers to stimulation of a named nerve via direct placement of a lead next to the nerve

Table 1. Applications of peripheral nerve field stimulation in treatment of low back pain

Author/year	Patients, n	Outcome
Paicius et al. [8], 2007	6	Case series – patients reported reduction in pain and analgesic use and increase in quality of life measures
Verrills et al. [9], 2009	13	An overall 50% reduction in pain was observed at an average follow-up of 7 months
Sator-Katzenschlager et al. [10], 2010	68	Case series – pain reductions were reported by 92% of patients, as well as significant reduction in their analgesic use
Verrills et al. [11], 2011	44	Consecutive case series – patients reported average reduction in pain of 3.3±2.3 NPRS; reduced analgesic use was reported in 72% of patients with improvement in functional scores and employment capacity

either via a percutaneous or open approach. In peripheral nerve field stimulation (PNFS), leads are subcutaneously placed to stimulate the region of affected nerves, cutaneous afferents, or the dermatomal distribution of the nerves which converge back to the spinal cord [7]. Sometimes, the two terms are used interchangeably in the literature or not defined at all, making it difficult to ascertain the neurostimulation technique used without close reading of the methods section (table 1).

Stimulation Principles

Much work remains to be done on determining how much of a pain area can reasonably be attempted to be covered by paresthesia from a subcutaneous cylindrical lead. It is generally considered to cover a small area the size of a credit card or palm of the hand, although it seems that more extensive coverage can be obtained by cluneal nerve stimulation [Dr. Peter Courteney, pers. commun.]. Therefore, it is important to think about how many leads will be required and in what position or array the leads will be placed. We refer the reader to the excellent atlas produced by Dr. Giancarlo Barolat [12] detailing real case planning of peripheral leads. For most pain conditions it would be typical to use 2–4 leads given current implantable pulse generator (IPGs) offer 2–4 channels of stimulation.

PNS for low back pain obviates the difficulty of generating paresthesia from the dorsal columns into the low back and allows direct activation of peripheral nerve fibers.

It has been postulated that the efficacy of PNFS is reliant on several key factors, including eliciting the appropriate sensation within the region of pain. In this context, understanding the effects of electrode placement, and specifically lead depth, on

Table 2. Sensation classification

Cutaneous fiber	Sensation
Aβ_FA	Tingling, tickling, vibrating, massaging, tapping
Aβ_SA	Hammering, pressure, cramping
Aδ	Pinch, stabbing, pin-pricking
C	Burning (hot), cool, Itching
C/Blk	Dull, numb

Underlined descriptors denote the most common reported sensations.

nerve types is crucial to achieving optimal outcomes for pain relief. Verrills et al. [13] investigated the stimulation of cutaneous nerves at different electrode lead depths, using the 'pin-drop' technique. Following measurements, patients underwent a series of 16 electrode programming combinations to compare lead depths with paresthesia felt at both maximum discomfort and at 70% of the usage range intensity. Patients were divided into four groups according to lead depth, ranging from superficial to deep leads (<10, 10–12, 12–20, >20 mm). Paresthesia descriptions were classified into 5 groups based on cutaneous fiber type: Aβ fast adapt (Aβ_FA), Aβ slow adapt (Aβ_SA), Aδ, C nociceptive fiber stimulation (C), and sensation block (C/Blk) and other (table 2).

For any depth, the most commonly experienced sensation was that typical of Aβ_FA fiber stimulation (tingling, tickling, vibration, etc.). Maximal Aβ_FA sensation was observed at depth range of 10–12 mm. Therefore, a depth of 10–12 mm from the surface maximizes the target sensation (Aβ_FA) of PNFS, which is believed to be effective for pain relief (fig. 1, 2).

Patient Selection Criteria for Peripheral Nerve Field Stimulation

Appropriate patient selection has also been suggested to be a key element in optimizing PNFS outcomes. Most of the patients selected for trials have either suffered from failed back surgery syndrome or had failed other minimally invasive and conservative treatments. The important inclusion criteria are described below:

- A clearly defined, discrete focal area of pain with a neuropathic (or combined somatic/neuropathic) pain component characterized by burning and increased sensitivity
- Failure to respond to other conservative treatments including medications, psychological therapies, physical therapies, surgery, and pain management programs
- Psychological clearance (including a psychologist ruling out major drug addictions or significant psychiatric disorders that might impact on successful treatment)
- Informed consent

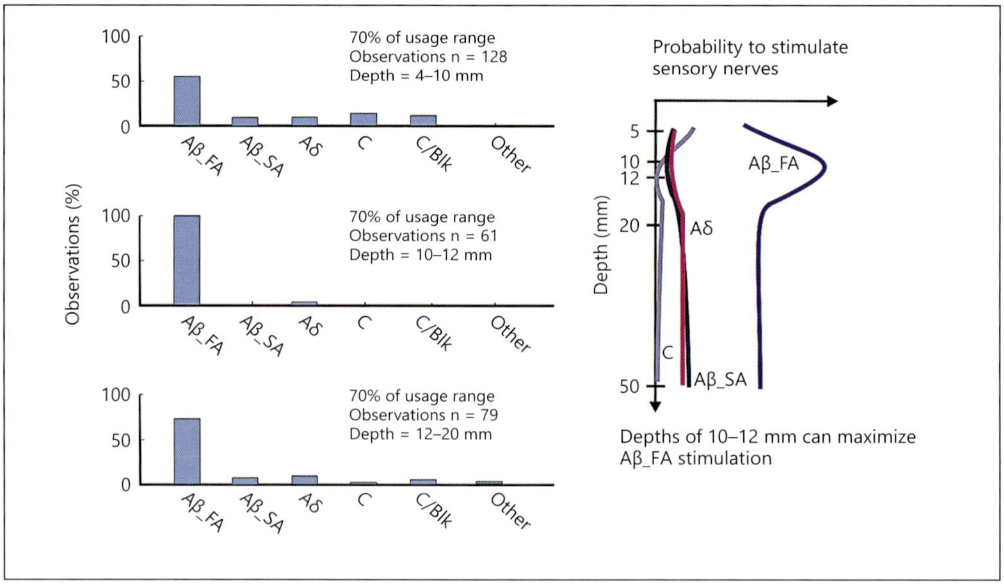

Fig. 1. Distribution of categorized sensations at 70% usage range.

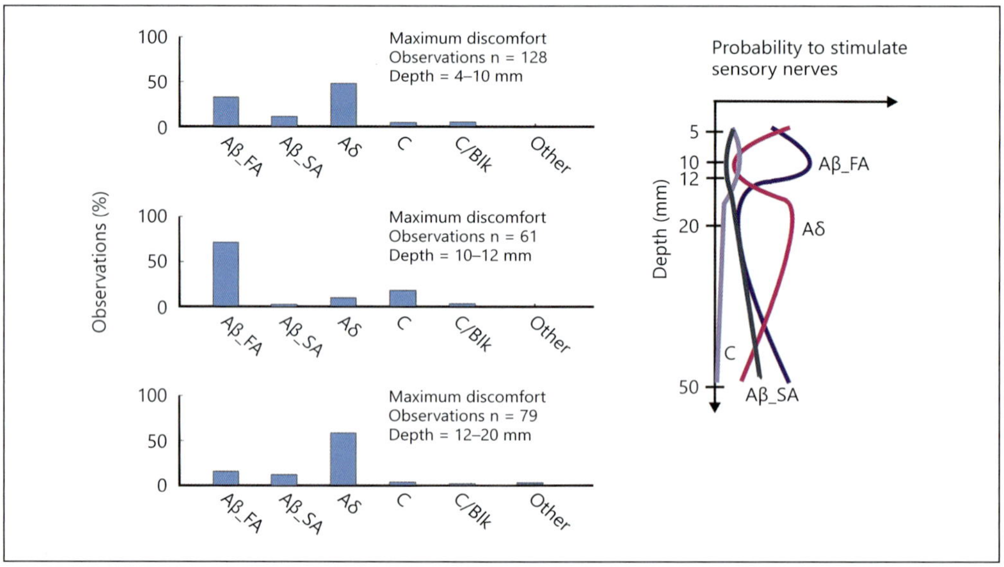

Fig. 2. Distribution of categorized sensations at maximum discomfort.

Trialing Procedure

All procedures are performed within a sterile operating room. Based on clinical assessment, the patient's area of pain is clearly outlined. Patients are minimally sedated and routinely given intravenous antibiotics (typically, 1 g cefazolin). Under live

C-arm fluoroscopy, octapolar leads are placed subcutaneously within the area of maximal pain using a 14-gauge vascular access catheter (e.g. Angiocath) and a small amount of lidocaine 1% at the insertion site. Between 1 and 4 leads may be used in the trial. On-table stimulation is performed to determine that paresthesia is felt in the area of pain and that it is comfortable. The leads are then sutured to the skin and dressings applied. Patients are monitored in the recovery suite, while initial stimulation parameters are programmed. The patient wears an external power source for 5–7 days attached to the leads (2 leads can be tested at a time), and careful monitoring occurs over the following days to determine whether adequate pain relief ensues. Verrills et al. [11], in a series of 100 patients, reported that 72% of all patients undergoing a PNFS trial achieved successful results of >50% pain reduction and progressed to a permanent implant.

Pulse Generator Implant Procedure

As with the trial procedure, the patient's skin is marked for area of pain, the position of successful trial leads, and placement of the IPG. A small incision is made outside the area of pain and the leads are inserted via a 14-gauge vascular access catheter (e.g. Angiocath). On-table stimulation is performed to confirm pleasant paresthesia coverage of the area of maximal pain. The leads are sutured to the deep fascia and tunneled to the site of the IPG where blunt dissection is used to create a tight pocket approximately half an inch deep. The most common site for IPG placement is the upper outer buttock (below the belt line but not impeding sitting positions). The leads are connected to the IPG, impedance is verified and leads are secured. Refinement of the stimulation parameters is performed over the following weeks.

Lead Depth

There appears to be an ideal depth for the placement of electrode leads to achieve effective stimulation of the affected nerves. Evidently, more superficial lead implantation in the dermal layers results in painful stimulation, while deeper tissue placement results in muscle recruitment and uncomfortable sensations. Though PNFS is one of the newest paradigms of neuromodulation – providing effective pain relief with low risks and minimal insult during a trialing phase – the ideal depth of the lead implant and its reproducibility are among several persisting issues that remain problematic [14, 15]. To date, there have been only a handful of published studies that have addressed this issue.

Most investigators describing subcutaneous lead implants in occipital nerve stimulation or PNFS do not report the lead depth; however, there is now a general consensus on the optimal depth of the electrode lead placement in PNFS. In a recent study,

Abejón et al. [16] utilized a radiofrequency probe (range of 0.5–1.0 V at 50 Hz) to identify optimal depth of the electrode lead in patients with PNFS for low back pain. This novel concept enabled greater reproducibility in achieving optimal stimulation with subcutaneous leads and has potential advantages over other techniques such as ultrasound guidance. However, this technique is invasive, requires additional equipment, and does not measure the electrode lead depth reliably enough.

In another study, presented in 2010, McRoberts and Cairns [17] measured the depth of the electrode lead implant in patients with PNFS for lower back pain using ultrasound guidance. Despite the authors reporting fairly accurate and comparable values for low back PNFS electrode lead depths, ultrasound is known to yield poor estimation of actual electrode depth because of tissue compression from the ultrasonic probe, as well as varied scatter from intervening tissues such as bone. These factors can potentially reduce this method's accuracy and reproducibility.

Verrills et al. [13] reported on lead depth measurements taken for 17 patients previously implanted subcutaneously with a PNFS system in their low back. The 'pin-drop' technique uses a device with freely moving multiple pins that sits on the skin directly above the implantation site. Using fluoroscopic imaging at 30° cephalad and caudad, the depth of each lead was estimated by measuring the depth between the contacts and the reference pins, with an accuracy of ~0.5 mm (fig. 3; table 3) [13]. Distribution of electrode lead depth ranged between 4 and 19 mm, with an average depth of 10.5 mm.

Across all three studies [13, 16, 17], which utilized different depth measurement techniques, the average electrode lead depth that delivered effective subcutaneous paresthesia in low back pain PNFS was found to be remarkably consistent and measured at 9.2–10.5 mm (table 4; fig. 4). Furthermore, the lead depth was found not to correlate with percentage pain relief achieved or BMI. The results of these studies corroborate the importance of having a unifying reference point for the depth of subcutaneous lead implantation with the goal of delivering the most adequate nerve stimulation.

Outcomes

Pain Indices

In a study of 44 low back pain patients, with a mean age of 60.6 years (33–88) and follow-up of 8.1 ± 4.7 months, a statistically significant reduction in pain was observed following lumbosacral PNFS with a reduction of 3.3 ± 2.3 pain scale points ($p \leq 0.001$) (fig. 5) [11]. To assess whether results obtained shortly after PNFS implantation were sustained over a longer period, patients were divided into two groups: those who were followed up for less than 8 months after treatment (average: 4.6 ± 1.4 months; range: 1–7), and those who were followed up for 8 months or longer (average: 12.3 ± 3.8 months; range: 8–23; fig. 6). Pre-PNFS pain scores were similar among the two groups,

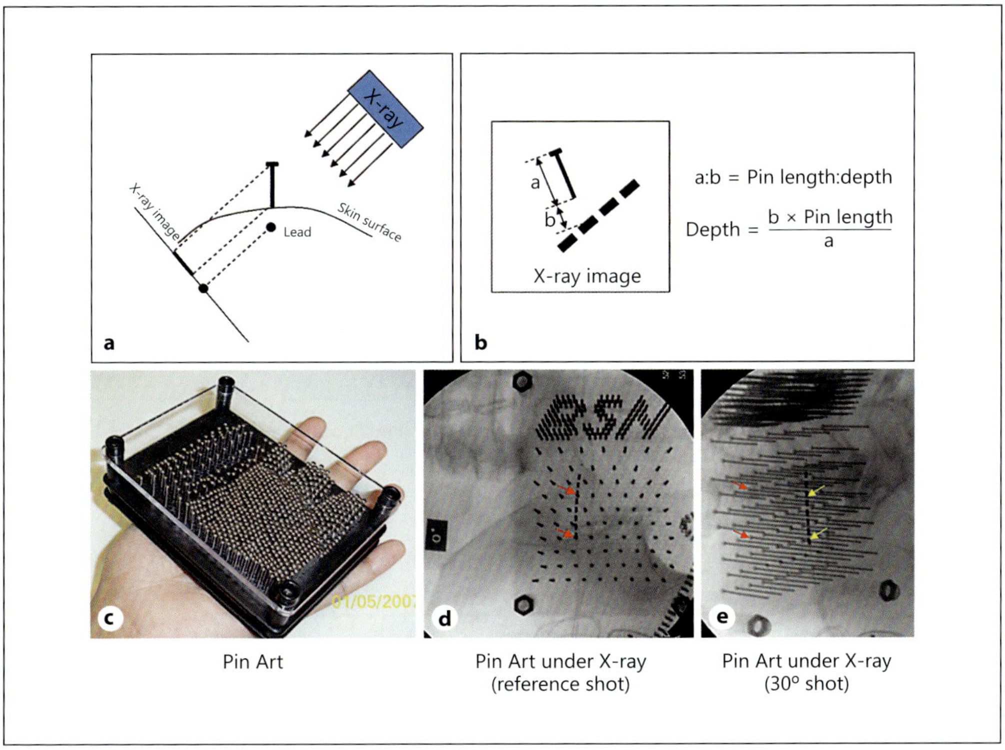

Fig. 3. Principles of lead depth measurement. **a** Under X-ray fluoroscope, a metal pin and electrode would be shown as a line and a square, respectively. The length of the pin image and the distance from the pin tip to contact would be proportional to real distances. Therefore, if we measure the real length of the pin (31 mm) and distance from the pin tip to contact of the X-ray image, we can estimate the depth of contact. **b** Mathematical equation to compute the depth of contact. Under X-ray image, length (a) of the pin image and distance (b) of the pin tip to contact should be measured. The lead depth can be estimated by the equation (b × pin length/a). **c** Pin Art device with multiple pins touching the surface of hand. Individual pin touches perpendicular to the surface of the skin. **d** X-ray image with 90° to identify reference pins (red/dark arrows) and contacts. **e** X-ray image with 30° rotation of fluoroscope. The identified pins (red/dark arrows) and contacts (yellow/light arrows) are used to measure the contact depth.

Table 3. Patient characteristics: PNFS for low back pain

Variable	Male	Female	All
Sample size, n	10	7	17
Age, years	65±18.7	46.9±13.4	57.4±18.6
Implant duration, months	12.6±11.8	17±12.2	14.4±11.8
Height, cm	176.2±9.7	167.5±9.6	172.5±10.4
Weight, kg	97.6±26.1	76±21.6	88.5±26.1

Table 4. Comparison of lead depth studies

Factor	Verrills et al. [13], 2013	McRoberts and Cairns [17], 2010	Abejón et al. [16], 2011
Depth measurement method	'Pin-drop' technique under c-arm fluoroscopy	Ultrasound	Radiofrequency probe to identify appropriate depth
Results	Average depth of 10.5 mm (4.0–19.3)	Average depth of 9.2 mm (5.6–15.1)	Average depth of 10.5 mm (9.8–11.3)

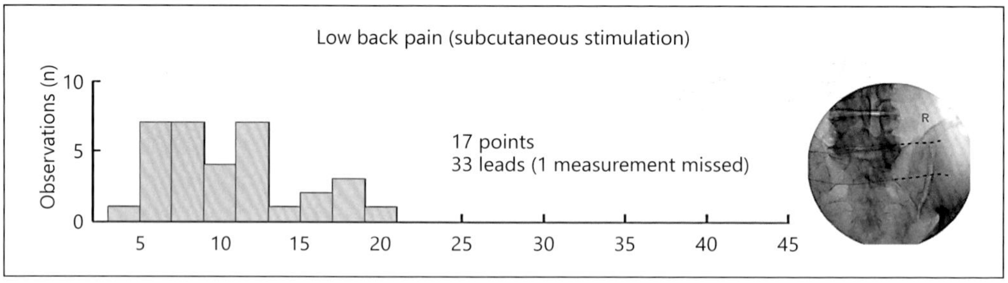

Fig. 4. Low back subcutaneous paresthesia was observed at an average lead depth of 9.2–10.5 mm.

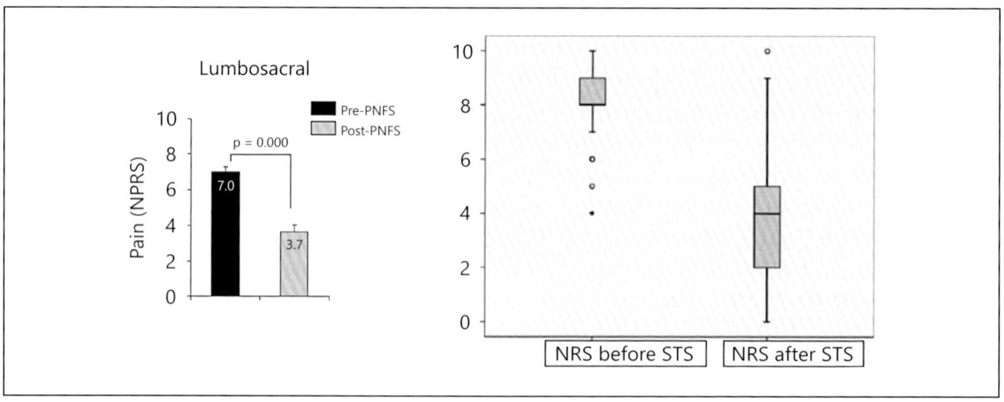

Fig. 5. PNFS significantly reduces Numeric Rating Scale (NRS) pain scores [10, 11]. Pain intensity score before and after PNFS (NRS; 0 = no pain, 10 = unbearable pain) (modified from Verrills et al. [11], with permission from John Wiley and Sons).

negating any potential impact on the follow-up results. Both groups demonstrated the same reduction in pain scores, confirming that there was no deterioration in therapeutic response over time [11].

In an Austrian PNFS series, Sator-Katzenschlager et al. [10] reported on patients with failed back surgery syndrome and low back pain (n = 68), with a mean age of

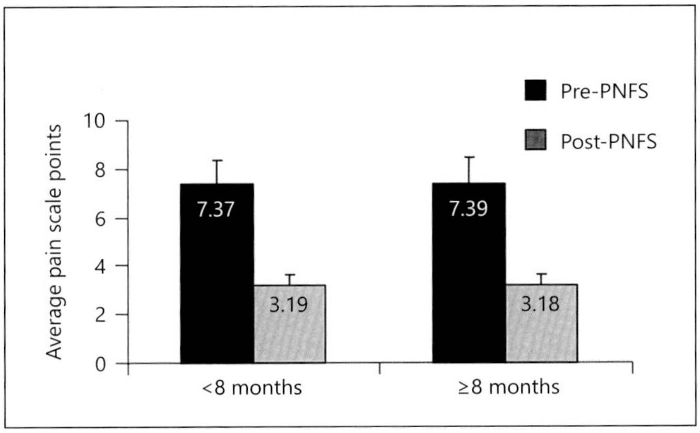

Fig. 6. Combined region pain scores following PNFS (n = 100): short-term pain relief is sustained. Pain scores of patients followed soon after PNFS implantation and up to 7 months of follow-up were compared with pain scores obtained from patients followed up for 8 months or longer. No difference was noted between the two groups. Data expressed as means ± SEM. Data were analyzed using the nonparametric Mann-Whitney U test, with p set at 0.05 (modified from Verrills et al. [11], with permission from John Wiley and Sons).

59 years and average duration of pain around 13 years, whose pain scores reduced in a similar proportion from 8.2 to 4.0. Patient age and gender were not predictors of outcome following PNFS.

Medication Use

Over 30% of patients report a decrease in their analgesic intake at 3 months following implant, with this number increasing to approximately 70% of patients at a follow-up duration of 8 months or greater. Approximately 20% of the patients state that their analgesic regimen is not altered following PNFS, with <5% reporting an increase [10, 11].

Satisfaction

Verrills et al. [11] showed that while 30% of all patients were completely satisfied with their outcome, a combined 86% of patients were satisfied, very satisfied, or completely satisfied with their results.

Function

In Verrills et al. [11], patients younger than 60 years were asked to assess their capacity for paid employment following PNFS. Overall, 43% of patients reported an increase in their capacity for paid employment, with half of this group assessing their improvement as extreme. No surveyed patients reported a decrease in their capacity for paid employment following PNFS, and only 14% of the cohort stated that capacity for paid employment was not applicable to their situation.

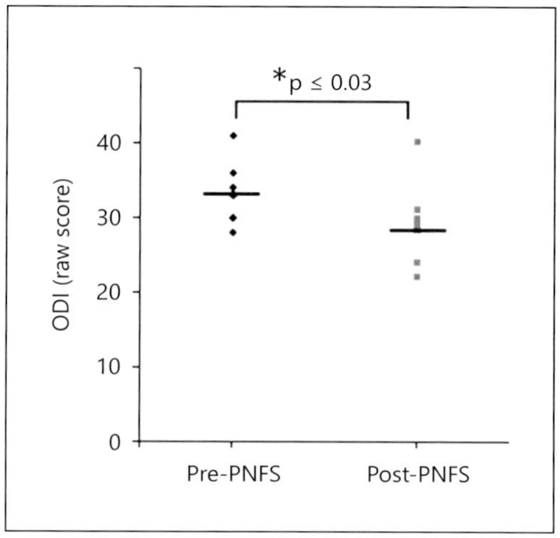

Fig. 7. PNFS significantly reduces ODI-assessed disability. Statistical differences were tested using a t test comparison of paired-means, with p set at 0.05 (modified from Verrills et al. [11], with permission from John Wiley and Sons).

Likewise, chronic low back pain patients receiving a PNFS implant in their lumbosacral region were assessed for degree of disability using the Oswestry Disability Index (ODI). These patients demonstrated a statistically significant reduction in their degree of disability as measured by the ODI (fig. 7).

Complications

Complication rates for PNFS have been reported to occur in 9–24% of patients, with lead migration and lead dislocation being the most frequent, affecting up to 13% of patients. Lead fractures and equipment failure occur in 2–5% of patients, infections in up to 6%, and lead erosions in approximately 5% of all PNFS patients [10, 11]. These results are in line with other large series of peripheral neurostimulation applications [18].

Conclusion

In patients with chronic low back pain, opioids have been shown to reduce pain by an average of 10 points on a 100-point pain scale, while having very little impact on improving the function or psychological condition [19]. Other drugs, such as tramadol, have been shown to provide moderate relief in 35% of patients; however, the observed time frame for efficacy was only 4 weeks [20]. In contrast to these observations, PNFS has been shown to provide pain relief with a mean decrease of 3.3–3.8 NPRS points, and a sustained effect observed in 8- to 23-month follow-up cohorts in the two key publications [10, 11]. In addition, up to 72% of patients are able to reduce their analgesic use following PNFS.

PNFS has a number of advantages over the traditional neuromodulation approach of SCS, namely that it does not carry the same neurological risks such as epidural hemorrhage, paralysis, and meningitis. Given the low invasiveness of PNFS and its reversibility, testability, and adjustability, it is also a preferable option when compared to the more intrusive surgical alternatives available. The main issue, as with any implantable device, is the risk of infection. Sator-Katzenschlager et al. [10] report an infection rate of only 6%, occurring during the first 2 weeks following implantation. Other complications such as lead migration and hardware failure are reported to have occurred in up to 13 and 5% of the patients, respectively, in the two key publications, with no patients reporting a serious or severe adverse event. This combined evidence suggests that PNFS is a safe and well-tolerated pain control option for intractable pain conditions [10, 11]. Notably, achieving efficacious pain relief relies on correct patient selection and the optimal placement of the leads, ensuring, in particular, a lead depth of 10–12 mm from the surface to maximize the target sensation (Aβ_FA) of PNFS, which is believed to be most effective for pain relief.

The future likely holds significant advances for both PNS and SCS, and hybrid techniques that combine the two are also a possibility. Optimization of parameters and implant strategies will determine how much of a role the PNFS approach will have.

References

1 Bell GK, Kidd D, North RB: Cost-effectiveness analysis of spinal cord stimulation in treatment of failed back surgery syndrome. J Pain Symptom Manage 1997;13:286–295.

2 Kumar K, Taylor RS, Jacques L, Eldabe S, Meglio M, Molet J, Thomson S, O'Callaghan J, Eisenberg E, Milbouw G, Buchser E, Fortini G, Richardson J, North RB: Spinal cord stimulation versus conventional medical management for neuropathic pain: a multicentre randomised controlled trial in patients with failed back surgery syndrome. Pain 2007;132: 179–188.

3 North RB: Spinal cord stimulation for intractable pain: long-term follow-up. J Spinal Disord 1990;3: 356–361.

4 North RB, Ewend MG, Lawton MT, Kidd DH, Piantadosi S: Failed back surgery syndrome: 5-year follow-up after spinal cord stimulator implantation. Neurosurgery 1991;28:692–699.

5 North RB, Kidd DH, Zahurak M, James CS, Long DM: Spinal cord stimulation for chronic, intractable pain: experience over two decades. Neurosurgery 1993;32:384–394.

6 North RB: Spinal cord stimulation for chronic, intractable pain. Adv Neurol 1993;63:289–301.

7 Slavin KV: Peripheral nerve stimulation for neuropathic pain. Neurotherapeutics 2008;5:100–106.

8 Paicius RM, Bernstein CA, Lempert-Cohen C: Peripheral nerve field stimulation for the treatment of chronic low back pain: preliminary results of long-term follow-up: a case series. Neuromodulation 2007;10:279–290.

9 Verrills P, Mitchell B, Vivian D, Sinclair C: Peripheral nerve stimulation: a treatment for chronic low back pain and failed back surgery syndrome? Neuromodulation 2009;12:68–75.

10 Sator-Katzenschlager S, Fiala K, Kress HG, Kofler A, Neuhold J, Kloimstein H, Ilias W, Mozes-Balla EM, Pinter M, Loining N, Fuchs W, Heinze G, Likar R: Subcutaneous target stimulation (STS) in chronic noncancer pain: a nationwide retrospective study. Pain Pract 2010;10:279–286.

11 Verrills P, Vivian D, Mitchell B, Barnard A: Peripheral nerve field stimulation for chronic pain: 100 cases and review of the literature. Pain Med 2011;12: 1395–1405.

12 Barolat G: Peripheral Subcutaneous Stimulation: A Photographic Surgical Atlas. Denver, Barolat Institute, 2009.

13 Verrills P, Nowesenitz G, Barnard A: Electrode lead depth distribution for peripheral nerve field stimulation and occipital nerve stimulation using a novel non-invasive 'pin-drop' technique. Neuromodulation 2013;14:567.
14 Aló KM, Abramova MV, Richter EO: Percutaneous peripheral nerve stimulation. Prog Neurol Surg 2011;24:41–57.
15 Abejón D, Krames ES: Peripheral nerve stimulation or is it peripheral subcutaneous field stimulation; what is in a moniker? Neuromodulation 2009;12:1–4.
16 Abejón D, Deer T, Verrills P: Subcutaneous stimulation: how to assess optimal implantation depth. Neuromodulation 2011;14:343–348.
17 McRoberts WP, Cairns K: A retrospective study evaluating the effects of electrode depth and spacing for peripheral nerve field stimulation in patients with back pain. Neuromodulation: Vision 2010. Proceedings of 14th Annual Meeting of North American Neuromodulation Society, Las Vegas, 2010; p 67.
18 Slavin KV: Technical aspects of peripheral nerve stimulation: hardware and complications. Prog Neurol Surg 2011;24:189–202.
19 Bogduk N: Pharmacological alternatives for the alleviation of back pain. Expert Opin Pharmacother 2004;5:2091–2098.
20 Schnitzer TJ, Gray WL, Paster RZ, Kamin M: Efficacy of tramadol in treatment of chronic low back pain. J Rheumatol 2000;27:772–778.

Paul Verrills, MD
Metro Pain Group
Level 1, 544 Hawthorn Road
Caulfield South, VIC 3162 (Australia)
E-Mail pverrills@metropain.com.au

Slavin KV (ed): Stimulation of the Peripheral Nervous System. The Neuromodulation Frontier.
Prog Neurol Surg. Basel, Karger, 2016, vol 29, pp 139–157 (DOI: 10.1159/000434667)

Peripheral Nerve Stimulation for Pain in Extremities: An Update

Jason E. Pope[a] · Jonathan D. Carlson[b, c] · William S. Rosenberg[d] · Konstantin V. Slavin[e] · Timothy R. Deer[f]

[a]Summit Pain Alliance, Santa Rosa, Calif., [b]The Pain Center of Arizona, Peoria Clinic, Phoenix, Ariz., [c]Midwestern Medical School, Glendale, Ariz., [d]Center for the Relief of Pain, Kansas City, Mo., [e]Department of Neurosurgery, University of Illinois at Chicago, Chicago, Ill., and [f]The Center for Pain Relief, Charleston, W.Va., USA

Abstract

Pain in extremities may occur in a variety of central and peripheral neuropathic and nociceptive syndromes, some of which may respond to central neuromodulation procedures. Peripheral neuromodulation techniques, either as a stand-alone therapy or as an adjuvant to spinal cord stimulation, may be particularly effective when the pain is localized to a part of a single extremity or when the source of the pain is related to the malfunction of a known peripheral nerve. Further, peripheral neuromodulation is used to treat disorders in which central simulation fails to provide discrete therapeutic paresthesia. Despite the fact that there are only a few neuromodulatory devices designed specifically for the periphery, clinical experiences are growing, and here we provide a clinical update on use of peripheral nerve stimulation (PNS) in management of chronic pain in extremities. Historical PNS strategies and innovative methods are reviewed and highlighted in this chapter. With the upcoming technological advances and new stimulation paradigms, along with clear updated guidelines statements, the utilization of PNS will likely continue to increase and improve the management of chronic pain syndromes in the extremities. The potential success of the novel devices specifically designed to target the peripheral nervous system is expected to positively impact and promote the use of PNS in treatment of chronic pain.

Chronic pain in extremities may present a challenge in terms of long-term management. One of the issues in the use of neuromodulation for pain in extremities is a frequently encountered inability to keep the stimulation field steady enough to match the area of paresthesia with the area of pain. Central neuraxial stimulation strategies often fail to discretely provide sustained therapeutic paresthesia overlying the patients' typical painful area, commonly resulting in 'bleed over paresthesia'. Although new central target and waveform offerings show some promise [1–7], it is important to appreciate that these aforementioned limitations alone may be an excellent reason to consider a more focused neuromodulation approach: peripheral nerve stimulation (PNS). Furthermore, not all neuromodulation performed in the periphery is PNS: peripheral nerve field stimulation (PNFS) is also frequently performed, and it is distinctly different from PNS. PNS and PNFS can be easily differentiated, as PNS requires stimulation of a named nerve, while PNFS does not. Several years ago, in a book on PNS [8], there was a comprehensive review of the stimulation of the peripheral nervous system for the painful extremity – it covered not only the historical use of neuromodulation for this indication, but also the technical aspects, patient selection, potential pitfalls, and solutions for implanting PNS devices for extremity pain [9].

In order to provide an update on this important topic, it may be important to look back on the origin of the modality. Pain in extremities was the main indication for PNS applications between the mid-1960s and late 1990s [10]. As a matter of fact, even though the first clinical application of PNS dates back to 1962 when it was used to treat neuropathic facial pain, the information about this experience was not presented until February 1967 and published in August 1967 [11]. By that time, the use of PNS for pain in the extremities had already been described in a series of patients reported by Wall and Sweet [12] in January 1967 in *Science*. This pioneering paper has always been considered a clinical confirmation of the 'gate-control' theory of Melzack and Wall [13] published a year earlier. Among 8 patients in the Wall and Sweet series, 7 had pain in their extremities, 3 in the arm/hand, and 4 in the leg/foot area. Of these 7 patients, 2 had their nerves stimulated via surface electrodes (preempting transcutaneous electrical nerve stimulation), 3 had nerve roots stimulated with a monopolar wire electrode inserted through a needle into the subarachnoid space [preempting subsequent pioneering intrathecal placement of the first spinal cord stimulation (SCS) electrode by Shealy et al. [14] that was published in July 1967], and 1 had stimulation of the ulnar nerve with a percutaneously inserted '20-gauge concentric bipolar hypodermic needle' that produced tingling in the ulnar nerve distribution and freedom of severe burning and lancinating pain [12]. Patient No. 1 in this series, a 26-year-old woman with chronic burning and stabbing pain and extreme tenderness in her hand following a fractured elbow, had a true PNS device implanted: the paper describes 'Silastic split-ring platinum electrodes ... implanted around the median nerve above the elbow with the leads being run through the skin of the antero-medial forearm' [12]. During stimulation with a frequency of 100 Hz and pulse width of 100 μs, this patient described a tingling and buzzing sensation and complete relief of her otherwise intractable pain, as well as the return of her ability to freely move the painful hand [12].

As time went on, SCS and other central neuromodulation approaches became a mainstream direction for chronic pain management, but multiple limitations remained. These challenges included the inability to create discrete stimulation fields, the need for perceived therapeutic paresthesia, potential complications of invading the structures of the central nervous system (including paralysis and death), the inability to offer neurostimulation in patients with a bleeding diathesis or inability to discontinue their therapeutic anticoagulation for neuraxial intervention, issues related to tunneling and placement of an implantable pulse generator (IPG) that requires a relatively large anatomic site, and postural intensity changes of the therapeutic stimulation. These challenges forced pain providers to have a more patient-centric look to the periphery. Although new central stimulation may mitigate the need for perceived therapeutic paresthesia [1], this solution needs to work in concert with innovation of neuromodulation in the periphery, as one does not cannibalize the other.

The term PNS refers to a direct electrical stimulation of named nerves along their course inside the body, outside of the neuraxis, directly inhibiting primary afferents. As experience and interest in neuromodulating the periphery grew, so too did the interest in making the procedure simpler, moving away from open dissection nerve identification [15–17] to image-guided or stimulation-targeting strategies [18–21]. These less invasive options may allow for minimally invasive options.

Although there is more robust literature and experience supporting the use of PNS, inherent challenges remain. First, the electrical cathodal stimulation of the nerves in the periphery is inconsistent, as anatomically the topography of the fascicles within the nerve is variable. This leads to an unpredictable response and requires testing, regardless of lead orientation to the nerve [22]. Second, PNS is performed with practitioner-modified, off-label use of equipment designed for the neuraxis, inherently creating challenges from the rigidity, size, shape, and length of the lead, along with their delivery [23–25]. Third, as PNS typically requires distal extremity placement to treat pain, a site suitable to accommodate IPG implantation to avoid extensive tunneling is difficult to identify. Fourth, tunneling leads across joints is less than ideal, as it may contribute to the incidence of the lead migration. Lastly, the cost of SCS hardware adapted to PNS introduces a cost burden, ranging between United States Dollars (USD) 30,000 and 40,000. It seems that equipment designed for the periphery, including a cheaper, smaller, and more 'peripheral friendly' equipment, would offer a therapeutic and economic advantage [26].

Update on Traditional Technology

Both percutaneous and paddle type electrodes continue to be used for PNS in extremities. Percutaneous PNS remains a less invasive option as it does not require surgical exploration of the stimulated nerve, lending itself to wider acceptance in the pain community. Expectantly, PNS stimulation follows the path of the named nerve stimulated, and PNFS creates paresthesia surrounding the lead.

Percutaneously Inserted Peripheral Nerve Stimulation in Extremities

The cases illustrated in figures 1–3 are examples of the percutaneous PNS approach. In the first illustrative case, the patient's pain was in her thigh in the distribution of the distal branches of the lateral femoral cutaneous nerve as this nerve was apparently

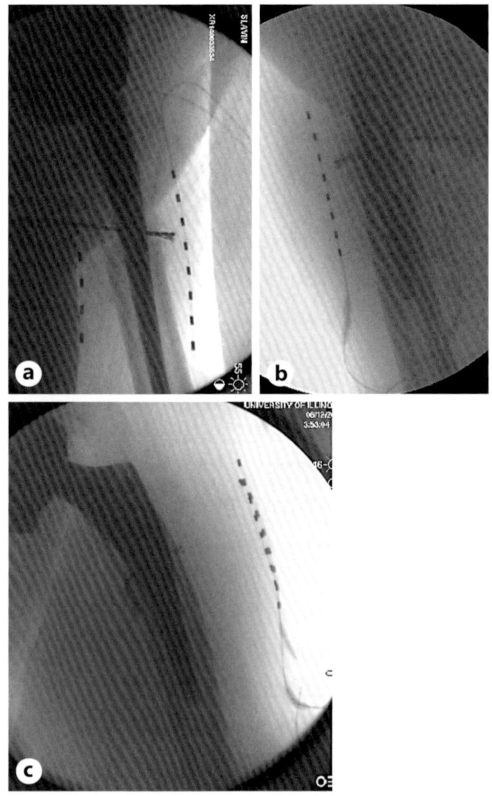

Fig. 1. Intraoperative radiographs of percutaneously implanted PNS electrodes in a patient with thigh pain due to iatrogenic injury of the lateral femoral cutaneous nerve. **a** The temporary PNS electrode leads are inserted in a 'proximal-to-distal' direction around the course of the lateral femoral cutaneous nerve and parallel to it. **b**, **c** Anteroposterior and lateral views of the permanent electrode lead location; the electrode leads are inserted in a 'distal-to-proximal' direction and anchored to the thick subcutaneous fascia.

damaged during a complicated partial hip arthroplasty. Here, the detached trochanter required additional pinning of the proximal femoral bone through the lateral approach, and the patient had a discrete area of medically refractory pain in the distribution of lateral femoral cutaneous nerve, with a point tenderness resembling a Tinel sign next to her surgical incision. After a successful week-long trial of PNS, a permanent device was implanted with two 8-contact electrodes placed parallel to the course of the lateral femoral cutaneous nerve (fig. 1).

In the second case, the patient's sharp and shooting pain was in the distribution of the saphenous nerve in the inner aspect of his shin and calf; it started after several interventions on the knee joint. Once again, the pain was relieved substantially during a week-long trial with percutaneously inserted cylindrical electrodes, so a permanent system was implanted with two 4-contact electrodes and a generator (fig. 2). Of note, correlating with the patient's pain pattern, the PNS-induced paresthesias were perceived in the distribution of the saphenous nerve rather than the field between the electrode contacts.

In the third case, the patient experienced significant pain and hyperesthesia surrounding the patella following a right total knee arthroplasty. After the patient responded to lumbar sympathetic blocks with excellent transient relief, she was

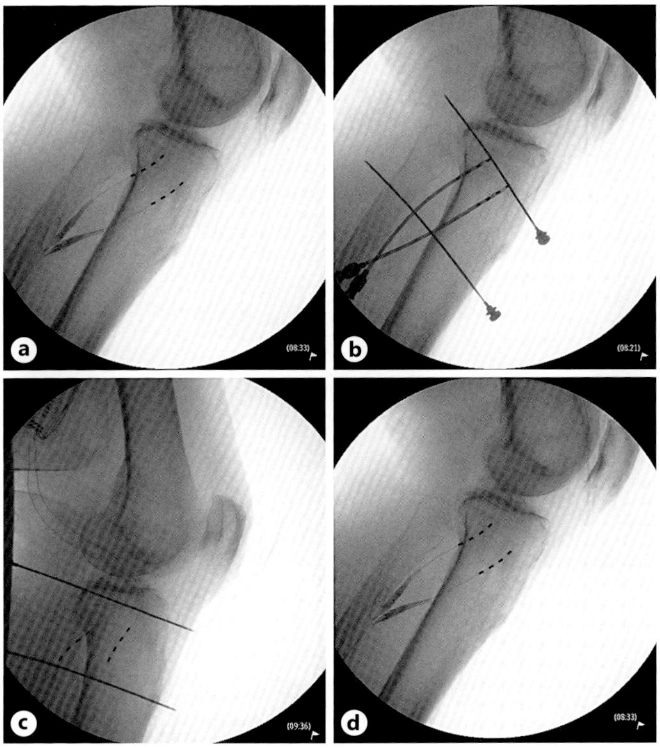

Fig. 2. Intraoperative radiographs of percutaneously implanted PNS electrodes in a patient with inner shin pain due to isolated postsurgical neuropathy of the saphenous nerve. **a** The temporary PNS electrode leads are inserted in a 'proximal-to-distal' direction around the course of the saphenous nerve and parallel to it. The needle stylets are inserted perpendicular to the needles through the same insertion point to facilitate lead tunneling using the 'needle-over-the-stylet' technique. **b** Final position of temporary PNS electrodes. Stylets are placed on the patient's skin to mark the ends of electrode arrays for external reference. **c** Insertion of permanent PNS electrode leads in a 'distal-to-proximal' direction. Stylets are placed on the patient's skin for external reference of the ideal lead location. **d** The electrode leads are anchored to the thick subcutaneous fascia.

trialed with two 8-contact percutaneous, cylindrical leads capturing both the superior lateral, inferior lateral, superior medial, and inferior medial genicular nerves (fig. 3). After a successful trial with greater than 80% pain reduction, she underwent second-stage surgery, with the IPG implanted in the lateral anterior thigh.

Three points are worth discussing in regard to percutaneously inserted PNS systems. First it is important to try positioning permanent PNS electrodes exactly where the trial (temporary) electrodes were located. However, to minimize risk of infection, the duration of the trial should be the shortest possible, once the patient has the confidence in assessing the outcome of the trial. Some providers intentionally insert the trial electrodes in the direction opposite to one that will be used for permanent

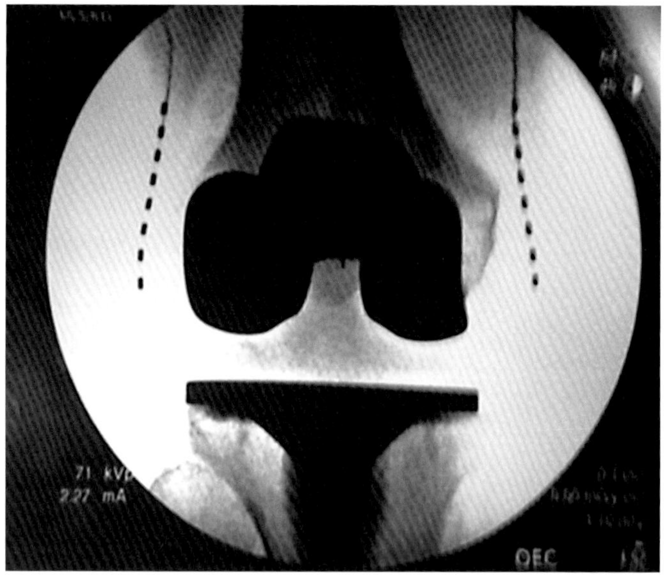

Fig. 3. Intraoperative radiograph of percutaneously implanted PNS electrodes in a patient with inferior and superior medial and lateral genicular neuralgia following total knee arthroplasty.

implantation. As seen in figures 1 and 2, the temporary electrodes in both cases were placed in a 'proximal-to-distal' direction, whereas permanent electrodes were inserted in a 'distal-to-proximal' direction. Others place the leads in the same trajectory and orientation for the trial, and if converted, the permanent therapy. Second, to minimize the risk of lead migration, we use standard anchors. However, regardless of anchor choice or if the decision is made to suture directly to the lead ('figure of 8' stitch), it is important to suture the anchors to a hard underlying fascia. In many referral cases for revision due to migration, the leads were either not anchored at all or anchored to the subcutaneous fat layer or the inner edge of the dermis, both of which are not strong enough to withstand repetitive tension observed in mobile extremities. Finally, the efforts of miniaturization of the hardware system allow the ability to place the IPG directly within the soft tissues of the stimulated extremity (fig. 4). This allows one to avoid crossing the joints with electrode leads and/or extensions, thereby reducing risk of device migration or fracture over time.

Paddle Lead Peripheral Nerve Stimulation in Extremities

An alternative to percutaneous leads is the insertion of a paddle lead directly over the nerve. This approach presents a number of advantages. Contacts on paddle leads are unidirectional and therefore focus all stimulation in the direction of the nerve, thereby avoiding potentially undesirable sensorimotor effects as well as reducing the necessary power requirements. Direct placement of these rectangular electrodes within the epineurium results in a very stable implant. In addition, the fixed configuration of

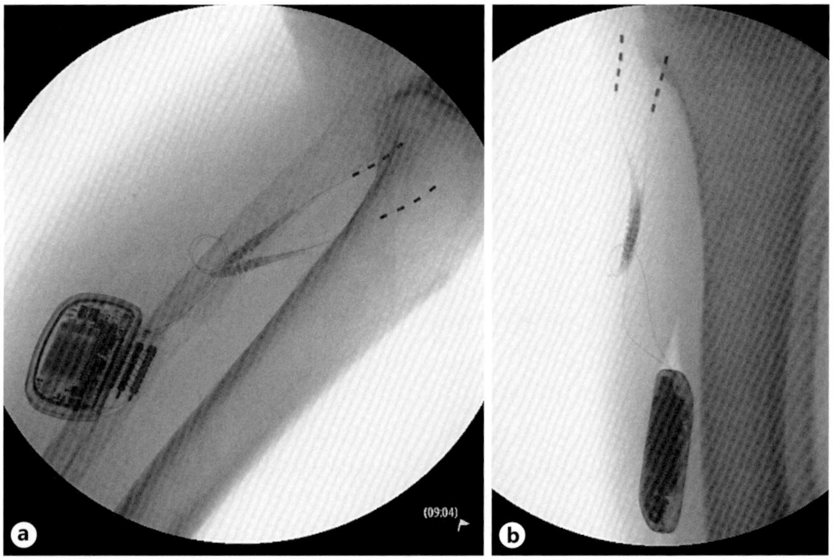

Fig. 4. Intraoperative radiographs of the entire PNS system (IPG and 2 electrode leads). Note the generator placement in the fascial intermuscular plane at the mid-calf level. **a**, **b** Oblique views of the implanted system.

contacts in a paddle lead can be deliberately oriented on multicomponent nerves (e.g. the peroneal and tibial components of the sciatic nerve). A disadvantage of this approach is the requirement for open placement (and removal in the case of a failed trial).

Peripheral nerve paddle stimulation is performed as a small, open cut-down onto the desired nerve, usually as an outpatient under general anesthesia, with the trial being conducted using a permanent lead placement. Unlike traditional peripheral nerve surgery, exposure of the nerve is kept to a bare minimum and circumferential exposure is avoided. Identification of the nerve is facilitated by intraoperative use of a nerve stimulator and electromyography monitoring, especially for sciatic nerve exposure through the hamstring musculature. In this case, after opening the fascia, it is possible to use a small nerve stimulator through the muscles to identify the location of the sciatic nerve and then gently separate the muscle fibers down to it. The entire breadth of the nerve is exposed, but longitudinal exposure is minimized and, as above, circumferential exposure is unnecessary. The epineurium is then gently opened and a plane carefully developed using a small blunt instrument in the desired direction of placement. The paddle is then introduced within the epineurium and slid into place with the contacts along the nerve. Electromyography monitoring during stimulation of the paddle contacts confirms proper placement; muscle activity should occur at a low amplitude using low-frequency stimulation. In the case of the sciatic nerve, a dual-column paddle is

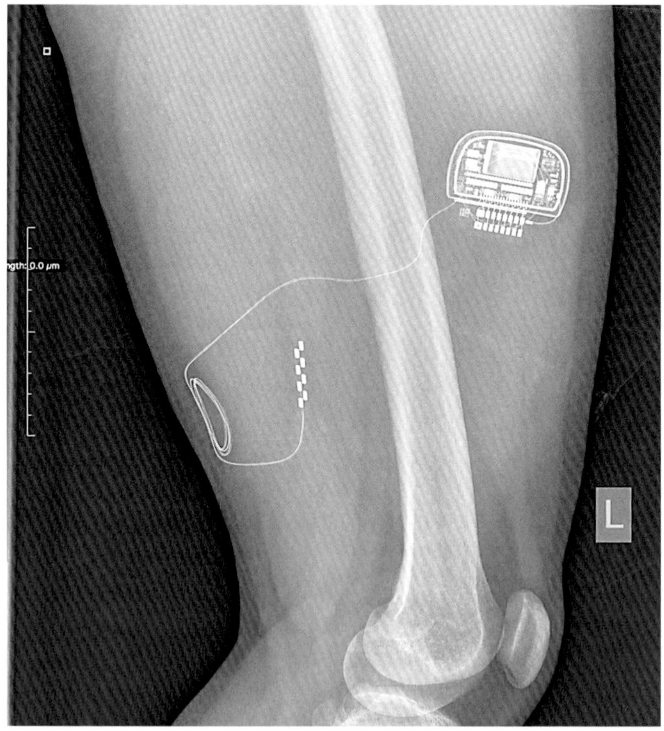

Fig. 5. Lateral radiograph of a permanent sciatic nerve paddle lead with multiple subcutaneous strain relief loops. It is placed in the thigh, an ideal location as the lead crosses no mobile articulations.

usually oriented to stimulate the peroneal component with one column and the tibial component with the other, resulting in optimization of the programming options. The paddle is secured to the epineurium with a single silk suture and a strain relief loop is developed in a subcutaneous pocket. A trial extension is brought out through a separate stab incision, planned to avoid the anticipated path of a permanent lead and IPG.

The trial is conducted for the shortest time necessary to ascertain success or failure. In the case of a successful trial, placement of the IPG is usually performed under general anesthesia. If leads or extensions are required to cross a joint, care is taken to plan and mark the center of the axis of rotation of the joint, placing the lead/extension in a position to minimize movement and stress. It is desirable to avoid crossing a joint (e.g. IPG placement in the thigh for a sciatic paddle lead; fig. 5), but this can be dependent on body habitus and other factors such as interference with clothing, etc.

The most common nerves treated with an implanted paddle lead are ulnar, median and sciatic nerves, although any nerve can be so treated if the exposure can be performed in a reasonably nondisruptive manner. In the case illustrated here (fig. 6), a prior ulnar nerve decompression resulted in chronic neuropathic pain. A quadripolar in-line paddle was successfully trialed and the IPG placed in the ipsilateral infraclavicular fossa. In a similar case, an ill-conceived spinal cord biopsy was performed,

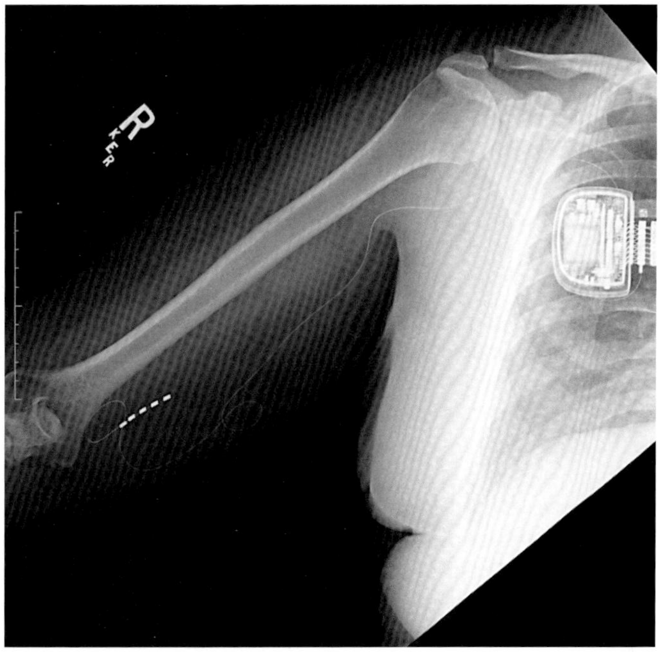

Fig. 6. Anteroposterior radiograph of a permanent right ulnar paddle lead and IPG. Note multiple strain relief loops in the course of the lead.

resulting in chronic neuropathic pain in an ulnar nerve distribution. An identical implant resulted in excellent, long-term pain relief, demonstrating the importance of precise paresthesia distribution over dogmatically placing the stimulating lead proximal to the injury. A similar type of paddle may be used in median nerve stimulation to treat chronic neuropathic pain as in a case that developed after carpal tunnel release surgery (fig. 7). Access to the nerve was most easily obtained by exposure just proximal to the prior surgery site. The IPG was also placed in the ipsilateral infraclavicular fossa.

A dual-column octopolar paddle may be used to stimulate sciatic nerve at the mid-shaft level of the femur as in figure 8. In this radiograph, the patient can be seen wearing his prosthesis for the first time in years, as it was impossible prior to PNS due to chronic stump and phantom limb pain. Redundant loops of the lead can be seen in the region of the greater trochanter, placed in the area of the axis of rotation, which allow for crossing this joint since the patient's thigh could not accommodate an IPG as shown in the earlier case (fig. 5).

Figure 9 shows bilateral foot pain after multiple orthopedic procedures successfully treated with bilateral PNS paddles (fig. 9). While the left paddle was placed over the distal sciatic nerve, the right paddle was positioned below the bifurcation on the proximal peroneal nerve. The need for this modification was discovered during trialing and the paddle was repositioned at permanent implantation.

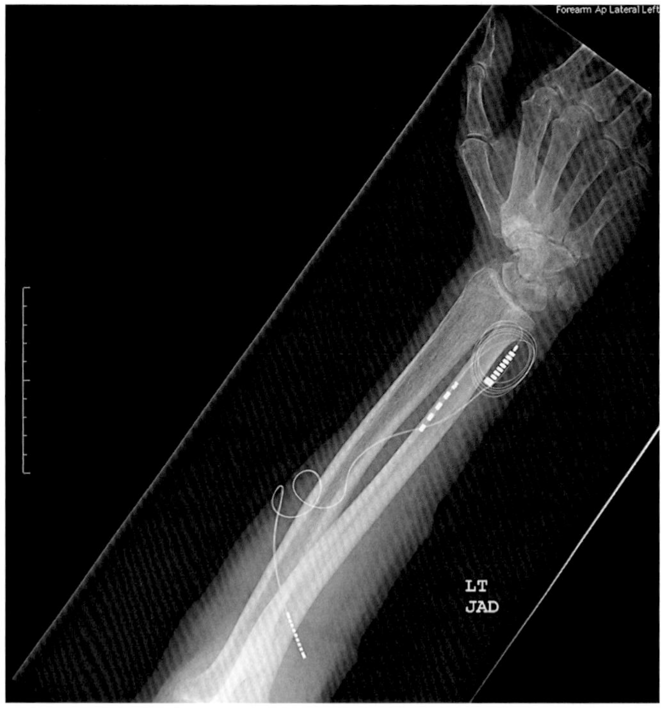

Fig. 7. Radiograph of a median nerve paddle trial. The multiple loops of the lead and extension header (just medial to the distal ulna) are within a subcutaneous pocket and the extension exits the skin just proximal to the loops at the mid-humerus. These loops and extension header are exposed at permanent placement, allowing for continued sterility of the lead.

Long-Term Follow-Up on Traditional Peripheral Nerve Stimulation and New Insights into Mechanism of Action

Since the publication of the last review on the use of PNS in extremities [9], new data has become available for an extraordinarily long-term follow-up in a cohort of PNS patients [27]. A group of 11 Belgian patients with neuropathic pain in the upper extremities was implanted with PNS devices in the 1980s [28]. All of the patients had an open placement of a circumferential electrode (Avery Biomedical, Cormack, N.Y., USA) around the proximal segment of the afflicted nerve in the upper limb with a receiver implanted in the pectoral region. During the subsequent decades, 4 devices were removed due to technical problems or infection and 1 patient died of unrelated causes; 1 patient continued to enjoy the benefits of stimulation but could not return for a follow-up assessment. The researchers were able to study the remaining 5 patients with an average of 23.2 years of follow-up (18–29 years after implantation), 2 with median and 3 with ulnar nerve stimulators, all of whom reported excellent pain relief with either regular or sporadic stimulation sessions [27, 28].

In these 5 long-term PNS patients, the neuropathic character of pain complaints was confirmed with quantitative sensory testing. PNS had no significant overall effect on any of the sensory modalities: tactile detection, cool, warm, cold pain and heat pain thresholds were not affected by PNS. The amplitude of laser-evoked potentials was lower (compared to age-matched controls) at baseline, but increased during PNS

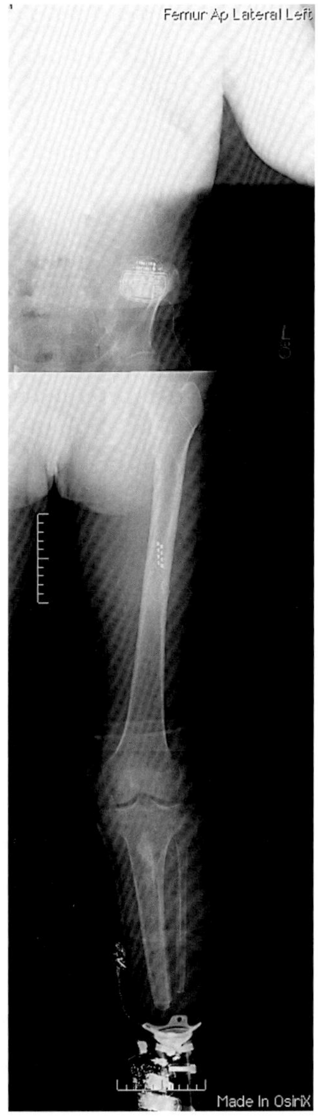

Fig. 8. Anteroposterior radiograph of a permanent sciatic nerve paddle (upper mid-shaft of femur). The IPG is placed in the upper buttock because it could not be accommodated in the thigh. There is a redundant lead in the region of the greater trochanter, a result of deliberately tunneling the lead through this axis of rotation and allowing for strain-free movement. The patient is seen standing on his prosthesis, which he has not worn for years, secondary to stump and phantom limb pain.

being turned on. This prompted the researchers to suggest a possibility of a pain relieving effect of PNS being in the counter-irritation mechanism and the consequent nociceptive inhibition that led to an increase in laser-evoked potential amplitude.

Finally, the positron emission tomography studies in these patients showed a significant increase in regional cerebral blood flow in the contralateral somatosensory cortex in response to PNS – something that is not observed in analgesia due to either spinal cord or deep brain stimulation, suggesting that the analgesic effects of PNS are at least partly different from those of central neuromodulation approaches. PNS also reduced spontaneous and heat-induced activity within the so-called 'pain matrix', which includes the posterior thalamus, insula, perigeniculate and subgenual cingulum,

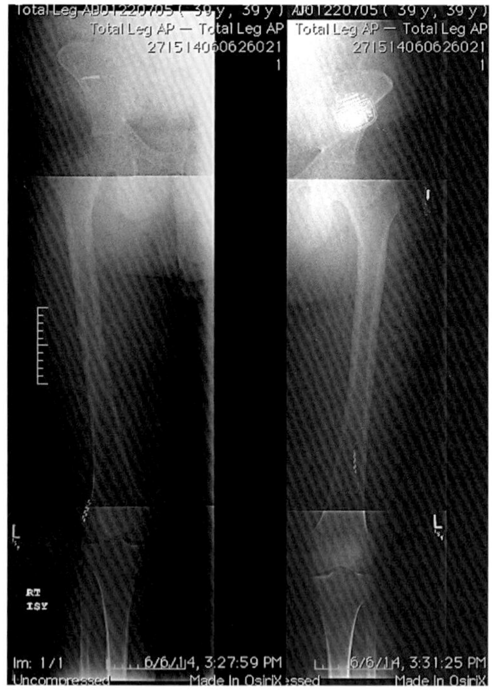

Fig. 9. Composite anteroposterior radiograph of permanent bilateral sciatic/peroneal paddle leads and IPG for bilateral foot pain following multiple orthopedic procedures. The IPG is in the left upper buttock and each lead crosses through the axis of rotation of the hip at the greater trochanter. The right lead is placed on the proximal peroneal nerve because it was this stimulation alone that resulted in pain relief during the trial.

caudate nucleus, and orbitofrontal cortex, and increased activation in areas involved in pain modulation, such as the anterior cingulate cortex. These local hemodynamic changes may reflect the areas mediating the analgesic effects of PNS [27].

Percutaneous Paddles

One of the limitations of percutaneous cylindrical electrodes is the omnidirectional nature of stimulation that may be counterproductive in cases where direction of stimulation is well defined. Traditionally, in SCS and PNS practice this issue has been resolved by using paddle-type electrodes that emit stimulation in one direction and are insulated both mechanically and electrically from other directions. The paddles, however, have always required open surgical exposure for proper lead placement. Recently, this has changed with introduction of percutaneously insertable narrow paddles (Lamitrode-S; St. Jude Medical, Plano, Tex., USA) and a special insertion tool (Epiducer; St. Jude Medical) [29].

To show the feasibility of using these new electrodes in PNS applications, a human cadaver study was performed specifically evaluating technical feasibility of ultrasound-guided percutaneous placement of the narrow paddle leads [30]. Based on experiments involving both the upper and lower extremities, the investigators concluded that although ultrasound localization of the upper extremity nerves (ulnar and median) was straightforward and clear, the procedural steps were technically easier in the lower extremities, where the saphenous (at distal thigh), sciatic (at the mid-thigh) and tibial nerves (at the proximal tarsal canal) were accessed. Fewer attempts were needed to maintain the lead in the desired tissue plane in lower extremity nerves, and the lead appeared to be more mechanically stable [30].

Emerging Technology

Multiple devices dedicated to PNS applications have been developed over the last decade to improve performance and function of the peripheral neuromodulation techniques.

StimRouter™

StimRouter (Bioness Inc., Valencia, Calif., USA) is a device where the lead is completely internalized under the skin near the target nerve and employs an external pulse generator (EPG) as its power supply. The EPG needs to be placed near the proximal end of the implanted lead. The lead system is markedly smaller than its conventional SCS counterpart, measuring 17 cm in length and 1.2 mm in diameter, with a 3-contact electrode array distally and a receiver on the proximal end [26]. After success with a small feasibility trial [31], a large, randomized, multicenter, comparative study was completed in 2014 and has been submitted to the FDA for consideration.

For the implantation procedure, and after assuming strict standard operative conditions, the target nerve is identified by either nerve stimulation or ultrasound guidance techniques. Once localization is performed, the point of entry is one that creates a trajectory where the final lead position is parallel to the target nerve [26]. The introducer is then placed, and the lead system is inserted and further testing is performed by gentle retraction of the sheath. Once appropriate testing has been performed, the sheath is retracted and the anchor deployed [26]. The proximal end of the lead is the buried using a modified tunneling strategy, taking into consideration that it must accommodate the external placement of the power generator (EPG; fig. 10).

Altius Electric Nerve Block™

An 'electrical nerve block' device developed by Neuros Medical (Altius Electric Nerve Block™; Willoughby Hills, Ohio, USA) utilizes the placement of a proprietary cuff lead around the target nerve. It is intended for use primarily in amputees for treatment of postamputation pain syndrome. It employs a high-frequency alternating current up to 30 kHz, creating a complete depolarization block.

Device placement requires an open surgical dissection, which is straightforward for neurosurgeons and other peripheral nerve specialists but has limited applicability for traditionally trained pain physicians. The cuff electrode is coiled around the trunk of the nerve that harbors distal amputation neuroma after an open dissection, similar

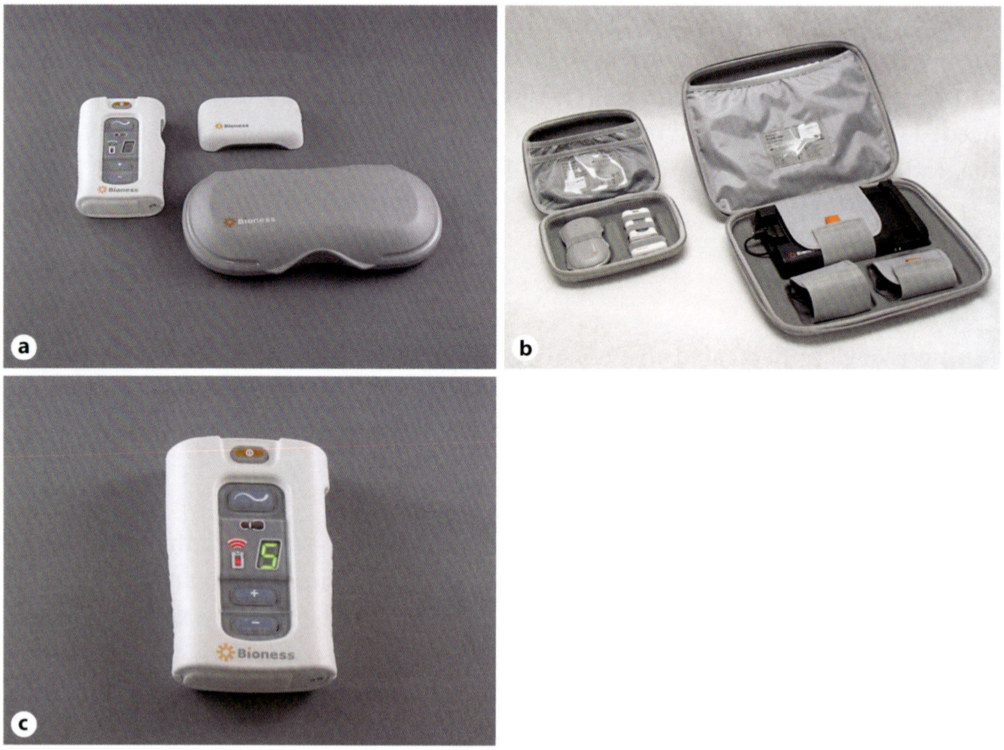

Fig. 10. Newly designed StimRouter device equipment: EPG (**a**), clinician programmer and externals (**b**), and patient programmer (**c**) (images courtesy of Bioness Inc.).

to the traditional PNS techniques, and then the lead is tunneled toward a single- or double-channel rechargeable IPG. Stimulation is delivered at a high frequency, usually on an on-demand basis, and the device is activated by the patients via a small remote control. For further information about this device please see the chapter by Soin et al. [this vol., pp. 158–167].

Freedom 4 and 8 Stimulators

Designed a few years ago by StimWave Technologies (Miami Beach, Fla., USA), this system utilizes an MRI compatible (at 1.5 T and 3.0 T) 'wireless' lead technology with an implantable lead that contains an integrated RF receiver.

At the time of print, this device has not been approved in the United States for PNS applications. The primary application is SCS; FDA approval for this was announced in December 2014. However, preliminary studies have been conducted to assess the viability of Freedom 4 and 8 Stimulators for PNS. The use of 'wireless' leads appears to be a promising treatment modality, as it can allow for placement of a lead with an integrated RF receiver for stimulation at the desired target nerve. The StimWave Freedom devices use an EPG to transmit the energy and programming to the stimulating lead/receiver assembly, but allows for longer distance between the two. The water-resistant, encapsulated external power unit lends itself to more flexibility and freedom for the patient to be active. For further information about this device, please see the chapter by Yearwood and Perryman [this vol., pp. 168–191].

SmartPatch^{TM} and MicroPulse® Technology

The concept of stimulating peripheral nerves with a percutaneously implanted very thin wire-like electrode that is placed relatively far from the stimulated nerve is the subject of investigations by SPR Therapeutics (Cleveland, Ohio, USA), a subsidiary of NDI Medical (Cleveland, Ohio, USA). The company plans to use both an external stimulator (SmartPatch) and a fully implantable (MicroPulse) long-term implant system.

The hypothesis behind these devices and principles is that positioning the electrode at a significant distance (0.5–3.0 cm) from the stimulated nerve may increase the threshold of nontarget fibers more than increasing the threshold of target fibers and that this difference would widen the therapeutic window and enable selective stimulation of the target fibers to produce comfortable paresthesias and pain relief [32, 33]. Decreasing the stimulus pulse width increases its amplitude threshold of the nontarget fibers because nontarget fibers have smaller diameters than target fibers.

Here, the fine-wire proprietary electrode lead is a helical coil wound from an insulated 7-strand stainless steel wire with a single anchoring barb and electrode contact (fig. 11). This lead is inserted under ultrasound guidance through a 20-gauge insulated hypodermic needle introducer within a 3-cm distance of the stimulated nerve after the nerve location is confirmed and paresthesias are mapped with a monopolar needle electrode [33]. This PNS electrode may then be connected to a skin-mounted percutaneous PNS system that is specifically designed for use in the periphery.

Initial Outcome Studies

Deer et al. [31] reported on the safety and feasibility of the StimRouter system. Eight patients with median nerve pain who failed surgical decompression at the carpal tunnel were enrolled. The lead was implanted and the patients underwent stimulation for 6 h/day for 5 days. All patients were implanted and no complications occurred. The patients reported a reduction in their pain scores of approximately 44%, and all patients indicated that they would have the implant if it were available outside of the study.

The feasibility study and 12-month pilot study look promising for the Neuros device [34–36]. Data on the Neuros 'electrical nerve block' cuff lead were derived from a pilot study of 9 patients. Over a 12-month period, 7 out of the 9 postamputation patients reported 50% or greater relief from the PNS cuff. They also demonstrated an average decrease in the NRS by 83% with over half discontinuing their opioid pain medication use during the study. There were no reported safety issues [36].

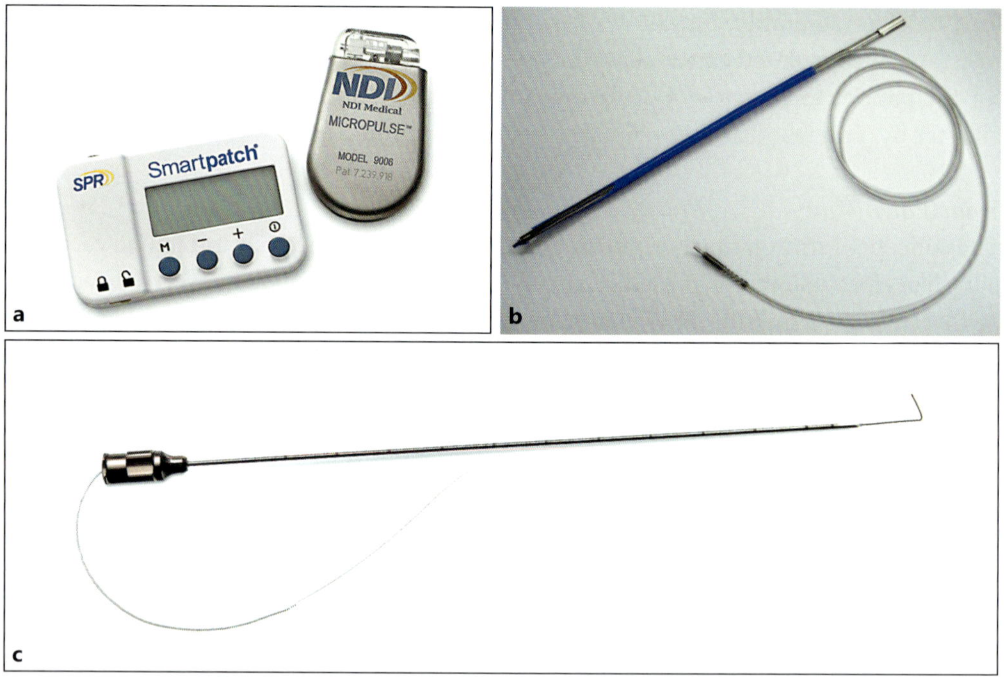

Fig. 11. PNS system from SPR Therapeutics: SmartPatch EPG and MicroPulse IPG (**a**), MicroPulse implantable lead and introducer (**b**), and SmartPatch percutaneous microlead (**c**) (images courtesy of SPR Therapeutics).

The 'wireless' lead system was utilized in a prospective, nonrandomized cohort study of 12 patients. It focused on the efficacy of its SCS application versus commercially available SCS products (Medtronic). The patients were serially implanted for a trial with both devices. The results demonstrated that the StimWave wireless lead was just as effective as its commercial counterpart [37]. The ability for PNS seems hopeful with this minimally invasive approach, as a case series has shown significant pain relief. A study analyzing the MRI exposure to 3.0 T or less demonstrated no apparent safety concerns with heat-related changes to the leads (<2.2°C) [38].

A feasibility trial for delivering PNS to patients with moderate-to-severe postamputation pain in the lower extremities using a fine-wire lead placed percutaneously under ultrasound guidance at a remote distance (0.5–3.0 cm) from either the sciatic or femoral nerve has been recently published [33]. This publication followed an earlier description of a single patient undergoing the procedure with encouraging short-term results [32]. Out of 16 patients selected for in-clinic testing, 14 responded to stimulation, reporting ≥75% paresthesia coverage and obtaining clinically significant pain relief. Five of these 14 patients did not complete the 2-week trial due to lead dislodgement, discomfort near the lead, and return of pain despite stimulation; the remaining 9 responders completed the trial and reported significant reductions in their mean daily postamputation pain (56 ± 26%), average residual limb

Table 1. PNS start-ups

Company	Strategy
Bioness	Small deployed lead with EPG
Neuros	High-frequency alternating current with cuff lead
StimWave	Implantable wireless radiofrequency transmitter
SPR Therapeutics	Short- and long-term PNS
Autonomic Technologies	Sphenopalatine ganglion stimulation
MicroTransponder	Vagus nerve stimulation with cuff lead
EnteroMedics	Vagus nerve blocking therapy

pain (72 ± 28%), average phantom pain (81 ± 28%), residual limb pain interference (81 ± 27%), phantom pain limb interference (83 ± 31%), and pain disability index (70 ± 38%) at the end of 2 weeks of stimulation. Most improvements continued for a long time after the PNS was stopped. At 4 weeks after the end of stimulation, the improvements remained quite impressive: there were reductions in their mean daily postamputation pain (56 ± 26%), average residual limb pain (42 ± 27%), average phantom pain (47 ± 48%), residual limb pain interference (53 ± 17%), phantom pain limb interference (56 ± 46%), and pain disability index (55 ± 32%) [33]. The authors of this industry-sponsored study concluded that achievement of significant pain relief and improvements in quality of life holds promise for this new minimally invasive method of PNS.

Discussion

Compared to the energy-consuming central neuromodulation strategies surrounding the neuraxis, PNS is gaining momentum with new and innovative therapies in development. Peripheral neuromodulation strategies may mitigate the challenges with central SCS and its inability to produce discrete, sustainable distal extremity coverage with perceived therapeutic paresthesia. PNS offers the ability to capture these areas more reliably, and at a lower cost to the system as a whole.

Table 1 demonstrates some of the efforts to fill the void in the peripheral neuromodulation space for pain care. However, it is certain that PNS is not without its own set of challenges. For example, the Altius (Neuros) cuff implantation requires extensive surgical skill and an open dissection, limiting its adoption by nonsurgically trained pain providers.

The StimRouter (Bioness) device is one that remedies the need for tunneling and is smaller and designed for the periphery, but it requires the placement of an EPG to be functional, which may not be acceptable in patients with adhesive sensitivities, regional anatomic barriers (i.e. hair, impaired skin integrity, etc.), or inadequate discretion with pain care treatment.

The Freedom 4 and 8 (StimWave) Stimulators require placement of the external battery to be worn around the torso or waist. This again may limit the usefulness of the therapy if discretion is desired. This therapy is MRI comparable, which may improve access to certain patient populations.

Conclusion

PNS continues to be an attractive option in the management of pain in extremities, and new innovative therapies will continue to improve performance and function of these devices. Wireless therapies, external patch strategies, and miniaturization of IPGs may also improve adoption into the pain care algorithm. The future looks bright for this facet of neuromodulation offerings, and further good-quality, prospective data will improve patient care.

References

1 Pope JE, Deer TR, Amirdelfan K, Kapural L, Verrills P: New concepts for waveform and current delivery for spinal cord stimulation: burst and high frequency. Minim Invasive Surg Pain 2015. http://southernacademicpress.com/misp-vol-3/new-concepts-waveforms-current-delivery-spinal-cord-stimulation-burst-high-frequency/.

2 Van Buyten JP, Al-Kaisy A, Smet I, Palmisani S, Smith T: High-frequency spinal cord stimulation for the treatment of chronic back pain patients: results of a prospective multicenter European clinical study. Neuromodulation 2013;16:59–65.

3 Al-Kaisy A, Van Buyten JP, Smet I, Palmisani S, Pang D, Smith T: Sustained effectiveness of 10 kHz high-frequency spinal cord stimulation for patients with chronic, low back pain: 24-month results of a prospective multicenter study. Pain Med 2013;15:347–354.

4 Tiede J, Brown L, Gekht G, Vallejo R, Yearwood T, Morgan D: Novel spinal cord stimulation parameters in patients with predominant back pain. Neuromodulation 2013;16:370–375.

5 Kapural L: SENZA-Clinical trials study; in: North American Neuromodulation Society: Celebrating 20 Years, 2014 Conference Program Book. Las Vegas, NANS, 2014, p 5.

6 De Ridder D, Vanneste S, Plaizer M, van der Loo E, Menovsky T: Burst spinal cord stimulation: toward paresthesia-free pain suppression. Neurosurgery 2010;66:986–990.

7 De Ridder D, Plazier M, Kamerling N, Menovsky T, Vanneste S: Burst spinal cord stimulation for limb and back pain. World Neurosurg 2013;80:642–649.e1.

8 Slavin KV (ed): Peripheral Nerve Stimulation. Basel, Karger, 2011.

9 McRoberts WP, Cairns KD, Deer T: Stimulation of the peripheral nervous system for the painful extremity. Prog Neurol Surg 2011;24:156–170.

10 Slavin KV: History of peripheral nerve stimulation. Prog Neurol Surg 2011;24:1–15.

11 Shelden CH, Pudenz RH, Doyle J: Electrical control of facial pain. Am J Surg 1967;114:209–212.

12 Wall PD, Sweet WH: Temporary abolition of pain in man. Science 1967;155:108–109.

13 Melzack R, Wall PD: Pain mechanisms: a new theory. Science 1965;150:971–979.

14 Shealy CN, Mortimer JT, Reswick JB: Electrical inhibition of pain by stimulation of the dorsal columns. Anesth Analg 1967;46:489–491.

15 Hassenbusch SJ, Stanton-Hicks M, Schoppa D, Walsh JG, Covington EC: Long-term results of peripheral nerve stimulation for reflex sympathetic dystrophy. J Neurosurg 1996;84:415–423.

16 Stanton-Hicks M, Salamon J: Stimulation of the central and peripheral nervous system for the control of pain. J Clin Neurophysiol 1997;14:46–62.

17 Stuart RM, Winfree CJ: Neurostimulation techniques for painful peripheral nerve disorders. Neurosurg Clin N Am 2009;20:111–120.

18 Klase D, Bischof A, Haendler G, Spuck S, Rasche D, Tronnier V: Peripheral nerve stimulation: lead position monitoring by reconstruction CT angiography – a technical report. Acta Neurochir (Wien) 2009;151:663–667.
19 Huntoon MA, Huntoon EA, Obray JB, Lamer TJ: Feasibility of ultrasound-guided percutaneous placement of peripheral nerve stimulation electrodes in a cadaver model: part one, lower extremity. Reg Anesth Pain Med 2008;33:551–557.
20 Huntoon MA, Hoelzer BC, Burgher AH, Hurdle MF, Huntoon EA: Feasibility of ultrasound-guided percutaneous placement of peripheral nerve stimulation electrodes and anchoring during simulated movement: part two, upper extremity. Reg Anesth Pain Med 2008;33:558–565.
21 Huntoon MA, Burgher AH: Ultrasound-guided permanent implantation of peripheral nerve stimulation (PNS) system for neuropathic pain of the extremities: original cases and outcomes. Pain Med 2009;10:1369–1377.
22 Grinberg Y, Schiefer MA, Tyler DJ, Gustafson KJ: Fascicular perineurium thickness, size, and position affect model predictions of neural excitation. IEEE Trans Neural Syst Rehabil Eng 2008;16:572–581.
23 Bittar RG, Teddy PJ: Peripheral neuromodulation for pain. J Clin Neurosci 2009;16:1259–1261.
24 Hayek SM, Jasper JF, Deer TR, Narouze SN: Occipital neurostimulation-induced muscle spasms: implications for lead placement. Pain Physician 2009;12: 867–876.
25 Slavin KV: Technical aspects of peripheral nerve stimulation: hardware and complications. Prog Neurol Surg 2011;24:189–202.
26 Deer TR, Pope JE, Kaplan M: A novel method of neurostimulation of the peripheral nervous system: the StimRouter implantable device. Techn Reg Anesth Pain Manage 2012;16:113–117.
27 Kupers R, Laere KV, Calenbergh FV, Gybels J, Dupont P, Baeck A, Plaghki L: Multimodal therapeutic assessment of peripheral nerve stimulation in neuropathic pain: five case reports with a 20-year follow-up. Eur J Pain 2011;15:161.e1–9.
28 Van Calenbergh F, Gybels J, Van Laere K, Dupont P, Plaghki L, Depreitere B, Kupers R: Long term clinical outcome of peripheral nerve stimulation in patients with chronic peripheral neuropathic pain. Surg Neurol 2009;72:330–335.
29 Deer T, Bowman R, Schocket SM, Kim C, Ranson M, Amirdelfan K, Raso L: The prospective evaluation of safety and success of a new method of introducing percutaneous paddle leads and complex arrays with an epidural access system. Neuromodulation 2012; 15:21–30.
30 Gofeld M, Hanlon JG: Ultrasound-guided placement of a paddle lead onto peripheral nerves: surgical anatomy and methodology. Neuromodulation 2014;17:48–53.
31 Deer TR, Levy RM, Rosenfeld EL: Prospective clinical study of a new implantable peripheral nerve stimulation device to treat chronic pain. Clin J Pain 2010; 26:359–372.
32 Rauck RL, Kapural L, Cohen SP, North JM, Gilmore CA, Zang RH, Boggs JW: Peripheral nerve stimulation for the treatment of postamputation pain – a case report. Pain Pract 2012;12:649–655.
33 Rauck RL, Cohen SP, Gilmore CA, North JM, Kapural L, Zang RH, Grill JH, Boggs JW: Treatment of post-amputation pain with peripheral nerve stimulation. Neuromodulation 2014;17:188–197.
34 Soin A: Surgical placement of a spiral cuff electrode in upper and lower extremities for the application of high frequency alternating current (HFAC) in the treatment of chronic pain disorders. Neuromodulation: Vision 2010, Proceedings of 14th Annual Meeting of North American Neuromodulation Society, Las Vegas, 2010, p 61.
35 Soin A, Kilgore K, Bhadra N, Fang ZP: Feasibility study on high-frequency electrical nerve block for amputation pain. Neuromodulation 2011;14:561.
36 Soin A, Fang ZP, Shah NS: Pilot study on high frequency electrical nerve block for post amputation pain: initial results. Neuromodulation 2013;16:e98.
37 Perryman LT, Speck B, Garcia CM, Rashbaum R: Injectable spinal cord stimulator system: pilot study. Tech Reg Anesth Pain Manag 2012;16:102–105.
38 Shellock FG, Audet-Griffin AJ: Evaluation of magnetic resonance imaging issues for a wirelessly powered lead used for epidural, spinal cord stimulation. Neuromodulation 2014;17:334–339.

Jason E. Pope, MD
President, Summit Pain Alliance
392 Tesconi Court
Santa Rosa, CA 95401 (USA)
E-Mail popeje@me.com

Slavin KV (ed): Stimulation of the Peripheral Nervous System. The Neuromodulation Frontier.
Prog Neurol Surg. Basel, Karger, 2016, vol 29, pp 158–167 (DOI: 10.1159/000434669)

Peripheral Neuromodulation to Treat Postamputation Pain

Amol Soin[a–c] • Zi-Ping Fang[d] • Jon Velasco[e]

[a]Department of Surgery, Wright State University, Dayton, Ohio, [b]Greene Memorial Hospital, Xenia, Ohio, [c]Soin Medical Center, Beavercreek, Ohio, [d]Neuros Medical, Willoughby Hills, Ohio, and [e]Kettering Medical Center, Kettering, Ohio, USA

Abstract

Some of the more common peripherally mediated pain disorders are postamputation stump pain and phantom pain. These disabling conditions have proven difficult to treat. Here we aim to illustrate an option to treat postamputation pain using peripheral neurostimulation techniques. Traditional peripheral neuromodulation techniques use standard stimulation parameters and work by stimulation of nerve tissues which are then felt by the patient as a tingling sensation or paresthesia. Recently introduced high-frequency (10 kHz) electrical nerve block [HFAC (high-frequency alternating current) block] via a surgically implanted peripheral nerve cuff electrode results in true conduction block which actually blocks action potentials emanating from the painful neuroma and thus suppresses pain without tingling or paresthesia felt by the patient. In a recently completed 10-patient pilot study, the average pain level decreased from a score of 5.7 to 1.4 (out of 10) after HFAC block therapy with 85% of all testing sessions yielding a >50% pain reduction; a very significant reduction in the use of opioid and other analgesics was also noted, with all tested patients either stopping or decreasing their analgesic intake significantly. Patients achieved meaningful and significant pain reduction throughout the study, and patients who had phantom pain (in addition to stump pain) that responded to local anesthetic injections also responded favorably with HFAC block, presumably because in these particular patients, the phantom symptoms were peripherally generated. Each of the tested patients reported that HFAC block provided the most significant amount of pain reduction they had ever experienced when compared to other pain modalities tried since their amputations. The high-frequency electric nerve block technique is currently investigational pending FDA clearance. The next step for this modality is a pivotal trial, with the goal of having this therapy available to the mass market upon FDA clearance.

One of the more common peripherally mediated pain disorders is postamputation stump and phantom pain. After an amputation, due to the severing of various peripherals nerves, patients often develop painful neuromas. These neuromas can generate two different types of pain conditions: residual limb pain and peripherally generated phantom limb pain.

These disabling conditions have proven difficult to treat despite many modern advancements in medicine. Here we aim to illustrate an option to treat postamputation pain using peripheral neurostimulation techniques.

It is estimated that residual limb pain is experienced by up to 76% of major limb amputees [1]. Currently there are approximately 2,000,000 patients in the United States who have major limb amputations, and approximately 185,000 new amputations are performed annually [2].

Some modalities to treat residual limb pain include opioid analgesics, nonsteroidal anti-inflammatory medications, physical therapy, spinal cord stimulation, and intrathecal drug delivery. Patients may also undergo amputation revision surgeries or a neurectomy to remove painful neuromas.

Pathophysiology

Postamputation pain is usually divided into two different types of painful conditions: phantom limb pain and residual limb pain. Residual limb pain presents at the end of the stump and may be exacerbated with palpation or pressure placed directly on a neuroma (e.g. when patients use their prosthetic devices), which can limit the patient's ability to maintain their activities of daily living.

After an amputation, a neuroma forms on the distal end of the severed nerve. This neuroma may fire abnormal action potentials which cause unpleasant sensations such as pain in the stump or in the missing part of the limb [3].

Spinal or central nervous system mechanisms may influence residual limb or phantom pain. Neuromas or damaged peripheral nerve tissue can lead to degeneration of C-fibers that project to the dorsal horn of the spinal cord and termination of A-fibers, which may subsequently branch into the same dorsal horn. The A-fiber inputs may then be reported as noxious stimuli, which may then lead to hyperexcitability of the spinal cord, thus producing chronic pain [4].

Additionally, peripheral mechanisms may influence postamputation pain conditions. As a neuroma forms at the end of a severed peripheral nerve, there is often a proliferation of sodium channels which can transmit significant abnormal and unwanted action potentials that can be perceived as a painful sensation. If these action potentials could somehow be blocked, then the painful condition could be eliminated. This is postulated as a mechanism of action of high-frequency electric nerve block resulting in pain reduction.

Types of Peripheral Neurostimulation Modalities

Peripheral nerve stimulation (PNS) of various types has been used to treat amputation stump pain. These modalities vary from percutaneously placing a linear electrode lead in the immediate vicinity of the offending peripheral nerve to surgical dissection and placement of paddle leads around or near peripheral nerves.

A recent case study demonstrated that percutaneous and remote placement of a lead >1 cm from the femoral nerve achieved a 60% reduction in residual limb pain during a 2-week home stimulation trial [5]. While promising, this report is insufficient to draw serious conclusions as larger sample sizes will be needed to determine efficacy, particularly considering the fact that the lead was not in direct contact with the peripheral nerve in question. The publication, however, does show that there could be potential promise in percutaneous PNS lead placement near a peripheral nerve in patients with residual limb pain.

These traditional peripheral neuromodulation techniques use stimulation parameters similar to other PNS modalities and work by stimulation of nerve tissues which are then felt by the patient as a tingling sensation or paresthesia. Recent advances in PNS include high-frequency conduction block which actually blocks action potential from the painful neuroma and thus no tingling or paresthesia is felt by the patient.

High-Frequency Electric Conduction Block

High-frequency (10 kHz) electrical nerve block [HFAC (high-frequency alternating current) block] via a surgically implanted peripheral nerve cuff electrode is one of the more recent and promising modalities to treat residual limb and peripherally generated phantom limb pain. In this technique the electrode is attached to a targeted nerve proximal to a neuroma located near the amputation stump to block the pain signals originating in the residual limb. By placing a nerve cuff electrode around a severed peripheral nerve proximal to a neuroma and administering HFAC, it is possible to block unwanted painful action potentials and prevent neurotransmission of the unpleasant stimuli [6–12].

Drs. Kevin Kilgore and Niloy Bhadra [13] from Case Western Reserve University showed that HFAC using sinusoidal waveforms can be used to block peripheral motor activity in an in vivo mammalian model. The block threshold amplitudes showed a linear relationship with frequency, with the lowest threshold being 5 kHz. They showed that HFAC block has three phases: an onset phase, a period of asynchronous firing, and then a period of steady-state complete nerve block. The onset response and the asynchronous firing can be minimized by using an optimal frequency-amplitude combination [14]. Achievement of a complete nerve block and prevention of neural transmission of pain signals is considered the mechanism of action for HFAC block application in humans with amputation stump pain.

Table 1. Eligibility criteria for peripheral stimulation for amputation pain

Inclusion criteria	
	Amputation of a lower or upper limb
	Chronic pain from amputation for ≥6 months
	Pain refractory to conventional medical management
	Severe pain in an amputated limb (worst pain intensity ≥7 on 0–10 NRS)
	Frequent occurrence of severe pain (≥2 episodes/week on average by recall and confirmed by screening diary of 2–4 weeks)
	Significant pain reduction (≥50% on NRS) after local anesthetic injection for temporary nerve block for HFAC block (additionally, no significant pain reduction after saline injection as a placebo injected prior to the anesthetic)
	Percutaneous linear lead trial for traditional peripheral stimulation
Exclusion criteria	
	Pacemaker or other implanted devices
	Debilitating pain other than pain in amputated limb
	Pregnancy
	Inability to accurately and consistently report pain intensity and related information
	High risk of infection due to comorbidity or compromised immune state, e.g. chemotherapy
	High risk of mortality for general anesthesia, e.g. severe cardiopulmonary
	Infectious etiology for amputation, e.g. osteomyelitis, cellulitis
	Uncontrolled diabetic vascular disease or neuropathy
	Skin graft or severe scarring over targeted implant site

Patient Selection

The eligibility criteria for amputation patients considered for peripheral neuromodulation with HFAC block are listed in table 1.

Since amide local anesthetics block action potentials [15], patients undergo screening using local anesthetic nerve blocks proximal to the neuroma as a 'trial' prior to surgical implantation of the nerve cuff electrode for high-frequency stimulation. HFAC block creates a complete depolarizing nerve block around the targeted peripheral nerve and its mechanism of action is very similar to that of amide local anesthetics in that HFAC also blocks action potential. Since the mechanism of action of HFAC block is different than that of spinal cord or traditional PNS modalities, it is not surprising that unlike spinal cord stimulation and traditional PNS techniques, no paresthesia is felt by the patient. The sensation felt by the patient after HFAC block is similar to that felt after a peripheral nerve block with local anesthetic.

The screening local anesthetic peripheral nerve blocks used as a 'trial' for HFAC block can be done under ultrasound guidance. This allows the practitioner to visualize the neuroma at the end of the severed nerve and identify the location, depth, and diameter of the targeted nerve to help facilitate surgical placement of a peripheral nerve cuff (fig. 1). However, other traditional modalities of peripheral nerve blocks including direct infiltration of local anesthetic proximal to the neuroma via the palpation technique or the usage of an echogenic needle (Stimuplex; B. Braun Medical Inc.,

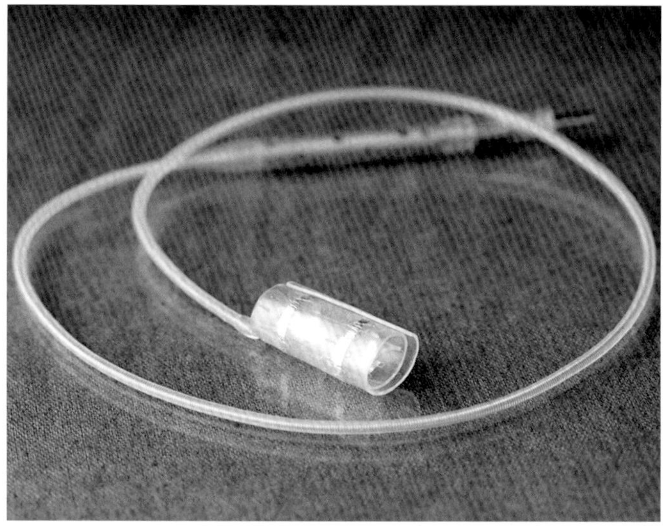

Fig. 1. An image of the peripheral nerve cuff electrode.

Bethlehem, Pa., USA) are also acceptable ways to complete the 'trial' local anesthetic block.

The location and placement of the cuff electrode depends on which of the severed peripheral nerves is/are transmitting the pain signals. Local anesthetic peripheral nerve blocks help to identify which nerves are involved in pain transmission. Once the practitioner achieves significant pain reduction after local anesthetic blocks to a nerve or group of nerves, he or she has a roadmap showing which nerves the nerve cuff electrode, paddle lead, or percutaneous lead have to be attached to in order to achieve effective pain relief. The metric of success is a >50% pain reduction after a diagnostic local anesthetic peripheral nerve block.

After the offending peripheral nerve is identified, peripheral nerve cuffs, percutaneous leads, or paddle leads are placed around the appropriate nerves. In below-the-knee amputation patients, painful neuromas typically occur near the common peroneal and tibial nerves (fig. 2). In above-the-knee patients (fig. 3), the sciatic nerve is usually the pain generator. For upper extremity amputations, painful neuromas typically occur around the radial, ulnar, median, or musculocutaneous nerves.

Implantation Technique

Electrode implantation for HFAC is achieved via surgical dissection for cuff electrodes. Traditional neurostimulation modalities may be done via open surgical dissection for paddle leads or percutaneously for linear lead placement. Caution must be taken when completing surgical dissection to ensure that vascular or adjacent nerve structures are not damaged when placing the peripheral nerve cuff. These risks can be

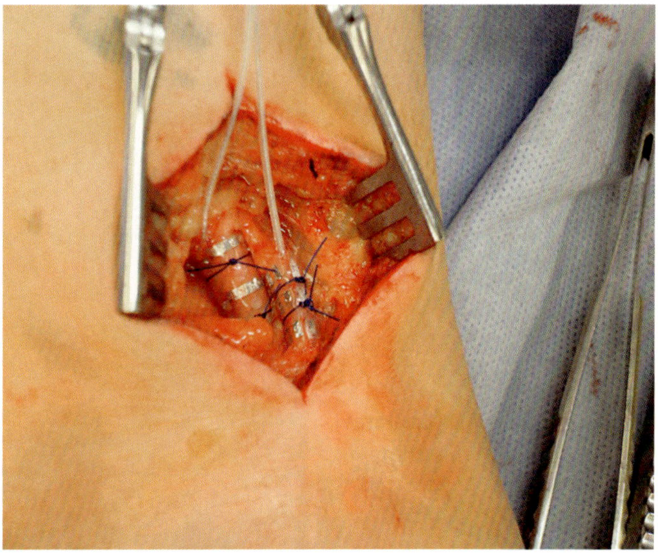

Fig. 2. Peripheral nerve cuffs placed around the common peroneal and tibial nerves in a below-the-knee amputee.

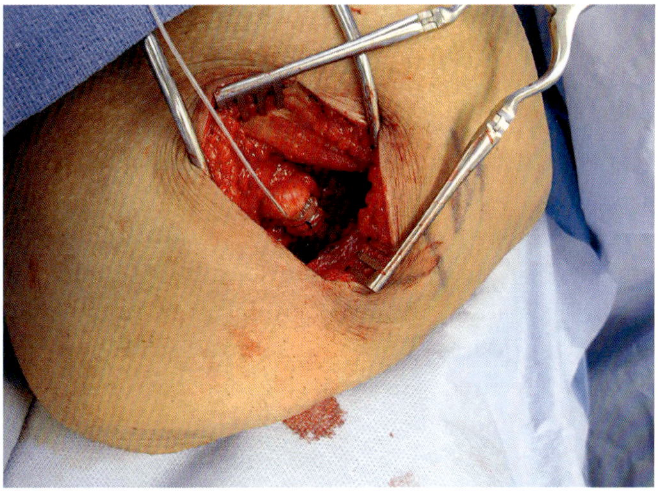

Fig. 3. A picture of the stimulating nerve cuff placed around the sciatic nerve in an above-the-knee amputee.

decreased by performing a perioperative ultrasound map of the patient's vascular and neural structures. In the clinical studies for HFAC cuff placement, a preoperative ultrasound was completed in the preoperative holding area to mark the location and depth of the targeted nerves. This technique allowed for faster and more efficient cuff placement, providing the implanting physician with an accurate nerve depth and location prior to incision. Additionally, during the preoperative ultrasound map, the surgeon can choose to inject 0.1 ml of methylene blue near the targeted nerve so that after the incision is made and dissection is carried out to the desired depth, the surgeon can see the methylene blue surrounding the targeted nerve. These techniques

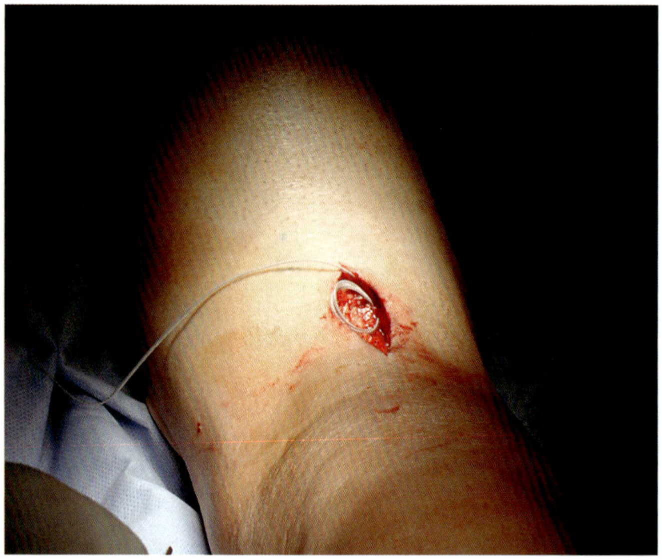

Fig. 4. Preoperative ultrasound mapping facilitates small incision size. Also note that a tension loop is created at the site similar to spinal cord stimulation implants.

allow for not only more rapid nerve exposure (average exposure time of the targeted nerve was <10 min in the HFAC trial), but also facilitated a smaller incision (fig. 4). While helpful, experienced surgeons may not need to complete ultrasound mapping on patients prior to implantation as the anatomy and locations of peripheral nerves are well documented.

Once the peripheral nerve is exposed, a cuff electrode is wrapped around it. The cuff electrode is sized to fit the appropriate nerve, and the diameter of the nerve is confirmed intraoperatively by direct measurement prior to placing the nerve cuff around the desired nerve. After cuff placement, an impedance check is completed and the cuff is secured with one or two nonabsorbable sutures around the diameter of the nerve. It is important to ensure that the sutures are not placed too tightly around the nerve. A tension loop is created with the lead similar to the loops used during implantation of a spinal cord stimulation lead (fig. 4), and the lead is then tunneled for connection with the pulse generator (fig. 5, 6).

Therapy Parameter Settings for High-Frequency Conduction Block

In our studies, the therapy parameters were set approximately 1–2 weeks after the implantation surgery. During the patient programming process, the amplitude of a 10-kHz waveform was gradually increased to achieve pain reduction without inducing a sensation of discomfort. This was achieved with a 5-min linear ramp-up followed by a 25-min plateau of stimulation with a plateau of 2–7 V. The total therapy session time was 30 min. Pain reduction was reported within a matter of minutes after the

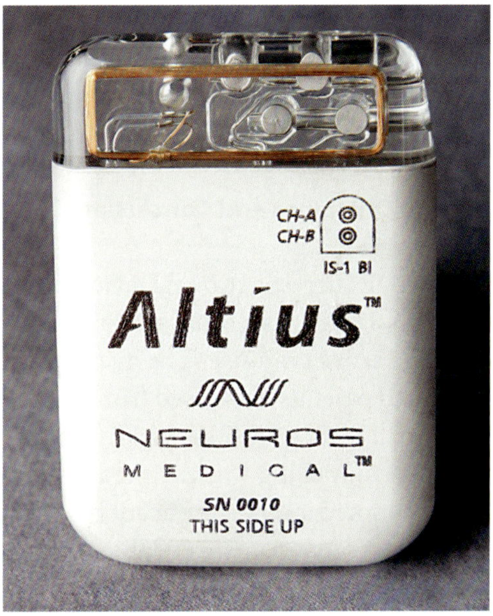

Fig. 5. An image of the internal pulse generator, which allows for up to two peripheral nerve cuff electrodes to be implanted in a patient.

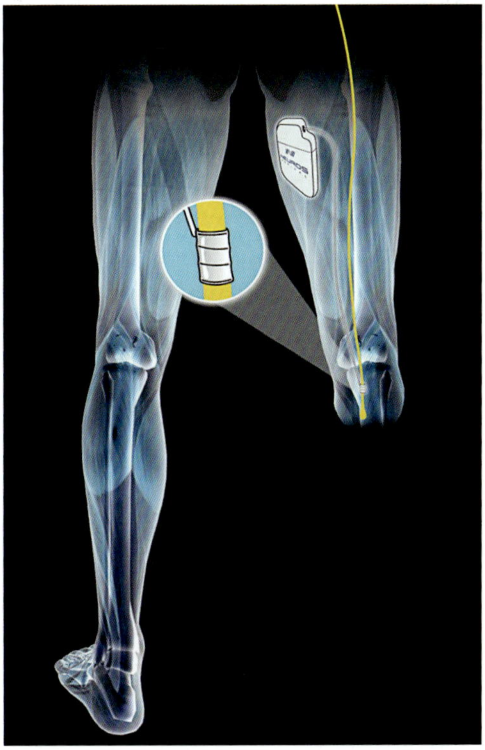

Fig. 6. A cartoon depiction of lead placement around a peripheral nerve attached to the internal pulse generator.

treatment session commenced. The duration of pain relief per therapy session mirrored the results of the local anesthetic peripheral nerve block screening using a rapid acting amide local anesthetic (e.g. 1% lidocaine without epinephrine).

Clinical Outcomes and Conclusions

In our IDE (Investigational Device Exemption)-approved pilot study [16], 10 patients were implanted with 9 patients receiving in-clinic testing and 7 patients progressing to long-term home-use. The average pain score on the Numeric Rating Scale (NRS) for tested patients decreased from 5.7 to 1.4 (out of 10) after HFAC block therapy with 85% of all testing sessions yielding >50% pain reduction.

Also compelling was the medication dose reduction patients experienced. Tested patients noted a very significant reduction in the use of opioid and other analgesics in which several patients were able to eliminate opioids and NSAID medications completely, and all tested patients were able to decrease their analgesic pill counts used per day significantly.

Patients achieved meaningful and significant pain reduction throughout the study, and patients who had phantom pain (in addition to stump pain) that responded to local anesthetic injections also responded favorably with HFAC block. This is presumably because in these particular patients, the phantom symptoms were peripherally generated. Each of the tested patients reported that HFAC block provided the most significant amount of pain reduction they had ever experienced when compared to other pain modalities tried since their amputations.

The HFAC block technique is currently investigational pending FDA clearance. The next step for this modality is a pivotal trial, with the goal of having this therapy available to the mass market upon FDA clearance.

References

1 Kooijman CM, Dijkstra PU, Geertzen JH, Elzinga A, van der Shans CP: Phantom pain and phantom sensations in upper limb amputees: an epidemiological study. Pain 2000;87:33–41.

2 Amputation Coalition of America: Amputation fact sheet: limb loss in the United States. http://www.amputee-coalition.org/fact_sheets/limbloss_us.html (accessed on January 2, 2015).

3 Ramachandran VS, Hirstein W: The perception of phantom limbs. The D.O. Hebb lecture. Brain 1998;121:1603–1630.

4 Cook AJ, Woolf CJ, Wall PD, McMahon SB: Dynamic receptive field plasticity in rat spinal cord dorsal horn following C-primary afferent input. Nature 1987;325:151–153.

5 Rauck RL, Kapural L, Cohen SP, North JM, Gilmore CA, Zang RH, Boggs JW: Peripheral nerve stimulation for the treatment of postamputation pain – a case report. Pain Pract 2012;12:649–655.

6 Peng CW, Chen JJ, Lin CC, Poon PW, Liang CK, Lin KP: High frequency block of selected axons using an implantable microstimulator. J Neurosci Methods 2004;134:81–90.

7 Baratta R, Ichie M, Hwang SK, Solomonow M: Orderly stimulation of skeletal muscle motor units with tripolar nerve cuff electrode. IEEE Trans Biomed Eng 1989;36:836–843.

8 Tanner JA: Reversible blocking of nerve conduction by alternating-current excitation. Nature 1962;195:712–713.

9 Abdel-Gawad M, Boyer S, Sawan M, Elhilali MM: Reduction of bladder outlet resistance by selective stimulation of the ventral sacral root using high frequency blockade: a chronic study in spinal cord transected dogs. J Urol 2001;166:728–733.
10 Cattell M, Gerard RW: The 'inhibitory' effect of high-frequency stimulation and the excitation state of nerve. J Physiol 1935;83:407–415.
11 Woo MY, Campbell B: Asynchronous firing and block of peripheral nerve conduction by 20 kc alternating current. Bull Los Angel Neuro Soc 1964;29:87–94.
12 Ishigooka M, Hashimoto T, Sasagawa I, Izumiya K, Nakada T: Modulation of the urethral pressure by high-frequency block stimulus in dogs. Eur Urol 1994;25:334–337.
13 Kilgore KL, Bhadra N: Nerve conduction block utilizing high-frequency alternating current. Med Biol Eng Comput 2004;42:394–406.
14 Gerges M, Foldes EL, Ackermann DM, Bhadra N, Bhadra N, Kilgore KL: Frequency- and amplitude-transitioned waveforms mitigate the onset response in high-frequency nerve block. J Neural Eng 2010;7:066003.
15 Park JS, Jung TS, Noh YH, Kim WS, Park WI, Kim YS, Chung IK, Sohn UD, Bae SK, Bae MK, Jang HO, Yun I: The effect of lidocaine · HCl on the fluidity of native and model membrane lipid bilayers. Korean J Physiol Pharmacol 2012;16:413–422.
16 Soin A, Fang ZP, Shah NS: Pilot study on high frequency electrical nerve block for post amputation pain: initial results. Neuromodulation 2013;16:e98.

Amol Soin, MD, MBA
The Ohio Pain Clinic
8934 Kingsridge Dr.
Centerville, OH 45458 (USA)
E-Mail drsoin@gmail.com

Slavin KV (ed): Stimulation of the Peripheral Nervous System. The Neuromodulation Frontier.
Prog Neurol Surg. Basel, Karger, 2016, vol 29, pp 168–191 (DOI: 10.1159/000434670)

Peripheral Neurostimulation with a Microsize Wireless Stimulator

Thomas L. Yearwood[a, b] · Laura Tyler Perryman[c]

[a]Comprehensive Pain and Rehabilitation, Pascagoula, Miss., [b]Department of Neurology, University of South Alabama, Mobile, Ala., and [c]Stimwave Inc., Fort Lauderdale, Fla., USA

Abstract

Implementation of wireless technology enables tremendous reduction in the size of implantable neurostimulator devices. Without the need for tethering to an implantable pulse generator, a multitude of clinical applications can be envisioned, utilizing safe, rapidly implanted, economical, and culturally sensitive methods. External pulse generators providing power to implanted microsize wireless leads and/or contact pairs can be incorporated into belts, fabric, jewelry, and other suitable and convenient accoutrements. Microsized wireless neurostimulator lead placements can provide neuromodulation therapies without mechanically compromising normal physiological function in numerous anatomical locations not so accessible now. Avoiding implantation of the pulse generator dramatically reduces the expense of these therapies and can potentially lead to wider global access of care for neuromodulation in general.

Brief Overview of Wireless Technology

In 1873, Scottish physicist James Clerk Maxwell was one of the first to describe electromagnetic energy in a series of mathematical relationships incorporating the relationship between light, magnetism, and electricity into a single unified field theory known as the Maxwell equations. This was the first major challenge to Newtonian mechanics and cannot be overestimated in its significance, both philosophically and practically. In the years that followed, the ideas came to fruition when Franz Hertz successfully transferred energy from one device to another using electromagnetic waves. Further developments rapidly ensued, and we now take for granted a life surrounded by myriads of electromagnetic wave generators and receivers used for communication (the transmission of data) and power (the transmission of energy).

Radio frequency radiation (RFR) occurs when a waveform is transmitted through a medium at a frequency within the radio frequency (RF) portion of the

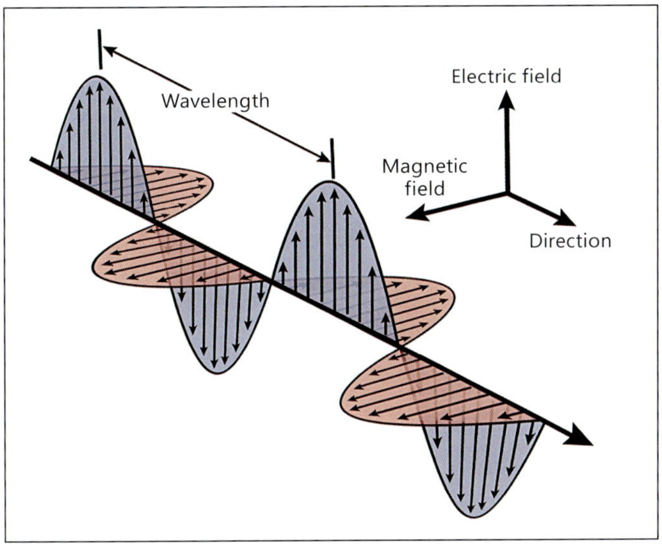

Fig. 1. Three-dimensional representation of the electromagnetic wave: magnetic and electric components of the waveform (modified from http://qph.is.quoracdn.net/main-qimg-5055566df5ba9809b22c262801246760?convert_to_webp=true).

electromagnetic spectrum: frequencies from 10 kHz to 300 GHz. The frequency range of RFR includes the most common frequencies used in transmitting data and power to medical devices. In general, electromagnetic waves include magnetic waves and electric waves that synchronously radiate at perpendicular angles to each other (fig. 1).

A narrower band of frequencies within the frequency range of RFR, from 100 to 500 kHz, is known as the inductive range. These frequencies tend to be the most efficient at creating an induced current by means of an electromagnetic flux passing across coiled circuits. Frequencies within the inductive range band are most commonly used to charge implanted medical devices. The Medical Implant Communication Services (MICS) band of frequencies from 402 to 405 MHz is specified by governmental agencies to be reserved for communications with medical implants. Uninterrupted communication with medical implants is absolutely essential to the well-being of the patient, which is why the MICS band must be safeguarded carefully. The primary safety concern with using inductive power is the amount of heating which can occur at the tissue interface. Thermal heating is a function of the specific absorption rate, which is the amount of absorbed energy measured in watts per kilogram of tissue (W/kg). Electromagnetic fields used for medical device implant power are classified as near fields, and are typically nonpropagating in nature, vary in strength rapidly over distance from the source, and are subject to interference with objects placed near the source.

With near fields, the trade-off for transmission power from the source is typically a balance between specific absorption rate, range of distance from the source of power (emitter) to coiled antenna (receiver), and power consumption. It should be noted it is a critical requirement for near-field power and communications transmission to maintain appropriate alignment of the emitting and receiving devices. As alignment of the emitter and receiver is varied, the efficiencies of power and communications

Table 1. Sensations associated with dermal and subdermal sensory fibers (modified from Verrills and Barnard [12])

Fiber types	Associated sensation
A-β: fast adapt	Tingling, tickling
A-β: slow adapt	Vibrating
A-δ	Sharp pain, stinging
C fibers	Burning, aching

Dermis: mostly A-δ. Subcutaneous tissue: more A-β. Optimal depth below dermal surface for A-β fast adapt: 10–12 mm.

transfer are altered, reaching a minimum at a 90° offset in any combination of three-dimensional space. The clinical importance of maintaining appropriate alignment governs the size, shape, and anatomic location of remotely powered implantable medical devices. In the inductive range, a more shallow location is needed for the receiver coils.

In this chapter we discuss various types of pulse generators that have been used in neurostimulation in order to understand the evolution that has led to the development of wireless pulse generators (WPGs) and their clinical applications.

Fundamentals of Neurostimulation Technology

External Pulse Generators

Transcutaneous Electrical Nerve Stimulation

Transcutaneous electrical nerve stimulation units are commonly used to elicit an electric field on the surface of the dermis in order to recruit sensory nerve fibers and muscle fibers near the electrodes. The dermis itself is particularly rich in unmyelinated C-nociceptive sensory fibers, with a variable population density of A-δ sensory nerves at certain locations. Deep to the dermis, in the subcutaneous fat between the dermis and the first fascial layer, there are numerous A-β sensory nerve fibers. Muscle fiber recruitment begins within the first fascial layer. Depending on the distance from the dermis to the first fascial layer, the intensity of the stimulation may be such that recruitment of the C-nociceptive unmyelinated fibers and the A-δ fibers becomes quite uncomfortable if a motor response is clinically indicated for this therapy. Table 1 demonstrates the typical human sensory perception for each of these different neuronal recruitments.

Transcutaneous electrical nerve stimulation is the most commonly used form of electroanalgesia, primarily due to the noninvasive nature of the therapy and its associated cost ('price point'). A transcutaneous electrical nerve stimulation device typically consists of externally placed electrode pads, from as few as 2 to 12 or more, wired

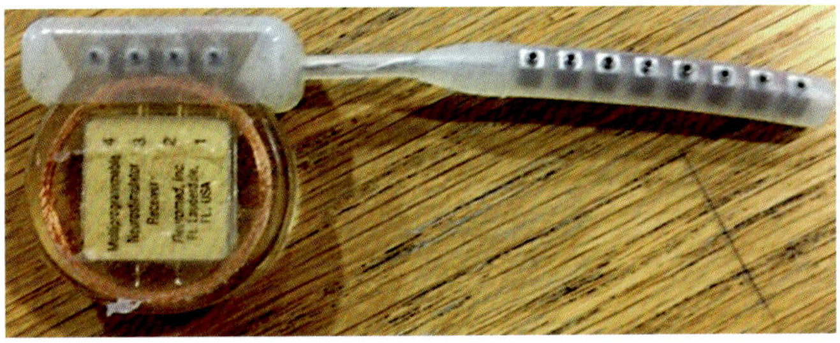

Fig. 2. Radiofrequency pulse generator. Note the presence of coils to convert power externally through the dermis by means of electromagnetic coupling using frequencies in the induction range.

to an external battery-powered electrical signal generator carried with the patient. This signal generator creates a biphasic waveform electric field with pulse widths from 10 to 1,000 μs (typically 50 μs), pulse rates (frequency) from 1 to 150 Hz, and at amplitudes of 10 to 30 mA. Skin irritation can occur in many patients from electrode adhesives or improperly applied electrode gel.

Radiofrequency Pulse Generator

Radiofrequency pulse generators (RPGs) are pulse generators powered by inductively coupled energy from outside the body. These devices contain a coil receiver (fig. 2), which receives power from an external pulse generator (EPG). Using RFR in the inductive range of frequencies, power is transferred through the dermis and subcutaneous tissues to the implanted RPG. The energy produced within the RPG receiver coils is routed to microelectronic circuitry, which generates a biphasic waveform pulse. This biphasic waveform pulse is then routed to a connector attached to a wired lead containing 4–8 individual electrode contacts, depending on the anatomy of the targeted neuronal pathways.

The RPG system has advantages and disadvantages for durable neurostimulation therapy. The potential advantage is a theoretical ability to upgrade the system software, and possibly even the firmware, without explanting part or all of the system, as advanced programming paradigms may become available. There is also an ease of changing or recharging the battery of an external RPG rather than replacing or recharging the implanted generator. The primary disadvantages of the RPG are concerns regarding patient acceptance, patient convenience, and patient compliance with therapy. In order to use the external device effectively, the antenna must be placed on the skin in exact alignment with the RF receiver. In the long run, RPG technology has faded from the marketplace in favor of implantable generators with fewer issues involving emitter-receiver alignment and patient compliance.

Implantable Pulse Generators

Implantable pulse generators (IPGs) are pulse generators that contain a stored power source (battery), which can consist of a primary cell battery, with a limited life span that must be explanted after 2–3 years depending on usage, or a rechargeable battery

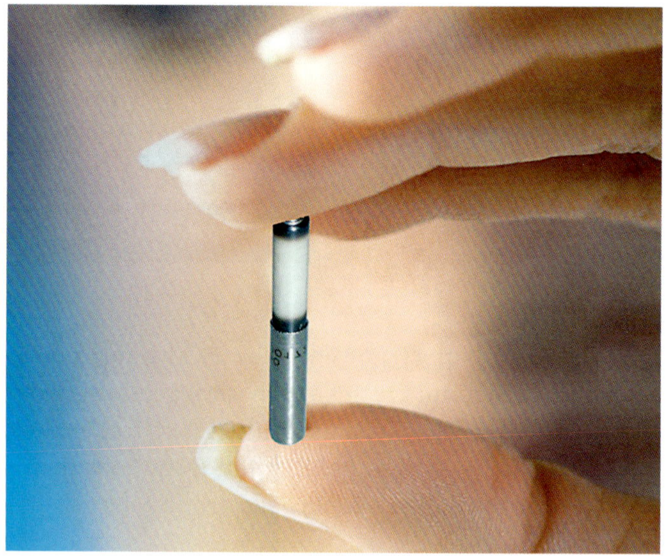

Fig. 3. BION implantable rechargeable pulse generator (photograph courtesy of Boston Scientific®).

(typically a lithium ion battery), with various recharging characteristics related to battery performance. Rechargeable batteries typically have lifespans of 5–10 years. All IPG batteries contain small amounts of toxic materials. As such, they must be hermetically sealed in containers, which must not be physically compromised over the lifetime of the implant. The amount of toxic material contained in most battery cells is proportional to the lifespan of the battery and the number of potential recharge cycles. As with the RPG, there is a need for hardwired connectivity between the pulse generator and the electrode array at the site of therapy.

The majority of IPGs have dimensions in the range of 25–35 mm × 15–25 mm. A notable exception is the BION® device, a miniaturized IPG which is 2–3 mm in diameter and 13–17 mm in length (fig. 3). It is powered by RF induction, which was developed by the Alfred Mann Foundation Inc. (Valencia, Calif., USA). BION includes an on-board power source in the form of a 10-mW rechargeable lithium ion battery, which is recharged by a 'lower frequency' (127 kHz) magnetic link with an external coil worn only during charging. The lithium ion battery was specified to have a cycle life of 2,000 cycles for a standard charge/discharge cycle, a considerably longer cycle life than most of the rechargeable batteries available at the time.

External Wireless Pulse Generation

What Makes a Wireless System 'Wireless'

The term 'wireless' has several uses in the English language. As a noun, 'wireless' is the British term for what Americans call 'radio'. As an adjective 'wireless' has at least two meanings: 'without wires' and 'the transmission of power or communications through any medium using electromagnetic energy rather than a "wired" connection'.

Within the context of implantable medical devices, the term 'wireless' is an adjective, meaning that an external WPG is simply a device that transfers the power required to create a pulsed electrical field at some distance from the source of power, with the capability of controlling the timing, amplitude, and character (or pattern) of that pulse. An RPG, as a medical device, may be powered externally through the dermis by means of electromagnetic coupling using frequencies in the induction range. In this case the implanted receiver must be just beneath the skin, but does not have a hardwired connection through the dermis. Because there is no wired connection through the dermis, this scenario could be mistaken for a wireless device, but in fact it is just a charging/recharging mechanism. One might be tempted to use the term 'wireless', as in 'not having a wired connection'. An RPG is simply a relay station to the site of meaningful bioelectric activity, with or without a rechargeable battery, and transfers both power and control communications via a wired connection to that site of action. Because it technically requires a wired connection between the source of power and the site of action, an RPG is not a wireless neurostimulator.

As medical devices have become more and more miniaturized, it is now possible to build a very small IPG with a rechargeable battery for implantation some distance from the dermis and at the site of bioelectrical activity, as in the case of BION. However, that does not necessarily make it a true wireless neurostimulation system: the battery will eventually need to be replaced, and the electrical contacts creating the clinical stimulation are hardwired to the battery (though over a very small distance). Nevertheless, this is not to suggest that a micro-IPG is not an entirely worthwhile and reliable source of neurostimulation; perhaps with more precision in stable power control than a true wireless system at the present stage of development, a micro-IPG has its advantages, but there are always tradeoffs when tackling difficult clinical problems. To be truly wireless, the power generation and the communication control of the system would need to depend completely on an electromagnetic radiofrequency field from a location external to the body.

Trends in Neurostimulation

The trend in neuromodulation has been towards a reduction in size, but battery lifetime has been a limiting factor. A new product implementation is an external WPG by Stimwave (Fort Lauderdale, Fla., USA), which utilizes a dipole antenna for the direct energy conversion method of electric field coupling. This electric field coupling is accomplished with high-frequency (GHz level), pulsed electromagnetic waves: 'microwaves', so termed because of the very short wavelength involved. The Stimwave device is based on the principle of powering microelectronic devices with radiative electric field coupling through tissues at microwave frequencies rather than the more commonly used lower frequencies (100–500 kHz) of the inductive range of frequencies, the electromagnetic field approach typical of most implanted medical devices.

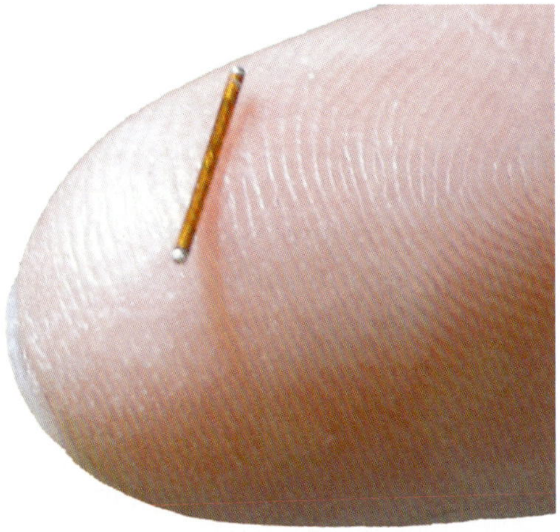

Fig. 4. Stimwave receiver/WPG for one electrode anode-cathode pair.

The advantages of using microwave technology over inductive technology include smaller implant sizes, reduced size of external circuitry, and significantly deeper implantable receiver placements.

There are much smaller electrical losses with this approach, as the dissipation of energy into tissue at these higher frequencies is governed by the inverse square root of the applied frequency, rather than the inverse cube root seen at lower frequencies with inductive coupling. This allows a superior transfer of power to much smaller implanted devices, as the microwaves are able to penetrate bone, fat, muscle, and white and grey matter with substantially less tissue absorbency and energy dissipation. The practical stimulation requirements of neuronal tissues vary: brain and dorsal root ganglion (DRG) stimulation may require smaller currents in the microampere (μA) range, while muscle stimulation and epidural spinal cord stimulation (SCS) require much higher currents in the mA ranges. This technology allows for implanted devices to be as small as 500 μm in diameter and yet still provide clinically appropriate intensities for both brain and muscle tissue. The typical packaging for these devices can be between 800 and 1,350 μm in diameter, which makes them substantially smaller than traditional IPG-based devices (fig. 4). The WPG is no larger than the typical lead body itself, with receiver and nanoelectronics embedded in the lead body. A WPG of this size can be placed in various lead body types, with multiple numbers of electrodes: 2, 4, 8, or more; in percutaneous or surgical paddle lead configurations (fig. 5).

Microwave-based neurostimulation uses small dipole antennae (the 'receiver') embedded within the device body that intercept high-frequency microwave electromagnetic fields, producing an oscillating electric field across the receiver to drive a current flow. For an antenna to be reasonably efficient in energy capture, Poon et al. [1] found the field frequency in the GHz range is more efficient. Since 2012, external WPGs have been available, designed to produce electrically balanced waveforms delivered to electrodes to induce a local electric field in tissue where it can act on nerve fibers.

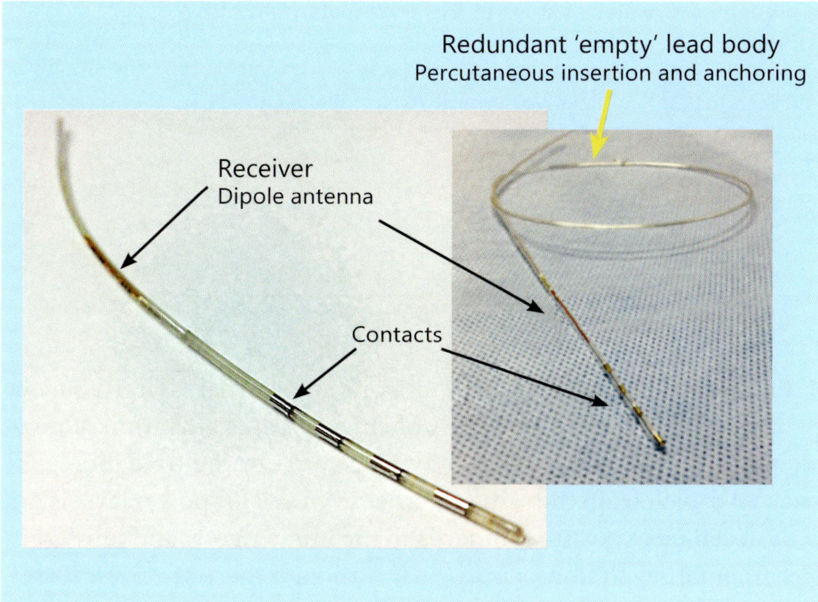

Fig. 5. Stimwave device: anatomy of a wireless lead assembly.

Anatomy and Function: The Components and Clinical Effects of a Wireless System

Device Design, Placement, and Function

The device construction, both in terms of design and material, is crucial to accomplishing the mission of the wireless neurostimulation device. The devices are in many respects identical to those found in more conventional IPG-based neurostimulation systems, but must be appropriately sealed to protect the antennae from tissue fluids. While the contents of the device are not toxic to the body, bodily tissues can damage the efficiency and functionality of the receiver over time.

The electrodes are formed from standard platinum-iridium materials and are connected to the receiver by means of braided wires soldered to the electrodes by laser. The antenna within the lumen of the device typically has a length of 2–8 cm. The length of the antenna can vary depending on the clinical application for the device. Electromagnetic energy is absorbed by various body tissues, and the amount of power received by the receiver is related to the amount of fat, muscle, bone, and vascular structures through which the electromagnetic energy must traverse. The deeper a device antenna is placed in tissue, the longer the antenna must be to receive sufficient power from the emitted microwave frequencies due to the wavelength of the electromagnetic energy. Embedded circuitry within the device body enables the production of charge-balanced waveforms emitted at the electrodes according to internalized addressing systems, a part of an application-specific integrated circuit which routes the power independently to each contact.

Table 2. Dielectric properties of various tissues at 915 MHz (data from http://niremf.ifac.cnr.it/tissprop/)

Tissue	Conductivity, μs/cm	Relative permittivity	Wavelength, cm
Fat	514	5.45	13.96
Muscle	9,481	55.00	4.35
Dry skin	8,716	41.33	4.90
Wet skin	8,502	46.02	4.70
Air			35.67

Placement of an implanted device at 2–6 cm from an external GHz frequency transmitting antenna can generate up to 20 mA of current. The generation of power for therapeutic treatment can be increased by placement of multiple dipole receivers in the tissue, all driven from the same external source. This power level is not particularly high by accepted exposure standards to the human body and fully complies with all governmental regulations worldwide. Although there are tissue losses, the power can be transferred efficiently to receivers placed at significant tissue depths.

Microwave fields do not normally cause any effect on nerve tissue because tissues are refractory to high frequencies oscillating at orders of magnitude faster than that required for activating cell membranes. Rectification of the pulsed microwaves, however, can produce pulsed currents over a wide range of stimulating frequencies (well into the kHz range) to generate an action potential response. The stimulation parameters of pulse width, amplitude, and repetition rate (frequency) are fully adjustable by harvesting the electrical current flows and producing the biphasic neurostimulation pulses used clinically.

Trade-offs can be made to achieve increased tissue penetration depths by employing novel dipole antenna designs to increase microwave energy capture and power output. For example, if antenna lengths are selected to be equal to half the wavelength of the electromagnetic energy through a particular medium, this improves the power transfer. In mixed soft tissue types, the typical wavelength of electromagnetic energy at a frequency of 915 MHz is roughly 8.5–9.0 cm, whereas in air this wavelength is approximately 36 cm (table 2). The amplitude, shape, pulse width, and frequencies of neuronal stimulation are all determined by the spatial envelope of the applied energy field, which is fully adjustable. Implant current generation depends not only on applied energy to the skin, but also on the impedance matching of the RF coupling of the EPG (emitting antenna) to the implanted device (receiving antenna).

As part of the verification for these concepts, Perryman et al. [2] developed a computer model (Ansoft HFSS) for a 915-MHz RF electric field distribution in tissue to examine tissue depth versus power output. While pulsed electromagnetic power can produce heating, the overall average tissue heating levels are lower than the regulatory guidelines, yet capable of providing effective clinical therapy at deeper tissue locations. There is a cosine relationship between emitting and receiving antenna orientations, such that the greatest energy transfer occurs when the antennae are parallel, falling to zero energy transfer when they are perpendicular. Even coupled with the RF scattering that normally occurs in tissue, pulsed microwave antennae could be off-parallel by up to 30° with only a minimal effect on the resulting energy transfer. This feature offers a tremendous advantage over induction-type devices operating at much lower frequencies in the kHz range. A great deal of attention has been devoted to examining the safety aspects of applying pulsed microwave energy to the skin of humans. There are a number of different guidance documents that govern such exposure and the limits vary depending on whether the exposures are to the general public or to a person who gains a therapeutic benefit from an electromagnetic powered device.

The microwave frequency bands utilized at 915 MHz and 2.45 GHz for clinical applications reside in the ISM license-free microwave band under rule Part 18 designated by the FCC for protocols other than those used in communications. Digital TV, cell phones, microwave ovens, and radar are all within this spectrum. It has only been since the early 1990s that the new miniature transistorized microwave equipment operating near or above 1 GHz became available at reasonable prices. Previously, the primary mode of microwave generation was bulky traveling-wave vacuum tubes. With communication technology driven by the wide use of cell phones, the generation of high frequencies in small device platforms has become commonplace.

External Pulse Generator

The EPG is a microwave transmitter containing typical cell phone electronics technology. The pulse output power achievable in the compact design can be as much as 1 W on average, depending on the pulse stimulation parameters and duty cycle required. The drain on batteries in the external transmitter is directly proportional to the total power delivered. The power drain is comparable to other microwave battery-powered commercial devices. Microwave antenna geometries are defined by the operating frequency and wavelengths utilized. The 915-MHz frequency range antenna designs can take on a variety of forms, are compact, flexible, and do not have to touch the skin like magnetic field-inductive coils. Parameters such as pulse width, repetition rate, and pulse waveform characteristics are controlled by the envelope of the transmitted waveform and can thus be programmed to a variety of combinations depending on the excitation needs of the particular neuronal tissue being targeted for stimulation.

The EPG is encased in a waterproof, lightweight, comfortable shell. The EPG is meant to be worn or kept near the body at all times. Its power supply is a rechargeable, off-the-shelf lithium ion polymer battery. The battery capacity can vary according to the indicated use depending on the amount of power required for clinically relevant use and whatever physical size requirements for normal use are needed in that application. Internal to the EPG is an RF transmitter that encodes stimulus waveforms into a microwave carrier signal based on the programming settings for amplitude, pulse width, shape, and rate of pulse generation. The RF transmitter functions alongside a microprocessor that controls settings, data communication, and event handling.

Controller

The EPG is programmed and given commands by a controller. The controller is linked to the EPG through Bluetooth technology, and contains a sophisticated user interface. The controller can be easily embodied as a software application on a smartphone or tablet device, and allows the clinician to develop programs for the patient within clinically relevant parameters. It also enables the patient to adjust the stimulation parameters as needed during use.

Clinical Application of Wireless Neurostimulation

Comparison with Traditional 'Wired' Neurostimulation Systems

Wireless neurostimulation offers a tremendous clinical advantage to the field of neurostimulation. Once the implanted array of electrical contacts has been freed from its tether to an IPG, the anatomical barriers to implantation diminish significantly. The complexity of the surgical implantation procedure is greatly lessened for any clinical application in which the IPG would ordinarily be expected to be at a distance and separated from this lead array (table 3). This is especially true when leads or lead extensions must traverse bony articulations and muscle bodies where they are subject to numerous biomechanical forces involving tension and compression of the leads. Specifically in the upper and lower extremities, with wireless technology it is no longer necessary to tunnel portions of the lead to an IPG across the wrist or elbow, ankle or knee to target specific peripheral nerves. There is no need for creating strain-relief 'loops' in subcutaneous leads to accommodate the large ranges of motion associated with normal joint biomechanics. Thus, a percutaneous 'injectable' implantation of a short contact array becomes a matter of a few minutes rather than the considerable operative time needed for tunneling and subcutaneous pocket creation for the IPG. This reduces patient exposure to postoperative infections, surgical complications, and the various forms of anesthesia that may be required for the implantation process. Additionally, with fewer biomechanical forces being exerted on the contact array as a result of traversing articulations, there is considerably less potential for contact migration.

With improvements in percutaneous anchoring systems used to deploy these wireless leads, multiple lead arrangements become feasible, potentially enhancing the clinical efficacy of a peripheral neurostimulation (PNS) system as a whole. Figure 6 demonstrates the concept of percutaneous anchoring, effectively eliminating the need for surgical incisions to facilitate placement and anchoring devices over the leads. The potential for wider field coverage using multiple wireless devices to surround a single

Table 3. Procedural differences between traditional IPG-based wired neurostimulation system implantation and wireless neurostimulation system implantation

Traditional, IPG-based wired neurostimulator implantation
Cut down from midline in placement
Introduce and place device(s)
Test device(s)
Attach extension cable
Add tension-relief loops and anchors in midline wound
Create subcutaneous pocket for IPG
Tunnel from midline wound to IPG pocket
Add tension relief loops and anchors
Connect device to IPG
Test connectivity
Irrigate and close surgical wounds (± wound drain depending on depth of wound)
Bandage patient
Transfer to postprocedure recovery area
Recover patient from anesthesia (local, regional, IV sedation, etc.)
Discharge patient with postoperative analgesics and instructions
Follow-up wound care
Wireless neurostimulator implantation
Percutaneous needle insertion(s)
Introduce and place device(s) into the posterior epidural space
Test device(s)
Inject anchor percutaneously
Bandage patient
Discharge patient with postoperative analgesics and instructions

peripheral nerve (PNS) is shown in figure 7, and overcomes the limiting effects of 'umbrage' or 'field shadow'. In this example, altering the axis of the contact array relative to the longitudinal axis of the nerve provides greater stimulation coverage along the nerve, as beautifully shown by Narouze et al. [3]. The simple addition of a second or third wireless lead array allows the opportunity to recruit an even greater number of fascicles for more complete stimulation of the nerve as a whole. Multiple wireless leads can also be distributed throughout an area of peripheral nerve field stimulation. For peripheral applications this adds a '3rd dimension' for contact distributions not possible with traditional linear arrays as originally developed for epidural neurostimulation applications.

Anatomical Sites for Wireless Neurostimulation

Table 4 lists sites of applications for wireless neurostimulation systems. To date, clinically relevant trials have been performed for SCS, DRG and transforaminal placements, and peripheral nerve stimulation applications (PNS and peripheral nerve field stimulation). Further clinical trials are presently being designed for stimulation of the stellate ganglion, the celiac plexus and splanchnic nerves, and elements of the lumbar sympathetic chain. In addition, a specific neural target is the vagus nerve, for both

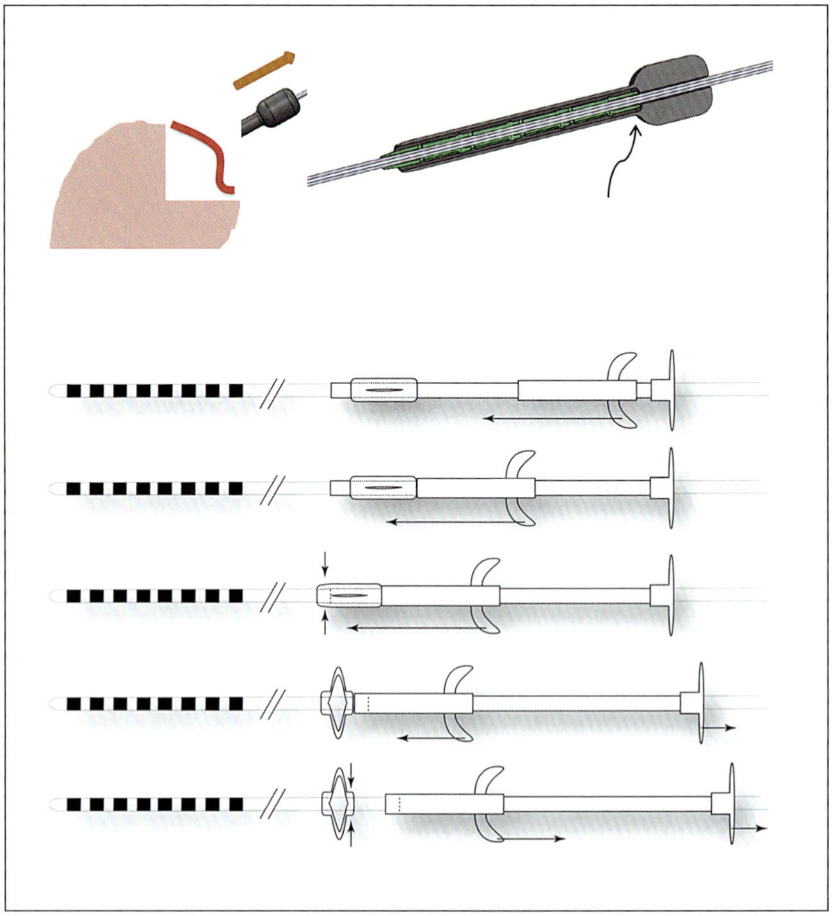

Fig. 6. A percutaneous anchor slips over 'empty' redundant tubing of the device body at some distance from the antennae, introduces anchoring 'wings', and clips excess tubing. The anchor sleeve is delivered over the empty tubing portion of the implantable device. When deployed, it clinches tightly over the device body diameter while simultaneously collapsing, creating a 'winged' shape which projects laterally from the device body. A 'clipping' mechanism trims the redundant empty tubing. This anchor is tightly bound around the device body to prevent migration.

epilepsy therapy and gastrointestinal related therapies. Additional long-range goals include the development of lead adapters for deep brain stimulation and motor cortex stimulation.

Wireless neurostimulation therapy can be employed at virtually any anatomical location, and is limited only by the appropriate surgical techniques necessary for device delivery to the target tissue. The surgical techniques to be employed include percutaneous, open surgical, or laparoscopic/endoscopic delivery systems. Radiological guidance for device delivery can include fluoroscopy, CT, ultrasound, or their combination. Thus, it is possible to consider wireless neurostimulation therapy in the intracranial space, the intra-abdominal space, the intraspinal space, and in multiple

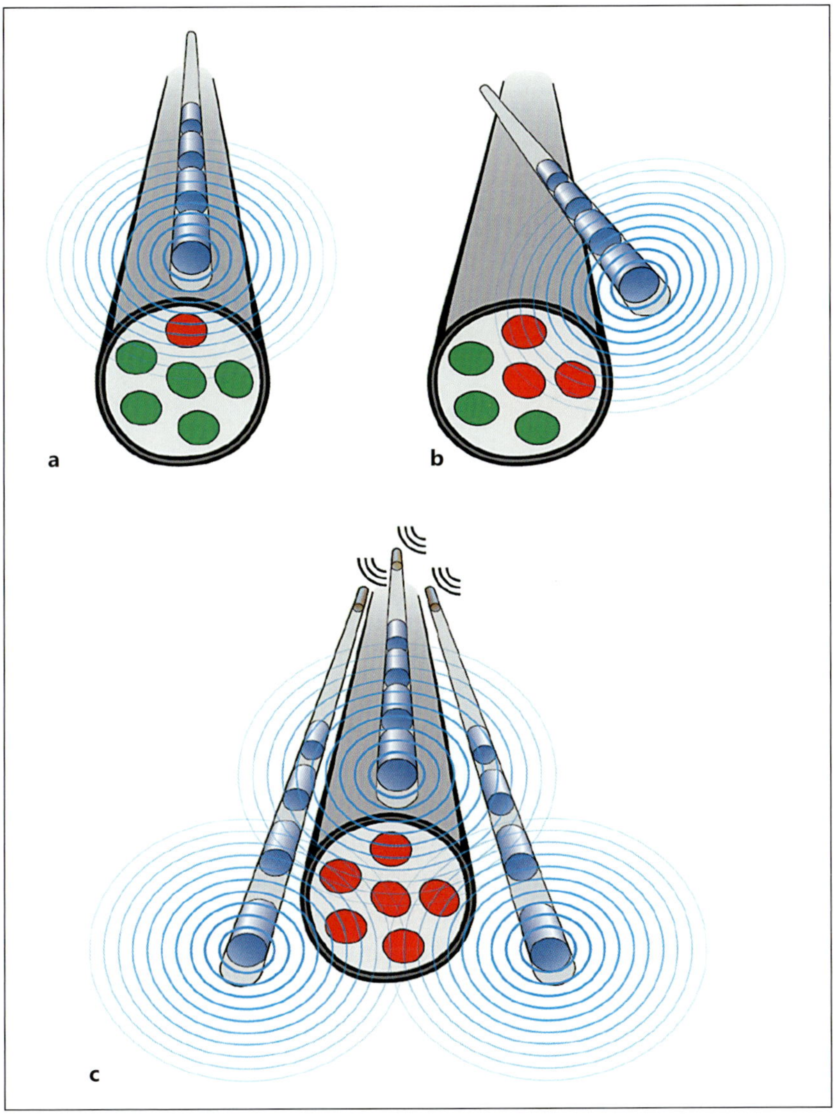

Fig. 7. Effect of device position on nerve coverage ('umbrage' concept). **a** Electrode is positioned along the nerve axis – maximal umbrage. **b** Electrode is off the nerve axis – the umbrage is reduced. **c** Multiple leads around the nerve – minimal umbrage. Red: stimulated fascicles within the field; green: unstimulated fascicles within the area of umbrage.

locations about the face, skull, trunk, and limbs. Intraperitoneal and retroperitoneal locations are excellent choices for wireless neurostimulation where a 'hardwired' connection to an IPG could be difficult and cumbersome.

A simple adapter can also now be easily connected to most commercially available leads to convert them to a wireless platform, minimizing implanter disruption by employing wireless technology in the more traditional applications of neurostimulation

Table 4. Sites for clinical application of wireless neurostimulation systems

Peripheral sites
Craniofacial
Extremities
Trunk
Skeletal muscle
Functional electrical stimulation
Central sites
Intraspinal
SCS, DRG, spinal nerve root
Paraspinal
Ganglion, plexus, nerve roots
Intracranial
Deep brain stimulation, motor cortex stimulation, SSCS
Visceral
Uterine, cardiac, pulmonary gastrointestinal, genitourinary, intervertebral disc

SSCS = Somatosensory cortex stimulation.

therapy. These adapters can contain not only the appropriate antennae needed for each contact on the device, but can also contain a miniature embedded application-specific integrated circuit, which may potentially enable subtle programming capabilities of parameters (such as frequency, pulse width, intensity, and timing or phase-lag) along with individually programmed power requirements for each contact. As shown in figure 8, the versatile capability of wireless programming greatly enhances the application of this technology to a wide variety of clinical needs. What had previously been limited in traditional hardwired IPGs can now be transformed into 'virtual' IPGs by wireless technology, creating independently functioning regions within any given contact array, as long as electrical neutrality is maintained at the end of each pulse cycle. This Virtual IPG Application™ potentially provides a level of programming flexibility heretofore unimaginable.

The programming capability and depth of tissue penetration of the EPG can easily accomplish a variety stimulating waveforms in these deeper areas, including high frequency (>5 kHz) applications. Where needed for a specific application, 'passive' or 'active' repeaters can be implanted to help steer and amplify the signal to an implanted device. A passive repeater acts as a 'stepping stone' for the activating signal, whereas an active repeater can behave more like a 'springboard' to amplify the signal in difficult to reach situations.

With the development of laparoscopic and endoscopic placement techniques, intra-abdominal, intravascular, and intraspinal applications can now also be contemplated. Without the need for hardwired connectivity to an IPG, stimulators can be laparoscopically placed at the walls of the large and small intestines for regulation of peristalsis, to the uterus or bladder to control smooth muscle contraction, and to many other viscera for regulation of their mechanical, hormonal, or metabolic func-

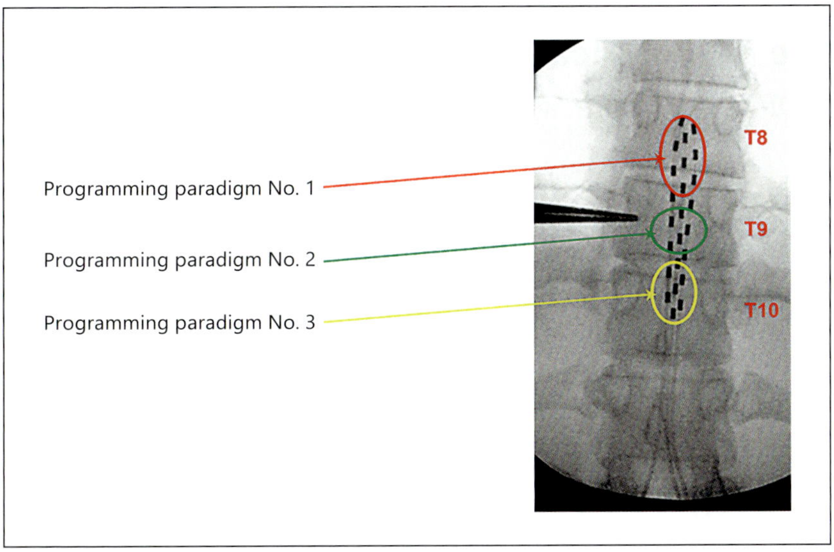

Fig. 8. The 'virtual' IPG concept: wireless technology creating multiple regions of neurostimulation within a given electrode array. By assigning an individual digital address to each contact pair, multiple regions of neurostimulation therapy can potentially be created along any particular lead arrangement, tremendously enhancing the versatility of therapy.

tions. In addition, ultrasound guidance greatly enhances the targeting capability, accuracy, and safety of wireless device placement near peripheral nerves, vascular structures, and articulations. Using wireless technology, many more clinical applications are now possible in a variety of anatomical locations.

Traditionally conceived peripheral device placements have been predicated on two overriding principles: (1) adaptation to the peripheral space of linear electrode arrays originally designed for epidural neurostimulation, and (2) 'fixed' contact spacing.

The anatomic features of the peripheral space are vastly different from the more traditional notions of neurostimulation in the epidural space. In general, the electrical fields generated for SCS behave more like a 'spotlight on a stage', producing a two-dimensional 'fabric of electrical field' across the surface of the cord. In the peripheral space, the field shape is more three-dimensional and the neurostimulator array is actually creating a 'volume of electrical field' through which nerves pass (fig. 9). Depending on the size of the nerve and the size of the field in question, there may be 'umbrage' or a 'field shadow' where a section of neurons within a named peripheral nerve receive no activation (figure 7). For much smaller microscopic nerves in the reticular networks of the subcutaneous space, the field may be many orders of magnitude larger than the individual nerves being stimulated (mm^3 vs. μm^3), which pass through a field volume defined by the ambient impedances of each specific tissue type (fat, vascular structures, neural structures, stroma, etc.) and the specific programming paradigm for the neurostimulation signal.

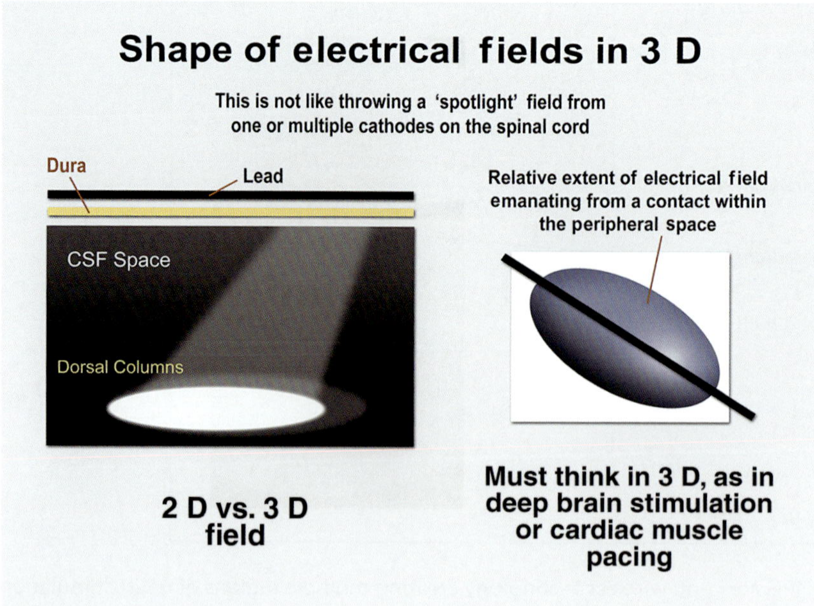

Fig. 9. Electrical fields for epidural applications vs. peripheral applications.

Wireless technology provides the opportunity to rethink the design and implementation of site-specific contact placement without the traditional lead design or 'fixed' contact arrangement. It is now possible to place independent, miniaturized, and individually programmable bipolar contacts at anatomically specific locations without the need for 'hardwired' connectivity to an IPG. Wireless neurostimulation of the future may look more like the night sky, with its myriad of shining stars, each carefully fitted to the anatomical and neurophysiological environment, and less like a telephone line or draped pearl necklace.

Clinical Examples

Trigeminal Neuropathic Pain

Many cases of chronic neuropathic craniofacial pain have been found to be very suitably treated with PNS [4–7]. There are many causes of chronic neuropathic craniofacial pain, some of which are listed in table 5, and there are reports which indicate that the prevalence of craniofacial pain and dysfunction in the United States ranges from 5 to 12% in the general population, with approximately 10.8 million adults experiencing craniofacial pain [8]. Recently, Perryman and Yearwood [9] reported on a very successful pilot study treating craniofacial pain with wireless neurostimulation therapy.

The authors conducted clinical trials in 10 patients with chronic craniofacial pain from one or more causes, including postoperative dental neuralgia, infection, classic

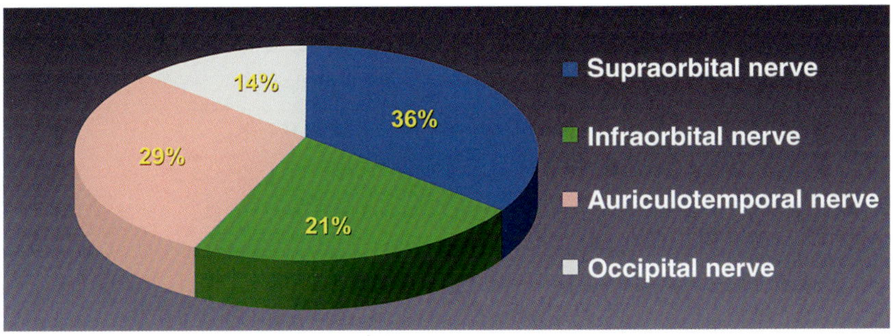

Fig. 10. Distribution of sites of craniofacial pain in a pilot study of treating craniofacial pain with wireless neurostimulation therapy.

Table 5. Causes of chronic neuropathic craniofacial pain

Trauma
Oral, facial, neurological, and dental surgeries
Infection (i.e. zoster)
Trigeminal neuralgias
Classic
Secondary
Referred craniofacial pain
Cervicogenic headache, temporomandibular joint dysfunction
Chronic headache of central origin
Migraine
Cluster
Trigeminal autonomic cephalalgia
Neoplasms

trigeminal neuralgia, whiplash, and failed neck surgery syndrome after C3-C4 anterior discectomy and fusion. The median age was 60 years, and 70% of the subjects were female. Figure 10 shows the neural anatomic distribution of craniofacial pain in these 10 patients. Clearly, multiple neuroanatomical distributions were noted in the majority of patients tested. The wireless neurostimulation devices used in this pilot study were 12 cm in length; the majority of the devices were purposefully redundant to allow appropriate, individual tailoring of the device implantation within the hairline whenever possible [9].

These wireless neurostimulator devices were placed within the subcutaneous space directly overlying branches of the trigeminal nerve(s) or the occipital nerve(s) using a 16-gauge bent tip Tuohy epidural needle or a 14-gauge vascular access catheter also with a bent tip. One or more quadripolar wireless neurostimulator leads with 3-mm contacts × 4-mm spacing were placed over the various indicated neural targets in each patient, tunneled beyond the margin of hairline, and anchored with a suture sleeve underneath the dermis via a 1-cm incision, after functional verification of paresthesia and pain relief. Programming utilized charge-balanced constant current with a pulse

Table 6. Clinical results of a wireless craniofacial pain pilot study

Clinical variable	Clinical result
Patients obtaining pain relief, %	100
Median paresthesia coverage, %	67
Median pain reduction, %	82
Patient experiencing sustained pain relief, %	100
Median visual analog scale score	
Baseline	9.17±1.77
End of study	1.56±0.35
≥50% reduction in oral pain medications, %	100
Patient stopping all pain medications during the trial, %	60
Patient acceptance and satisfaction, %	100
Lead fracture	None
Migration	None
Infection	None
Skin erosion	None

width of 160 μs and frequency of 60 Hz. The trial duration was 30 days, after which the devices were explanted. The EPG was placed in the lining of a standard baseball cap, and patients were monitored at 3 days, 2 weeks, 4 weeks, and as the circumstances required.

Results of this 'first-in-human' pilot study of wireless neurostimulation therapy for craniofacial pain are shown in table 6. The average time to implant each device in this pilot study was less than 10 min. It is anticipated that this implantation time will be further reduced in the future with the use of the percutaneous anchor instrument. All of the patients indicated they would certainly pursue permanent implantation when it becomes available. This study indicates that wireless neurostimulation therapy for the craniofacial area is not only minimally invasive, but is also rapid, safe, effective, cosmetically acceptable, and enables direct implantation in the pain generator locations along neural pathways to more central locations with therapeutic benefit.

Wireless PNS therapy in the craniofacial area appears to be a practical and simplified therapy that provides a viable treatment option without requiring intricate tunneling in the head and neck, or cumbersome IPG implantation. The complications are few and operating time is drastically reduced.

Dorsal Root Ganglion Stimulation for Failed Back Surgery Syndrome-Related Lumbar Radiculitis

The DRG and other areas of the exiting nerves in the lumbar spine can be sites of chronic pain neuromodulation in cases of neuropathic mechanical or chemical disorders in patients with failed back surgery syndrome. Recently, there have been considerable efforts in targeting the DRG for neurostimulation therapy in these and many other cases. It is quite clear that the DRG is an excellent site for interventional neurostimulation therapy. Great care, however, must be taken to avoid recruiting motor axons, and meticulous care must be taken to appropriately place the device contacts and ensure stability of the anatomical placement. Further, the mechanical properties of the device should include miniaturization and flexibility, so as to minimize biomechanical stress that can result in the development of postimplantation scarring and fibrosis. All implanted 'foreign bodies' will induce the normal tissue response of encapsulation, but this encapsulation may well be a function of the relative rigidity of implanted device, and producing a device with minimal biomechanical resistance to the surrounding tissues during normal activities of daily living should ultimately be a significant concern. Additionally, stabilizing the device should certainly not interfere with the anatomy of the DRG or the nerve roots in the paraforaminal region.

We have recently reported on DRG stimulation using a wireless device in 10 patients to treat chronic low back pain associated with failed back surgery syndrome [10]. Under C-arm fluoroscopy, an 18-gauge bent tip Tuohy epidural needle was used to place the stimulator device through the Kambin triangle [11], directly dorsal to the DRG inferior to the targeted pedicle. A 4-contact wireless miniature stimulator device was placed percutaneously along the exiting nerve root, and was anchored with a percutaneously injected 'winged' anchor, as described above. The implanted device was powered and EPG-embedded in a belt, and was programmed using Bluetooth technology with a remote programmer. In this initial pilot study, there was some difficulty in maintaining a fairly dorsal placement to the DRG, but a suitable number of contacts were capable of sensory stimulation without motor axon recruitment in each case. Results of the 6-week trial of neurostimulation demonstrated average pain reduction of 45% from baseline over the low back areas involved in a power level equivalent to 2 mA distributed across 4 contacts.

There was only minimal device migration noted during the study in 4 of the 6 patients; 2 of the 6 patients experienced migration of 3 and 6 mm, respectively, attributable to implanter error while becoming familiar with the use of the percutaneous anchoring device. Several design alterations have been made in this device as result of this pilot study, and further design considerations are ongoing to develop more appropriate and easier delivery of wireless neurostimulator systems for clinical applications about the DRG. Nevertheless, this pilot study shows placement of a wireless neurostimulator percutaneously through a Coudé-type Tuohy needle directly to the dorsal area of the L2 DRG and exiting nerve root to be a viable alternative approach to pain management to treat low back pain [10].

As in all other clinical pilot studies performed with wireless neurostimulation therapy thus far, intraoperative time and patient acceptance have been enormously enhanced. With the development of improved percutaneous anchoring devices, it is anticipated this technology will blossom in its implementation and substantially increase patient accessibility to neurostimulation therapy for the control of chronic neuropathic pain.

Future Concepts

The Future of Clinical Application

Wireless neurostimulation can be used for a wide variety of therapies in addition to the treatment of chronic pain. Any specific organ tissue or anatomical structure directly or indirectly controlled by the nervous system is a potential target for wireless neurostimulation therapy. This includes applications in functional electrical stimulation to assist in the treatment of movement disorders, influencing subtle alterations in hormone production and release, visceral organ function, vascular and pulmonary regulation, epilepsy, and neurobehavioral phenomena such as appetite suppression and depression. Freed from 'hardwired tethering' to an IPG, the possibilities of placement for therapeutic intervention local to the affected area are tremendously increased. Table 7 presents a sample list of some modalities currently under investigation using wireless neurostimulation technology.

The Future of Lead Design

Lead design benefits from wireless neurostimulation since the traditional mechanical and functional constraints are removed, enabling novel designs that may include (1) printed circuits on thin, pliable sheets of film that can be controlled wirelessly with minimal biomechanical tissue impact, (2) multiple, independently implantable, independently programmable electrode arrays in a wide variety of shapes and surfaces that can be developed for specialized applications, and (3) highly flexible leads. These leads, the size of sewing thread, can be embedded in dissolvable compound polymers with percutaneous or endoscopic implantation within vascular, bronchial, retinal, adrenal, pancreatic, brain, or spinal cord tissues to be wirelessly powered and controlled for neuromodulation of metabolic, hormonal, or other physiologic processes. The compound polymer structures containing these flexible, thread-like leads would eventually melt at body temperature and be absorbed in the surrounding tissues, leaving the lead behind, with biomechanical properties having low-to-none tissue impact. Encapsulation of these leads under these circumstances could be expected to be minimal, and they would conform to mobile biological surfaces with great ease and less tethering by postoperative scarring and fibrosis.

The Future of Programming

Advanced programming paradigms can be greatly enhanced and easily upgraded with the advent of Virtual IPG Application™. This advanced programming feature is capable of providing multiple, independently operational sectors of any given contact

Table 7. Sample list of clinical applications currently under investigation or development using wireless neurostimulation technology

Clinical condition	Targets, methods, etc.
Metabolic disorders	Diabetes (pancreatic regulation) Hypo-/hyperthyroidism (thyroid regulation)
Labor and delivery	Pain control during labor Feedback pain control with tocodynamometer Feedback control of uterine contractions with fetal heart rate monitoring
Cancer pain	Disposable neurostimulation therapy for end-of-life care
Obesity	Vagus nerve stimulation (intra-abdominal)
Epilepsy and depression	Vagus nerve stimulation (cervicothoracic junction) Trigeminal nerve stimulation
Chronic headache of central origin	Chronic daily headache, cluster headache, trigeminal autonomic cephalalgia
Chronic widespread hyperalgesia syndrome ('fibromyalgia')	C2-C3 nerve distribution stimulation
Chronic pelvic pain	Sacral nerve stimulation Pudendal nerve stimulation
Bowel and bladder dysmotility	Sacral nerve stimulation Posterior tibial nerve stimulation
Movement disorders	FES
Sleep apnea	Hypoglossal nerve stimulation FES in the oropharynx FES in the neck
'Virtual leads' and 'virtual pulse generators'	Independently programmable and controlled contacts within electrode arrays using RFID digital addressing
Wireless transmission of neurostimulation data via Internet	Central servers for patient and clinician documentation: – Documentation of neurostimulation usage (specific programs used; duration of usage) – Documentation of patient activity levels with neurostimulation (couple with accelerometer) Central servers for documentation of system performance: – Battery discharge and recharge parameters – Contact impedance – Contact migration Protecting patient identity in the digital age Encryption technology

FES = Functional electrical stimulation.

combination, with each sector capable of running several contact configurations (e.g. 'Stim-Sets', 'areas', 'programs'). With the absence of hardwired connections to an IPG, high-speed WPG technology enables multiple different types of charge-balanced programming paradigms across any set of lead arrays. Figure 8 shows an example of this for epidural neurostimulation, but the Virtual IPG Application™ programming capability is certainly applicable to PNS therapy.

Updates for software and firmware within the EPG could reasonably be expected to be less expensive and minimally impacting on both patients and clinical staff. Thus, the patient could receive 'cutting edge' programming technology as it becomes available.

The use of an EPG in a variety of anatomical locations to power the implant enables the use of wearable medical device technology embedding the EPG into various functional forms of clothing and accessories. In addition, because of the EPG, the 'price point' for wireless neurostimulation technology is expected to be substantially lower than other neurostimulation systems, creating a larger adoption rate on a global basis for wireless neurostimulation technology. In Western societies, the cost of wireless neurostimulation therapy can be expected to fall within the range of 'self-pay' medical treatment options, and the traditional healthcare providers who perform neurostimulation implantation may find themselves strategically poised to adopt the same business model well known to plastic surgeons and cosmetic dentists/orthodontists. In other societies, implementation of this therapy could actually reduce national healthcare costs secondary to a decrease in medication requirements and an increase in patient productivity and functionality. In both scenarios, global use of neurostimulation technology is expected to increase.

The Future of the Wireless Neurostimulation Industry

Wireless technology appears to have substantial cost advantages. The price differences entailed in these designs compared to the more traditional implantable systems make the wireless alternative an extremely affordable option for lowering the cost of healthcare and improving its societal impact. Third-party payers and government-sponsored healthcare programs should realize substantial financial benefits from implementation of this technology. Reductions in medication usage brought about by rechargeable wireless neurostimulation therapies allow greater patient access to this therapy, with compounding financial implications. Compared to older and more expensive implantable options, the market sustainability of wireless neurostimulation technology would certainly appear to be excellent on a global perspective.

Patient acceptance of this technology will in part depend on fashionable and culturally sensitive incorporation of the EPGs within convenient and familiar construction of appropriate garments. Examples of fashionable accessories include socks, shoes, sandals, scarves, sweaters, shirts, shorts, smartphone cases, belts, undergarments, watch bands, necklaces, bracelets, anklets, earrings, various forms of head wear, various jewelry items, and even eyeglasses, many of which are currently under development.

Conclusion: Miniaturization, Versatility, and Sustainability

Wireless neurostimulation enables greater flexibility for therapy than traditional hardwired neurostimulation technology in terms of device design, anatomical device placement, and the use of multiple contact programming paradigms for the electrode arrays. Suitable targets of neurostimulation which are anatomically difficult to reach and do not lend themselves well to the use of tunneled leads can now be accessed with greater ease, less risk, and shorter operating times with the use of wireless technology. Miniaturization and freedom from tethered connectivity to a power source allows greater access to internal organs and other structures previously thought to be mechanically ‘off limits’. In more peripheral locations with highly mobile surfaces such as the face, where facial expression is so important, this feature is highly desirable to achieve improved pain control without compromising cosmesis.

References

1 Poon AS, O’Driscoll S, Meng TH: Optimal operating frequency in wireless power transmission for implantable devices. Conf Proc IEEE Eng Med Biol Soc 2007;2007:5674–5679.

2 Perryman LT, Larson P, Glaser J: Tissue depth study for a fully implantable, remotely powered and programmable wireless neural stimulator. NANS 2012: From Innovation to Reality, Las Vegas, 2012, p 4.

3 Narouze SL, Zakari A, Vydyanathan A: Ultrasound-guided placement of a permanent percutaneous femoral neurostimulator leads for the treatment of intractable femoral neuropathy. Pain Physician 2009; 12:E305–E308.

4 Weiner RL, Reed KL: Peripheral neurostimulation for control of intractable occipital neuralgia. Neuromodulation 1999;2:217–221.

5 Johnson MD, Burchiel KJ: Peripheral stimulation for treatment of trigeminal postherpetic neuralgia and trigeminal posttraumatic neuropathic pain: a pilot study. Neurosurgery 2004;55:135–142.

6 Slavin KV, Colpan ME, Munawar N, Wess C, Nersesyan H: Trigeminal and occipital peripheral nerve stimulation for craniofacial pain: a single-institution experience and review of the literature. Neurosurg Focus 2006;21:E5.

7 Slavin KV, Wess C: Trigeminal branch stimulation for intractable neuropathic pain: technical note. Neuromodulation 2005;8:7–13.

8 Management of temporomandibular disorders. National Institutes of Health Technology Assessment Conference Statement. J Am Dent Assoc 1996;127: 1595–1606.

9 Perryman L, Yearwood T: Peripheral nerve stimulation (PNS) for chronic craniofacial neuropathic pain with a novel wirelessly powered miniature implantable neurostimulator electrode array. Neuromodulation 2013;16:e168.

10 Perryman L, Yeung A: Targeted sensory nerve stimulation of the dorsal aspect of the dorsal root ganglion with a novel wireless injectable miniature stimulator for FBSS and sciatic back and leg pain. Neuromodulation 2013;16:e162.

11 Park JW, Nam HS, Cho SK, Jung HJ, Lee BJ, Park Y: Kambin’s triangle approach of lumbar transforaminal epidural injection with spinal stenosis. Ann Rehabil Med 2011;35:833–843.

12 Verrills P, Barnard A: The effect of electrode lead depth distribution on paresthesias in peripheral nerve field stimulation and occipital nerve stimulation. Neuromodulation 2011;14:566.

Thomas L. Yearwood, MD, PhD
Comprehensive Pain and Rehabilitation
4105 Hospital St., Suite 108
Pascagoula, MS 39581 (USA)
E-Mail tyearwood@nopaindr.com

Slavin KV (ed): Stimulation of the Peripheral Nervous System. The Neuromodulation Frontier.
Prog Neurol Surg. Basel, Karger, 2016, vol 29, pp 192–199 (DOI: 10.1159/000434671)

Sacral Neuromodulation for Genitourinary Problems

Mai Banakhar[a] · Magdy Hassouna[b]

[a]Faculty of Medicine, King Abdulaziz University, Jeddah, Saudi Arabia; [b]Department of Urology, Toronto Western Hospital, University Health Network, University of Toronto, Toronto, Ont., Canada

Abstract

Sacral neuromodulation (SNM) is a minimally invasive therapeutic option for many voiding dysfunction conditions. It is approved by the US FDA for refractory overactive bladder with and without incontinence and nonobstructive retention. Since SNM has shown a favorable response for these approved indications, other therapeutic applications have been proposed for various conditions such as painful bladder syndrome, chronic pelvic pain and neurological voiding dysfunction in both adult and pediatric age groups. SNM therapy with the most commonly used dedicated SNM device (InterStim) involves insertion of electrode(s) in the third and/or fourth sacral foramen next to the nerve root. The electrode is then connected to a battery-operated pulse generator. All patients need to have a test trial period before definitive device insertion. Here we discuss SNM therapy in functional urinary disorders and the technique of device insertion with the potential pitfalls.

History of Sacral Neuromodulation in Urology

The concept of nerve stimulation in urology was introduced as early as 1878 by Saxtorph who used intravesical electrical stimulation for urinary retention patient [1]. Tanagho, Schmidt and colleagues were the first to study the effects of sacral root stimulation [2–5]. In 1988, Schmidt [6] used the sacral nerve stimulation (SNS) device and described steps of the insertion procedure followed by several clinical trials for urinary incontinence and nonobstructive retention [7–9]. In 1997, SNS was approved by the

US FDA as a treatment for refractory overactive bladder (OAB) and urgency-frequency syndrome. Two years later, the use of SNM was approved for nonobstructive urinary retention.

Procedure and Technique

Before permanent implantation, all candidate patients for the therapy should undergo a stimulation test trial to determine patient eligibility for further SNS therapy. Test trials may be performed in an office – this is called percutaneous nerve evaluation (PNE) – or done as a staged implant that requires operating facilities. The patient is considered a candidate for SNM if he/she shows 50% or more subjective and/or objective improvement in one or more of the voiding parameters. Objective and/or symptomatic assessment is done by comparing the voiding diary filled out by the patient for 3–5 days before the test trial (baseline) with a second voiding diary filled out during the test trial period.

Percutaneous Nerve Evaluation Test

This is an outpatient, or office-based, test trial that is done under local anesthesia. During the procedure, the patient is positioned prone, and then the third and/or fourth sacral foramen is localized under fluoroscopy control and using a standard sterile technique. Local anesthetic (1% plain lidocaine solution) is injected in the skin overlying the 3rd sacral foramen down to the periosteum of the sacrum. With the help of an 18-gauge needle, cannulation of the appropriate sacral foramen is performed under fluoroscopy guidance. Electric monopolar stimulation of the third sacral root is done using an external generator starting with low-amplitude current delivered until the patient starts feeling a pulse or vibration sensation. Ideally, the sensation should be felt centrally at the perineum (scrotal/vaginal or rectal area). The procedure is done bilaterally and the site with more central sensation and lower threshold for sensation is selected for temporary electrode insertion. The electrode is then connected to an external pulse generator and the patient undergoes stimulation for 3–5 days during which time the patient is encouraged to fill in a voiding diary to document any changes in the voiding parameters such as number of voids per day, voided volume, degree of incontinence and postvoid residual volumes.

The main disadvantage of the PNE approach is the issue of electrode migration which may produce false-negative results. From our experience, patients who express loss or change of location of sensation require an X-ray of the sacrum that will help document migration. Such patients are offered either to repeat the PNE procedure or go for a 'staged' test trial. On the other hand, if patients express ≥50% improvement in one or more of the voiding parameters based on the voiding diary, they are considered good candidates for this modality and undergo the complete SNS device implantation.

Stage One Test Trial (Staged Procedure)

Patients who could not tolerate PNE and those who developed temporary electrode migration are offered the staged procedure. This procedure is done in the operating room under general anesthesia in the prone position using fluoroscopy guidance for foramen localization. The anesthesiologist is reminded to avoid any long-acting muscle relaxants which may negatively impact the motor response during the test stimulation of sacral nerve(s). The confirmation of the S3/S4 nerve root location is performed by virtue of the motor response detection. The typical motor responses for S3 stimulation is bellow action of the perineum (inwards contraction) and plantar flexion of the ipsilateral great toe. The unwanted motor responses are those of S2 such as anteroposterior motion of the anal sphincter, calf muscle contraction, plantar flexion of the foot and lateral rotation of the ipsilateral heel [10].

After radiographic and physiological confirmation of the third sacral nerve root, the needle is kept in position and a guide wire is introduced through the needle. A special dilator is introduced over the guide wire under fluoroscopic control that provides a lateral view of the sacrum. The dedicated tined lead electrode (Medtronic, Minneapolis, Minn., USA) is introduced via a dilator trough the appropriate sacral foramen (fig. 1, 2). Motor response testing is used to ensure the proper location of the electrode lead. After this, the electrode is attached to a long extension that is tunneled under the skin to the contralateral side where it is connected to the external pulse generator. The staged test offers a better trial than the PNE test since the tined electrode lead minimizes the risk of electrode migration and allows for a longer duration of stimulation (2 weeks compared to 3–5 days in PNE).

Among the limitations of the staged procedure is its dependence entirely on the motor response to select the appropriate location for the SNM rather than sensory response in PNE. Peters et al. [11] reported that sensory response assessment during the test trial reduced the reoperation rate from 43 to 0%. If the patient shows a favorable response, a second-stage procedure which includes the insertion of internal pulse generator (IPG) and its connection to the tined electrode lead is performed 2 weeks later in the operating room. In case of a poor response, the electrode is removed in the operating room as well.

Stage Two/Internal Pulse Generator Implantation

The implantation of IPG is done either as a second stage that follows a successful first stage, or as a part of the complete procedure along with insertion of a tined lead. A subcutaneous pocket is created under the skin of the buttock area of the patient's choice. It is important to maintain enough subcutaneous fat between the IPG and the surface of the skin in order to avoid any discomfort at the site of the implant. The quadripolar tined electrode is tunneled subcutaneously toward the pocket area and connected to the IPG. The wound is irrigated with antibiotic solution in sterile water

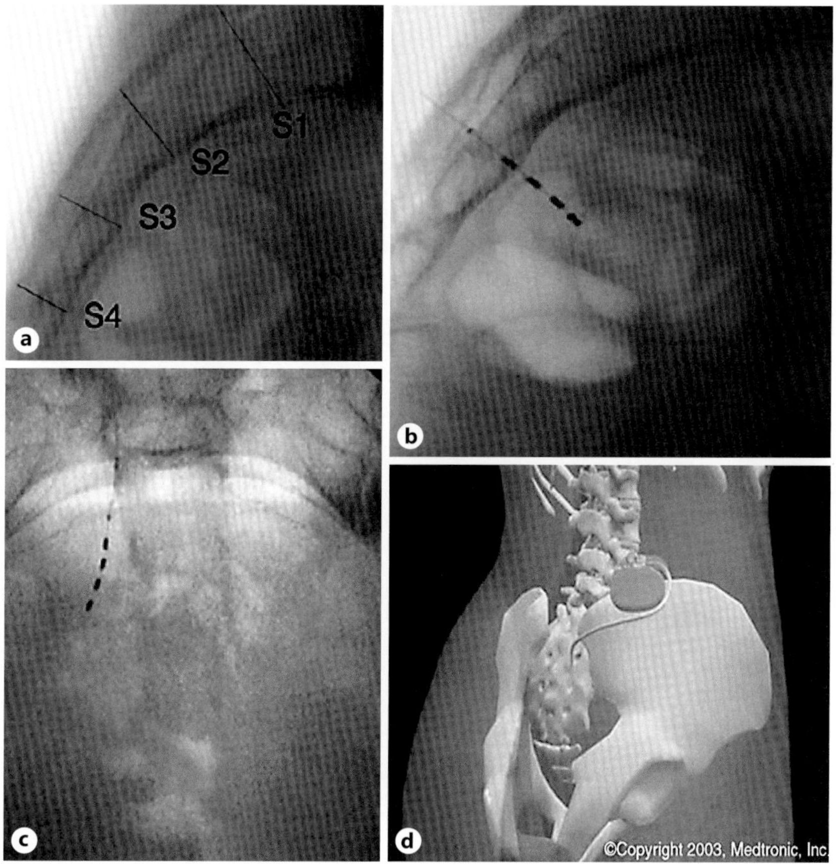

Fig. 1. a Lateral sacral radiograph with foramen localization. **b** Lateral radiograph for position of tined quadripolar electrode. **c** Anteroposterior view of electrode position. **d** Electrode and generator location. Reprinted with permission of Medtronic Inc.

(not saline) to reduce any electronic malfunction of the connections. The programming of the IPG is performed while the patients are fully awake in the postoperative period to help in the selection of their preferred program of stimulation.

Sacral Neuromodulation Therapy

SNM is approved for refractory OAB, frequency-urgency syndrome and nonobstructive retention [12–17].

Off-Label Uses of Sacral Nerve Stimulation

Neurological Conditions. Multiple sclerosis and spinal cord injury patients have shown benefit from SNM therapy in multiple reports [18–20].

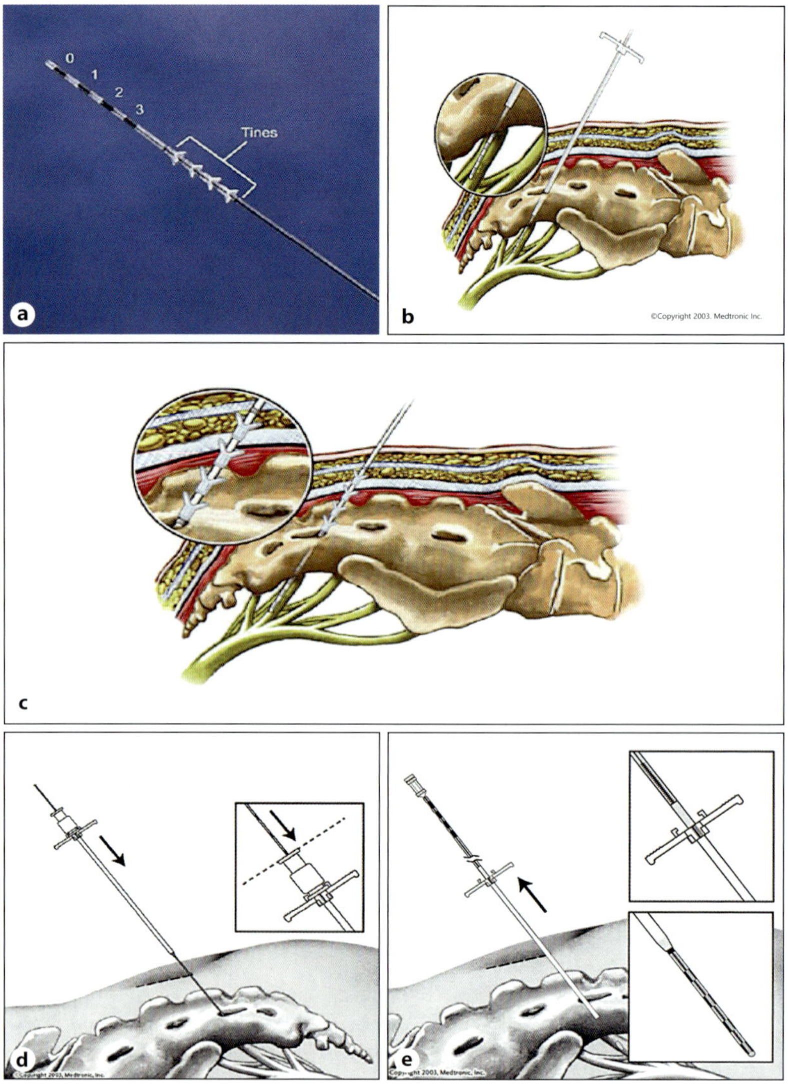

Fig. 2. a Quadripolar tined lead. **b–e** Steps of electrode insertion. **b**, **d** Dilator and guide wire. **c**, **e** The electrode is introduced through the dilator. Reprinted with permission of Medtronic Inc.

Interstitial Cystitis and Genitourinary Pain. Several reports have shown symptom control in interstitial cystitis patients and pelvic pain with improved quality of life and decreased narcotic requirement [11, 21–25]. Patients with chronic genitourinary pain have shown pain control while on SNM therapy. For chronic epididymitis, chronic epididymo-orchalgia and chronic nonbacterial prostatitis, Feler et al. [26] reported 75% pain control in a group of 44 patients.

Effect of SNM on Sexual Function. Few reports claim beneficial effect of SNM on sexual function in both male and female patients using IEF-5 and the Female Sexual

Function Index (FSFI). The majority of these reports were assessing the sexual effect in patients with voiding dysfunction [27–30].
SNM Use in Children. Humphreys et al. [31] reported the use of SNM in the pediatric age group with symptom improvement of 73–75% in urinary retention and incontinence while 83% improved in terms of nocturnal enuresis.

Contraindications to Sacral Neuromodulation
SNM is contraindicated in sacral agenesis as the bony deformity makes the procedure difficult. Other contraindications include the patient's inability to perform the programming (mental or psychiatric reasons) and unsuccessful stimulation test trial.

Controversial Issues in Sacral Neuromodulation Therapy

A few issues have arisen with the increasing adoption of SNM therapy.
Continuous versus Intermittent Stimulation. There are no reports in the literature that compare the effect of continuous versus intermittent use of stimulation on the outcome of the therapy itself. However, there is a tendency to prolong the battery life with the intermittent stimulation.
Unilateral versus Bilateral Stimulation. There is no clinical evidence of any additional beneficial effect of bilateral versus unilateral stimulation of the sacral nerve roots. In our center, we prefer to reserve the second side stimulation to those who lose benefit or develop decreased efficacy of unilateral SNM.
MRI. MRI is not allowed in patients undergoing SNM. The current recommendation is to avoid pelvic MRI until a new generation of MRI-friendly devices becomes commercially available [32].
Pregnancy. Most of the patients implanted for SNM are young females of childbearing age. There is no clear guideline about its use in pregnancy; however, there are published cases that reported safe delivery of healthy babies. It is probably safer for the female patient to plan her pregnancy and to keep her device turned off during the first trimester of gestation.
Intravesical Botulinum Toxin A. SNM and the use of intravesical botulinum toxin A have been studied in a limited number of studies. According to Smits et al. [33], the previous usage of Botox A in patients with OAB does not preclude the success of SNM to control their symptoms. In a study about decision analysis, it was found that both SNM and intravesical Botox A are both reasonable and effective strategies with similar outcomes [34].
Posterior Tibial Nerve Stimulation. This has been applied with success in patients with OAB. The limiting factor of posterior tibial nerve stimulation being a 'sustainable' therapy is the lack of a commercially available and implantable device. Currently, posterior tibial nerve stimulation, which requires 12 weekly sessions, is offered as a temporary therapy to control OAB [35].

References

1 Madersbacher H: Conservative therapy of neurogenic disorders of micturition (in German). Urologe A 1999;38:24–29.

2 Heine JP, Schmidt RA, Tanagho EA: Intraspinal sacral root stimulation for controlled micturition. Invest Urol 1977;15:78–82.

3 Schmidt RA, Bruschini H, Tanagho EA: Urinary bladder and sphincter responses to stimulation of dorsal and ventral sacral roots. Invest Urol 1979;16: 300–304.

4 Tanagho EA, Schmidt RA: Bladder pacemaker: scientific basis and clinical future. Urology 1982;20: 614–619.

5 Tanagho E: Neural stimulation for bladder control. Semin Neurol 1988;8:170–173.

6 Schmidt RA: Application of neurostimulation in urology. Neurourol Urodyn 1988;7:585–592.

7 Tanagho EA: Electrical stimulation. J Am Geriatr Soc 1990;38:352–355.

8 Tanagho EA: Neuromodulation in the management of voiding dysfunction in children. J Urol 1992;148: 655–657.

9 Shaker HS, Hassouna M: Sacral root neuromodulation in idiopathic nonobstructive chronic urinary retention. J Urol 1998;159:1476–1478.

10 Bullock TL, Siegel SW: Sacral neuromodulation for voiding dysfunction; in Statskin D (ed): Atlas of Bladder Disease. Philadelphia, Springer, 2010, pp 1–12.

11 Peters KM, Carey JM, Konstandt DB: Sacral neuromodulation for the treatment of refractory interstitial cystitis: outcomes based on technique. Int Urogynecol J Pelvic Floor Dysfunct 2003;14:223–228.

12 Abrams P, Andersson KE, Birder L, Brubaker L, Cardozo L, Chapple C, Cottenden A, Davila W, de Ridder D, Dmochowski R, Drake M, Dubeau C, Fry C, Hanno P, Smith JH, Herschorn S, Hosker G, Kelleher C, Koelbl H, Khoury S, Madoff R, Milsom I, Moore K, Newman D, Nitti V, Norton C, Nygaard I, Payne C, Smith A, Staskin D, Tekgul S, Thuroff J, Tubaro A, Vodusek D, Wein A, Wyndaele JJ; Members of Committees; Fourth International Consultation on Incontinence: Fourth International Consultation on Incontinence Recommendations of the International Scientific Committee: evaluation and treatment of urinary incontinence, pelvic organ prolapse, and fecal incontinence. Neurourol Urodyn 2010;29:213–240.

13 Knüpfer S, Hamann M, Naumann CM, Melchior D, Jünemann KP: Therapy-refractory overactive bladder: alternative treatment approaches (in German). Urologe A 2011;50:806–809.

14 Apostolidis A: Neuromodulation for intractable OAB. Neurourol Urodyn 2011;30:766–770.

15 Al-Shaiji TF, Banakhar M, Hassouna MM: Pelvic electrical neuromodulation for the treatment of overactive bladder symptoms. Adv Urol 2011;2011: 757454.

16 Abrams P, Blaivas JG, Fowler CJ, Fourcroy JL, Macdiarmid SA, Siegel SW, Van Kerrebroeck P: The role of neuromodulation in the management of urinary urge incontinence. BJU Int 2003;91:355–359.

17 Siegel SW, Catanzaro F, Dijkema HE, Elhilali MM, Fowler CJ, Gajewski JB, Hassouna MM, Janknegt RA, Jonas U, van Kerrebroeck PE, Lycklama a Nijeholt AA, Oleson KA, Schmidt RA: Long-term results of a multicenter study on sacral nerve stimulation for treatment of urinary urge incontinence, urgency-frequency and retention. Urology 2000;56(6 suppl 1): 87–91.

18 Ruud Bosch JL, Groen J: Treatment of refractory urge urinary incontinence with sacral spinal nerve stimulation in multiple sclerosis patients. Lancet 1996;348:717–719.

19 Hassouna MM, Siegel SW, Nÿeholt AA, Elhilali MM, van Kerrebroeck PE, Das AK, Gajewski JB, Janknegt RA, Rivas DA, Dijkema H, Milam DF, Oleson KA, Schmidt RA: Sacral neuromodulation in the treatment of urgency-frequency symptoms: a multicenter study on efficacy and safety. J Urol 2000;163:1849–1854.

20 Vastenholt JM, Snoek GJ, Buschman HP, van der Aa HE, Alleman ER, Ijzerman MJ: A 7-year follow-up of sacral anterior root stimulation for bladder control in patients with spinal cord injury: quality of life and users' experiences. Spinal Cord 2003;41:397–402.

21 Lukban JC, Whitmore KE, Sant GR: Current management of interstitial cystitis. Urol Clin North Am 2002;29:649–660.

22 Everaert K, Devulder J, De Muynck M, Stockman S, Depaepe H, De Looze D, Van Buyten J, Oosterlinck W: The pain cycle: implications for the diagnosis and treatment of pelvic pain syndromes. Int Urogynecol J Pelvic Floor Dysfunct 2001;12:9–14.

23 Siegel S, Paszkiewicz E, Kirkpatrick C, Hinkel B, Oleson K: Sacral nerve stimulation in patients with chronic intractable pelvic pain. J Urol 2001;166: 1742–1745.

24 Comiter CV: Sacral neuromodulation for the symptomatic treatment of refractory interstitial cystitis: a prospective study. J Urol 2003;169:1369–1373.

25 Peters KM, Konstandt D: Sacral neuromodulation decreases narcotic requirement in refractory interstitial cystitis. BJU Int 2004;93:777–779.

26 Feler CA, Whitworth LA, Fernandez J: Sacral neuromodulation for chronic pain conditions. Anesthesiol Clin North America 2003;21:785–795.

27 Lombardi G, Mondaini N, Macchiarella A, Cilotti A, Del Popolo G: Clinical female sexual outcome after sacral neuromodulation implant for lower urinary tract symptom (LUTS). J Sex Med 2008;5:1411–1417.
28 Lombardi G, Mondaini N, Giubilei G, Macchiarella A, Lecconi F, Del Popolo G: Sacral neuromodulation for lower urinary tract dysfunction and impact on erectile function. J Sex Med 2008;5:2135–2140.
29 Pauls RN, Marinkovic SP, Silva WA, Rooney CM, Kleeman SD, Karram MM: Effects of sacral neuromodulation on female sexual function. Int Urogynecol J Pelvic Floor Dysfunct 2007;18:391–395.
30 Banakhar M, Gazwani Y, Kelini ME, Al-Shaiji T, Hassouna M: Effect of sacral neuromodulation on female sexual function and quality of life: are they correlated? Can Urol Assoc J 2014;8:E762–E767.
31 Humphreys MR, Vandersteen DR, Slezak JM, Hollatz P, Smith CA, Smith JE, Reinberg YE: Preliminary results of sacral neuromodulation in 23 children. J Urol 2006;176:2227–2231.
32 Elkelini MS, Hassouna MM: Safety of MRI at 1.5Tesla in patients with implanted acral nerve neurostimulator. Eur Urol 2006;50:311–316.
33 Smits MA, Oerlemans D, Marcelissen TA, Van Kerrebroek PE, De Wachter SG: Sacral neuromodulation in patients with idiopathic OAB after initial botulinum toxin therapy. J Urol 2013;90:2148–2152.
34 Shepherd JP, Louder JL, Leug WW, Smith KJ: InterStim sacral neuromodulation and Botox botulinum-A intradetrusor injections for refractory urge urinary incontinence: a decision analysis comparing outcomes including efficacy and complications. Female Pelvic Med Reconstr Surg 2011;17:199–203.
35 Gupta P, Ehlert MJ, Sirls LT, Peters KM: Percutaneous tibial nerve stimulation and sacral neuromodulation: an update. Current Urol Rep 2015;16:479.

Prof. Magdy Hassouna, MD, PhD
Department of Urology, Toronto Western Hospital
University Health Network, University of Toronto
399 Bathurst Street
Toronto, ON M5T 2S8 (Canada)
E-Mail magdy.hassouna@uhn.on.ca

Slavin KV (ed): Stimulation of the Peripheral Nervous System. The Neuromodulation Frontier.
Prog Neurol Surg. Basel, Karger, 2016, vol 29, pp 200–212 (DOI: 10.1159/000434672)

Sacral Nerve Stimulation in the Treatment of Bowel Disorders

Johan Nordenstam[a] · Anne-Marie Boller[b] · Anders Mellgren[a]

[a]Division of Colon and Rectal Surgery, Department of Surgery, University of Illinois at Chicago, and [b]Department of Surgery, Northwestern University Feinberg School of Medicine, Chicago, Ill., USA

Abstract

Defecation problems occur in patients of all ages, but are more prevalent in the elderly, postpartum women, and patients with chronic and debilitating medical conditions. Most of the time, these problems respond to medical therapy and nonsurgical options, but it is not uncommon for patients to require surgical intervention. Sacral nerve stimulation (SNS) presents an alternative for patients with bowel dysfunction combining proven therapeutic benefits and limited surgical risks. Here we describe the common indications for SNS, patient selection, technical details of the procedure, published outcomes, and complications that can arise. Based on our review, SNS is an effective treatment option for fecal incontinence and may reduce the patients' clinical symptoms and help restore their quality of life. Future research studies may expand the role of this modality for other bowel disorders.

Defecation problems are common in the general population, with an increased prevalence in the elderly, postpartum women, institutionalized patients, and those with chronic, debilitating medical disorders [1–3]. Medical therapy or a nonsurgical option, including pelvic floor exercises with biofeedback, is sufficient in some patients. Surgical sphincter repair or repair of rectal prolapse will help some patients, but others will improve only temporarily or not at all after surgical repair. Additionally, many patients with fecal incontinence do not have a localized injury amenable to surgical repair. Sacral nerve stimulation (SNS) is an effective treatment alternative for patients with bowel dysfunction with limited surgical risks and proven therapeutic benefits.

Fecal Incontinence

Fecal incontinence, involuntary loss of control of feces, is a handicapping condition that is associated with significant social embarrassment. The reported prevalence varies widely in the literature (2–21%) [2, 4–7]; in postmenopausal women, the incidence rate for handicapping fecal incontinence symptoms is about 10%. Fecal incontinence symptoms may be the result of a variety of reasons, including childbirth, neurologic condition, rectal prolapse, gastrointestinal disorders affecting stool consistency, etc.

Therapy of fecal incontinence usually starts with dietary, lifestyle modifications, and medical therapy. The addition of fiber supplements and/or medications that modifies stool consistency, i.e. loperamide, may improve bowel control.

Pelvic floor exercises with biofeedback are often a beneficial addition. The biofeedback therapist educates the patient regarding pelvic floor muscle control, recognition of sensory thresholds, and optimal pelvic floor habits [8–11]. Biofeedback may be beneficial in treating patients with varying types of fecal incontinence, but patients with urge incontinence usually respond better than patients with passive fecal incontinence (leakage without forewarning) [12]. Interestingly, the effect of the biofeedback component varies between studies. In one study [13], it was found that biofeedback did not offer any additional benefit to patients when compared to those offered standard care (advice on diet, fluids, evacuation techniques, bowel training, and antidiarrheal medications). In a more recent study, Heymen et al. [14], found that biofeedback was more effective than pelvic floor exercises alone.

Patients with a localized anal sphincter injury, usually after childbirth or previous surgery, may benefit from an overlapping sphincteroplasty with repair of the injured segment of the muscle. This procedure is relatively straightforward and usually requires a short hospital stay. A majority of patients develop a limited localized infection with a superficial wound dehiscence. This usually heals with conservative management and short-term results may be satisfactory in up to two thirds of patients. However, results tend to deteriorate over time and are less satisfactory at longer follow-up [15, 16].

Patients with a weak or disrupted internal anal sphincter may benefit from treatment with injectable biomaterials and success has been demonstrated in both the short and long term [17, 18]. For patients with gross, passive fecal seepage, the usage of anal plugs has been utilized with variable success. The anal plugs can be difficult to tolerate, but available data suggests that they are useful in selected patient groups [19].

Patients with significant fecal incontinence who do not have a localized sphincter injury may benefit from a neosphincter procedure, such as a muscular transposition or placement of an artificial sphincter. Dynamic graciloplasty involves the transposition of the gracilis muscle to the perineum, where it encircles the anal canal. The muscle is artificially stimulated with an external electric generator. Several studies have reported clinical improvement of incontinence symptoms [20, 21], but the complication rate is high. The use of dynamic graciloplasty is limited and the procedure is not available in the United States [22–24].

Another option is placement of an artificial bowel sphincter, which is an approved treatment option. Some reports have shown satisfactory results with good functional outcome and a significant improvement in patients' quality of life [25, 26]. Complication rates, especially in inexperienced hands, are high and morbidity includes infection, skin erosion, and other issues that may require explantation [27]. A new alternative to artificial bowel sphincter, is a magnetic sphincter (FENIX™ Continence Restoration System; Torax Medical, Shoreview, Minn., USA) [28, 29]. This method is not yet approved in the United States, but has shown promise in early limited trials and is currently undergoing further assessment in Europe.

Patients who have failed other treatment alternatives are candidates for a diverting colostomy. This operation is unpopular among patients, although it offers them an increased level of autonomy.

Constipation

Constipation can be related to slow transit through the colon or difficult evacuation associated with outlet obstruction. Studies have shown that 3–15% of the general population are affected by constipation [30, 31]. In a self-reporting questionnaire, 1,833 eligible residents 65 years or older were surveyed in Minnesota. The study reported an overall age- and gender-adjusted prevalence of 40.1% for both functional and outlet obstruction constipation [32]. Outlet delay, but not functional constipation, was more frequent in women, while functional constipation was associated with advancing age.

As with fecal incontinence, treatment for constipation begins with medical management and lifestyle changes, such as dietary changes, including fibers and adequate daily water intake, laxatives, suppositories, and enemas. Biofeedback has been successfully utilized in the treatment of idiopathic constipation and may offer improvement in constipation symptoms and decreased need for laxative usage [33].

Some patients will continue to have persistent symptoms despite conservative therapy and selected patients may benefit from surgical intervention. A few patients with severe slow-transit constipation may benefit from a subtotal colectomy with ileorectal anastomosis, but it is not always successful [34]. Patients may have persistent symptoms or difficulties with diarrhea and some patients report abdominal pain and/or bloating [35]. Some patients with outlet obstruction may respond favorably to repair of a potential rectocele. Selected patients with constipation may also respond favorably to new surgical procedures, such as laparoscopic ventral rectopexy [36–38] or stapled transanal rectal resection [39].

Development of Sacral Nerve Stimulation for Bowel Disorders

SNS was initially developed for use in urinary dysfunction [40]. The first stimulators were implanted in 1981 for urinary urge incontinence and nonobstructive urinary retention [41]. Since that time, several additional clinical benefits have been discovered, including reestablishment of pelvic floor muscle awareness, resolution of pelvic floor muscle tension and pain, symptomatic improvement of vestibulitis and vulvodynia, decrease in bladder pain (interstitial cystitis), and normalization of bowel function [42].

In 1995, Matzel et al. [43] were the first to report the benefits of SNS in fecal incontinence. Initially, SNS treatment for fecal incontinence was restricted to patients with an intact external sphincter. However, over time it has become evident that SNS may also be beneficial in patients with sphincter injuries, constipation, and other bowel disorders [44–52].

Mechanism of Action of Sacral Nerve Stimulation for Bowel Disorders

The exact mechanism behind SNS is unclear. SNS applies a low-amplitude electrical current to a sacral nerve through an electrode which is placed through a corresponding sacral foramen. The stimulation of the sacral nerves may lead to recruitment of the pelvic floor musculature and pelvic organs, leading to improvement in pelvic floor function [53–55].

There is heterogeneity of data pertaining to the effects of SNS on anorectal and colonic functions. The initial hypothesis that the mechanism of SNS is primarily peripheral motor neurostimulation is not supported by the majority of more recent studies. SNS effects extend beyond the anorectum and therefore it appears that the influence of SNS on anorectal function occurs at a pelvic afferent or central level [56]. The S2–S4 nerves stimulated during SNS contain somatic fibers from the pudendal nerve, afferent sensory fibers from the anal sphincter/pelvic floor, and autonomic fibers primarily from the pelvic nerves. Activation of afferent neurons is suggested by EMG studies and anal sphincter contraction observed during SNS can be the result of an afferent-mediated response [57].

Sacral Nerve Stimulation Implant Technique for Bowel Disorders

SNS for bowel disorders is usually applied in a similar way as for urinary dysfunction and a two-stage approach is normally used. The effect is assessed using a bowel diary, which is usually filled out before the first stage (baseline diary) and between the first and second stage (level of symptoms with SNS applied). A reduction of 50% of fecal incontinence symptoms is usually required to proceed to implant.

The first stage can be accomplished with a temporary peripheral nerve evaluation lead ('basic evaluation') or with implantation of a long-term lead that is connected to

Table 1. Available neurostimulators and leads

External neurostimulators	
	Medtronic Model 3625
	Medtronic Model 3531
Implanted neurostimulators	
	Medtronic Model 3023
	Medtronic Model 3058 (InterStim II)
Tined leads	
	Medtronic Model 3093
	Medtronic Model 3089

an externalized extension ('advanced evaluation'). The temporary peripheral nerve evaluation lead is usually trialed for 7 days before it is removed, while the long-term lead can be trialed for up to 2 weeks. The procedure is usually performed under local anesthesia and sedation. With the patient in prone position, several of the S2–S4 foramina are cannulated and tested for optimal response [58, 59]. Fluoroscopy is routinely used to confirm the position of the electrode(s). The best response is frequently found in the S3 foramen; the typical S3 response is characterized by plantar flexion of the patient's ipsilateral first toe and the 'bellows response' of the pelvic floor [58, 59]. A portable external stimulator is utilized to stimulate the implanted electrode during the 1–2 weeks of testing [59].

The second stage is completed in the operating room under local or general anesthesia. The procedure is performed with the patient in the prone position. If the first stage was accomplished with a long-term lead ('advanced evaluation'), the percutaneous extension cable is removed and a generator is implanted in the gluteal region. If the first stage was accomplished with a temporary peripheral nerve evaluation lead ('basic evaluation'), the patient needs to undergo renewed testing to find an optimal lead location and thereafter a long-term lead and a generator are implanted.

The implantable pulse generator can be activated and controlled by using an external programmer or via a hand-held device [59]. Battery life for the implantable pulse generator depends on the amount of energy needed for stimulation. For the new smaller second generation of implantable pulse generators (InterStim II; Medtronic, Minneapolis, Minn., USA), battery life is estimated at 3–5 years, depending on the strength of stimulation used. Currently available devices are listed in table 1 and illustrated in figures 1 and 2.

Results of Sacral Nerve Stimulation in Fecal Incontinence

Several studies have investigated the efficacy of SNS in fecal incontinence. The majority of the studies are case series from specialized centers whose patients had failed conservative management and experienced at least one episode of fecal incontinence

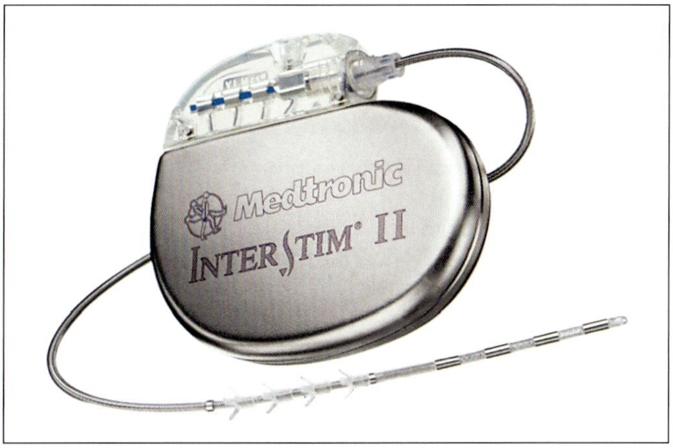

Fig. 1. InterStim II 3058 (courtesy of Medtronic Inc.).

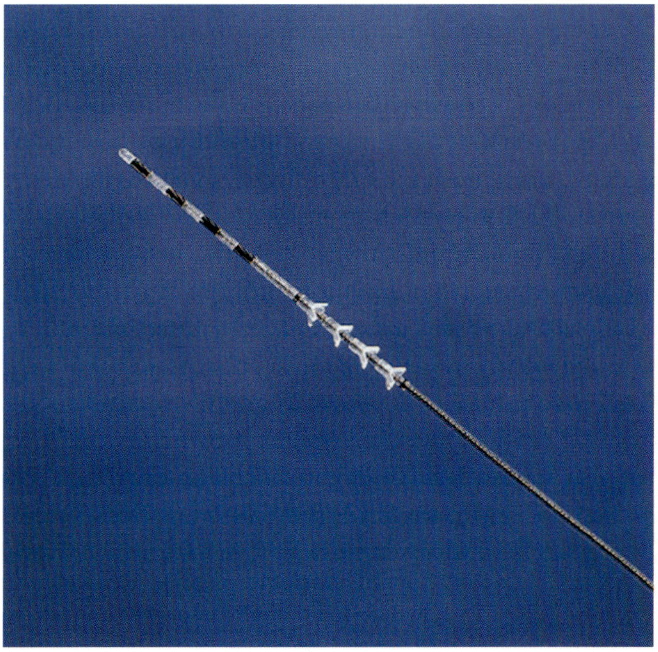

Fig. 2. Tined Lead Model 3889 (courtesy of Medtronic Inc.).

each week [54, 55]. Table 2 summarizes common inclusion and exclusion criteria in different studies. An intact external sphincter was required in most initial studies and common exclusion criteria included congenital anorectal malformations, untreated external rectal prolapse, chronic bowel disease with diarrhea, neurologic disease, and increased risk of infection or bleeding.

SNS is an effective treatment for the majority of patients in most studies [54, 55]. Approximately 80–90% of patients usually qualify for a permanent implant [44, 54, 55, 60, 61]. The majority (70–90%) of included patients are female and the follow-up period ranges from 1 month to more than 8 years [54, 55].

Table 2. Common patient selection criteria for SNS

Inclusion criteria
Signed informed consent
Age 18–75 years
One or more episode of fecal incontinence per week (assessed by means of a baseline bowel habit diary)
Intact external sphincter with or without previous repair
Failed conservative therapy (antidiarrheal and biofeedback)
Able to fill in questionnaires and attend clinics
Exclusion criteria
Congenital anorectal malformations
Rectal surgery within previous 12 months (within 24 months for cancer)
Present external rectal prolapse
Chronic bowel diseases (e.g. inflammatory bowel disease)
Chronic diarrhea, unmanageable by diet or drugs
Altered bowel habit associated with abdominal pain
Stoma present
Neurological diseases (e.g. diabetic neuropathy, multiple sclerosis, or Parkinson's disease)
Bleeding complications
Pregnancy
Anatomical limitations preventing placement of an electrode
Skin disease risking infection (e.g. pyoderma, pilonidal sinus)
Psychiatric or physical inability to comply with study protocol
Patients for whom information was not available in a language understood by the patient

Improvements in several continence parameters have been registered. In one study, participants increased the ability to defer defecation from a median of 1 min to 10 min [54, 55]. More than 75% of the study participants reported a more than 50% improvement in continence episodes, and 41–75% of patients reported complete continence to liquid and solid stool [44, 54, 55, 60, 61]. A moderate increase in anal pressures and improved sensory function to rectal distension have been reported in some studies.

Leroi et al. [62] studied 34 patients following SNS for fecal incontinence. Patients were randomized, following implantation of the electrode, to 'on' or 'off' stimulation for periods of 1 month. While patients were blinded, they chose which period they preferred. Without unblinding the study, the patients then continued in the preferred mode for 3 additional months. Participants receiving stimulation experienced a significant reduction in symptoms compared with the 'off' group. Stimulation led to a decrease in fecal incontinence episodes and symptom severity, and improved quality of life scores. Vaizey et al. [63] reported similar results in a study with similar design, but their study included only 2 participants.

In one study, Tjandra and colleagues [59, 64] randomized patients with fecal incontinence to receive either SNS or the best supportive therapy including pelvic floor exercises, bulking agents, and dietary modification. The study arms were evenly randomized and patients were followed for a period of 12 months. Patients randomized to receive SNS appreciated a significant improvement in quality of life scores, and incontinence episodes and benefits were sustained throughout the follow-up period, while those treated with supportive therapy did not experience any significant benefit from their treatment regimen.

The North American SNS Trial [65] is one of the largest and best controlled studies evaluating the effect of SNS for the treatment of fecal incontinence. This FDA controlled trial recruited 133 patients who underwent test stimulation with a 90% success rate. One hundred and twenty patients received chronic implantation. At 12 months, 83% of the subjects achieved therapeutic success and 41% achieved 100% continence. Therapeutic success was 85% at 24 months.

SNS can maintain a persistent clinical benefit in the long term. In an assessment of the medium- and long-term results of SNS for fecal incontinence, the North American multicenter study found that the therapeutic effect and improved quality of life for fecal incontinence were maintained [66, 67]. Seventy-six patients were followed for a minimum of 5 years and 89% of these patients had ≥50% improvement of their fecal incontinence, while 36% had complete continence. A group from St. Mark's recently evaluated their long-term outcome of SNS for fecal incontinence [68]. They evaluated the results of chronic SNS in 23 patients who had gone through more than 8 years of therapy. Data were collected prospectively by the use of bowel habit diaries and St. Mark's continence scores. Over a median follow-up of 114 months, full continence was maintained in 12 out of 23 patients, and 2 patients lost efficacy at 48 and 60 months after permanent implantation. A Danish study evaluated the outcome of SNS at 5 years after implantation and identified predictors of sustained efficacy [69]. In this study, 60 out of 101 patients reported a favorable outcome (43% on intention to treat and 56% per protocol). Age was a negative predictive factor for sustained efficacy. Positive predictors for sustained efficacy included improvement of urge incontinence episodes during the test phase and improvement of incontinence scores at 6 months.

Several studies have specifically evaluated possible predictors of success of SNS. After implantation, 10–25% of patients failed to respond to the SNS for unknown reasons. It has been difficult to identify predictors of success, besides the improvement during test stimulation. In a French multicenter study [70], 200 consecutive patients underwent permanent implantation for fecal incontinence. While fecal incontinence severity and quality of life scores were improved, the clinical outcome was not affected by age, gender, duration of symptoms, baseline quality of life, main causes of fecal incontinence, anorectal manometry, or endoanal ultrasound results. Only loose stool consistency and low stimulation intensity were associated with favorable outcomes. In a smaller more recent study, Roy et al. [71] could not identify any factors that would predict the 3-year clinical outcome of SNS based on pre- and postimplantation assessments.

The strength of SNS stimulation can be below the sensory threshold. In a blinded crossover study evaluating the effect of SNS at or below the sensory threshold in 18 patients, it was found that SNS was equally effective at different stimulation settings and patient satisfaction was high at all amplitude settings [72].

SNS can be an effective modality even if other neuromodulatory modalities, such as percutaneous tibial nerve stimulation, fail. Percutaneous tibial nerve stimulation is a new treatment method using temporary electric stimulation of the tibial nerve; it is usually administered in an outpatient setting by specially trained nurses. Patients undergo weekly sessions followed by 'tapering' treatments. In a recent study, Hotouras et al. [73] demonstrated that SNS is still effective in a majority of patients who did not gain an adequate therapeutic benefit from percutaneous tibial nerve stimulation.

Sacral Nerve Stimulation in the Treatment of Other Bowel Disorders

Dinning et al. [52] were the first to show that SNS can increase antegrade colonic propagating waves in patients with slow-transit constipation. Recently, the same group compared suprasensory SNS, subsensory SNS, and 'sham SNS' in patients with slow-transit constipation [74]. They concluded that only suprasensory SNS induced colonic propagating sequences as compared to 'sham'. Contrary to this, in a study from 2010 involving 62 patients, Kamm et al. [75] found a significant increase in evacuations per week as well as a decreased time spent toileting as a result of SNS in patients with chronic constipation. A recent systematic review included 13 studies evaluating SNS as a treatment for chronic constipation [76]. Three of these studies involved pediatric patients and 10 involved adults. Eighty-seven percent of patients treated by permanent SNS showed improvement in symptoms at the 28-month follow-up. SNS appears to be an effective therapy for chronic constipation, but significant research needs to be completed before the appropriate role of SNS in patients with idiopathic constipation can be determined. Long-term studies will be needed to more fully elucidate the benefits and adverse effects, and standardized outcome measures need to be adopted to make studies comparable.

New applications of the SNS technology continue to arise. Recently, Dudding et al. [51] reported on applying SNS to patients with functional anorectal pain in the absence of an organic cause. SNS has also been suggested as a therapy for patients with irritable bowel syndrome (IBS). In a recent crossover study, Fassov et al. [77] demonstrated that SNS significantly reduces IBS symptoms and improves quality of life in some patients. Diarrhea-predominant or mixed-IBS patients were randomized to have the stimulator 'on' or 'off' for 1 month, and then the opposite for another month. Investigators and patients were not informed of the setting. IBS-specific symptoms and quality of life were assessed through bowel diaries and validated questionnaires. IBS-specific symptoms and quality-of-life scores improved significantly during stimulation.

Sacral Nerve Stimulation Complications

Clinical studies of SNS in fecal incontinence have demonstrated limited morbidity. In 6 clinical series reviewed by Jarrett et al. [54], 10 adverse events were reported after temporary lead placement, with the lead dislodgement occurring in 9 patients and superficial skin infection in 1. After permanent implantation, 19 adverse events were noted in 6 studies. Again, the most frequent complications were lead migration (n = 8), pain problems (n = 6), wound infections (n = 3), and wound dehiscence (n = 1). No urinary or sexual dysfunction was reported.

In the FDA-controlled North American SNS Trial, Wexner et al. [65] reported a large number of adverse events. Investigators were required to report all adverse events over the course of the study and vast majority were mild and self-limiting. Among 120 patients, there were 5 events of implant site pain, 2 hematomas, 3 lead fractures, 2 lead migrations or dislodgements, and 2 episodes of extremity pain. Thirteen patients (11%) experienced implant site infection, of which 7 patients needed surgical intervention.

Faucheron et al. [78] evaluated 87 patients to investigate the causes of surgical revision following SNS. Thirty-six patients needed surgical revision and the most common causes included partial or total loss of clinical efficacy (n = 9), adverse stimulation with pain (n = 7), infection (n = 4), dysfunction owing to impedance increase of the system (n = 4), electrode displacement (n = 2), and electrode breakage (n = 2).

Conclusions

SNS is an effective treatment option for fecal incontinence and may reduce patients' clinical symptoms and help restore their quality of life. Future research studies may expand the role of SS for other bowel disorders.

References

1 Thomas TM, Ruff C, Karran O, Mellows S, Meade TW: Study of the prevalence and management of patients with faecal incontinence in old people's homes. Community Med 1987;9:232–237.

2 Nelson R, Norton N, Cautley E, Furner S: Community-based prevalence of anal incontinence. JAMA 1995;274:559–561.

3 Chassagne P, Landrin I, Neveu C, Czernichow P, Bouaniche M, Doucet J, Denis P, Bercoff E: Fecal incontinence in the institutionalized elderly: incidence, risk factors, and prognosis. Am J Med 1999; 106:185–190.

4 Ho KS, Ho YH: Diagnosing and managing faecal incontinence. Ann Acad Med Singapore 1999;28:417–423.

5 Kalantar JS, Howell S, Talley NJ: Prevalence of faecal incontinence and associated risk factors; an underdiagnosed problem in the Australian community? Med J Aust 2002;176:54–57.

6 Siproudhis L, Pigot F, Godeberge P, Damon H, Soudan D, Bigard MA: Defecation disorders: a French population survey. Dis Colon Rectum 2006;49:219–227.

7 Brown HW, Wexner SD, Segall MM, Brezoczky KL, Lukacz ES: Accidental bowel leakage in the mature women's health study: prevalence and predictors. Int J Clin Pract 2012;66:1101–1108.
8 Madoff RD: Surgical treatment options for fecal incontinence. Gastroenterology 2004;126:S48–S54.
9 Hosker G, Norton C, Brazzelli M: Electrical stimulation for faecal incontinence in adults. Cochrane Database Syst Rev 2007;2:CD001310.
10 Norton C, Hosker G, Brazzelli M: Biofeedback and/or sphincter exercises for the treatment of faecal incontinence in adults. Cochrane Database Syst Rev 2000;2:CD002111.
11 Norton C, Cody JD, Hosker G: Biofeedback and/or sphincter exercises for the treatment of faecal incontinence in adults. Cochrane Database Syst Rev 2006; 3:CD002111.
12 Norton C, Kamm MA: Outcome of biofeedback for faecal incontinence. Br J Surg 1999;86:1159–1163.
13 Norton C, Chelvanayagam S, Wilson-Barnett J, Redfern S, Kamm MA: Randomized controlled trial of biofeedback for fecal incontinence. Gastroenterology 2003;125:1320–1329.
14 Heymen S, Scarlett Y, Jones K, Ringel Y, Drossman D, Whitehead WE: Randomized controlled trial shows biofeedback to be superior to pelvic floor exercises for fecal incontinence. Dis Colon Rectum 2009;52:1730–1737.
15 Malouf AJ, Norton CS, Engel AF, Nicholls RJ, Kamm MA: Long-term results of overlapping anterior anal-sphincter repair for obstetric trauma. Lancet 2000; 355:260–265.
16 Bravo Gutierrez A, Madoff RD, Lowry AC, Parker SC, Buie WD, Baxter NN: Long-term results of anterior sphincteroplasty. Dis Colon Rectum 2004;47: 727–732.
17 Graf W, Mellgren A, Matzel KE, Hull T, Johansson C, Bernstein M; NASHA Dx Study Group: Efficacy of dextranomer in stabilised hyaluronic acid for treatment of faecal incontinence: a randomised, sham-controlled trial. Lancet 2011;377: 997–1003.
18 Mellgren A, Matzel KE, Pollack J, Hull T, Bernstein M, Graf W; NASHA Dx Study Group: Long-term efficacy of NASHA Dx injection therapy for treatment of fecal incontinence. Neurogastroenterol Motil 2014;26:1087–1094.
19 Deutekom M, Dobben AC: Plugs for containing faecal incontinence. Cochrane Database Syst Rev 2012; 4:CD005086.
20 Baeten CG, Geerdes BP, Adang EM, Heineman E, Konsten J, Engel GL, Kester AD, Spaans F, Soeters PB: Anal dynamic graciloplasty in the treatment of intractable fecal incontinence. N Engl J Med 1995; 332:1600–1605.
21 Baeten CG, Bailey HR, Bakka A, Belliveau P, Berg E, Buie WD, Burnstein MJ, Christiansen J, Coller JA, Galandiuk S, LaFontaine LJ, Lange J, Madoff RD, Matzel KE, Pahlman L, Parc R, Reilly JC, Seccia M, Thorson AG, Vernava AM 3rd, Wexner S: Safety and efficacy of dynamic graciloplasty for fecal incontinence: report of a prospective, multicenter trial. Dynamic Graciloplasty Therapy Study Group. Dis Colon Rectum 2000;43:743–751.
22 Penninckx F; Belgian Section of Colorectal Surgery: Belgian experience with dynamic graciloplasty for faecal incontinence. Br J Surg 2004;91:872–878.
23 Müller C, Belyaev O, Deska T, Chromik A, Weyhe D, Uhl W: Fecal incontinence: an up-to-date critical overview of surgical treatment options. Langenbecks Arch Surg 2005;390:544–552.
24 Koch SM, Uludağ O, Rongen MJ, Baeten CG, van Gemert W: Dynamic graciloplasty in patients born with an anorectal malformation. Dis Colon Rectum 2004;47:1711–1719.
25 Lehur PA, Glemain P, Bruley des Varannes S, Buzelin JM, Leborgne J: Outcome of patients with an implanted artificial anal sphincter for severe faecal incontinence. A single institution report. Int J Colorectal Dis 1998;13:88–92.
26 Wong MT, Meurette G, Wyart V, Glemain P, Lehur PA: The artificial bowel sphincter: a single institution experience over a decade. Ann Surg 2011;254: 951–956.
27 Ruiz Carmona MD, Alós Company R, Roig Vila JV, Solana Bueno A, Pla Martí V: Long-term results of artificial bowel sphincter for the treatment of severe faecal incontinence. Are they what we hoped for? Colorectal Dis 2009;11:831–837.
28 Lehur PA, McNevin S, Buntzen S, Mellgren AF, Laurberg S, Madoff RD: Magnetic anal sphincter augmentation for the treatment of fecal incontinence: a preliminary report from a feasibility study. Dis Colon Rectum 2010;53:1604–1610.
29 Pakravan F, Helmes C: Magnetic anal sphincter augmentation in patients with severe fecal incontinence. Dis Colon Rectum 2015;58:109–114.
30 Thompson WG, Heaton KW: Functional bowel disorders in apparently healthy people. Gastroenterology 1980;79:283–288.
31 Drossman DA, Li Z, Andruzzi E, Temple RD, Talley NJ, Thompson WG, Whitehead WE, Janssens J, Funch-Jensen P, Corazziari E, et al: U.S. householder survey of functional gastrointestinal disorders. Prevalence, sociodemography, and health impact. Dig Dis Sci 1993;38:1569–1580.
32 Talley NJ, Fleming KC, Evans JM, O'Keefe EA, Weaver AL, Zinsmeister AR, Melton LJ 3rd: Constipation in an elderly community: a study of prevalence and potential risk factors. Am J Gastroenterol 1996;91:19–25.

33 Chiotakakou-Faliakou E, Kamm MA, Roy AJ, Storrie JB, Turner IC: Biofeedback provides long-term benefit for patients with intractable, slow and normal transit constipation. Gut 1998;42:517–521.

34 van der Sijp JR, Rasing L, Kamm MA, Akkermans LM, van Vroonhoven TJ: Surgical management of severe idiopathic constipation: a review. Neth J Surg 1991;43:29–35.

35 Kamm MA, Hawley PR, Lennard-Jones JE: Outcome of colectomy for severe idiopathic constipation. Gut 1988;29:969–973.

36 Cullen J, Rosselli JM, Gurland BH: Ventral rectopexy for rectal prolapse and obstructed defecation. Clin Colon Rectal Surg 2012;25:34–36.

37 Evans C, Ong E, Jones OM, Cunningham C, Lindsey I: Laparoscopic ventral rectopexy is effective for solitary rectal ulcer syndrome when associated with rectal prolapse. Colorectal Dis 2014;16:O112–O116.

38 Wahed S, Ahmad M, Mohiuddin K, Katory M, Mercer-Jones M: Short-term results for laparoscopic ventral rectopexy using biological mesh for pelvic organ prolapse. Colorectal Dis 2012;14:1242–1247.

39 Jayne DG, Schwandner O, Stuto A: Stapled transanal rectal resection for obstructed defecation syndrome: one-year results of the European STARR Registry. Dis Colon Rectum 2009;52:1205–1214.

40 Tanagho EA, Schmidt RA: Bladder pacemaker: scientific basis and clinical future. Urology 1982;20: 614–619.

41 Mowatt G, Glazener C, Jarrett M: Sacral nerve stimulation for faecal incontinence and constipation in adults. Cochrane Database Syst Rev 2007;3: CD004464.

42 Pettit PD, Thompson JR, Chen AH: Sacral neuromodulation: new applications in the treatment of female pelvic floor dysfunction. Curr Opin Obstet Gynecol 2002;14:521–525.

43 Matzel KE, Stadelmaier U, Hohenfellner M, Gall FP: Electrical stimulation of sacral spinal nerves for treatment of faecal incontinence. Lancet 1995;346: 1124–1127.

44 Rosen HR, Urbarz C, Holzer B, Novi G, Schiessel R: Sacral nerve stimulation as a treatment for fecal incontinence. Gastroenterology 2001;121:536–541.

45 Ganio E, Luc AR, Clerico G, Trompetto M: Sacral nerve stimulation for treatment of fecal incontinence: a novel approach for intractable fecal incontinence. Dis Colon Rectum 2001;44:619–631.

46 Ganio E, Ratto C, Masin A, Luc AR, Doglietto GB, Dodi G, Ripetti V, Arullani A, Frascio M, BertiRiboli E, Landolfi V, DelGenio A, Altomare DF, Memeo V, Bertapelle P, Carone R, Spinelli M, Zanollo A, Spreafico L, Giardiello G, de Seta F: Neuromodulation for fecal incontinence: outcome in 16 patients with definitive implant. The initial Italian Sacral Neurostimulation Group (GINS) experience. Dis Colon Rectum 2001;44:965–970.

47 Matzel KE, Stadelmaier U, Bittorf B, Hohenfellner M, Hohenberger W: Bilateral sacral spinal nerve stimulation for fecal incontinence after low anterior rectum resection. Int J Colorectal Dis 2002;17:430–434.

48 Malouf AJ, Wiesel PH, Nicholls T, Nicholls RJ, Kamm MA: Short-term effects of sacral nerve stimulation for idiopathic slow transit constipation. World J Surg 2002;26:166–170.

49 Uludağ O, Koch SM, van Gemert WG, Dejong CH, Baeten CG: Sacral neuromodulation in patients with fecal incontinence: a single-center study. Dis Colon Rectum 2004;47:1350–1357.

50 Conaghan P, Farouk R: Sacral nerve stimulation can be successful in patients with ultrasound evidence of external anal sphincter disruption. Dis Colon Rectum 2005;48:1610–1614.

51 Dudding TC, Vaizey CJ, Jarrett ME, Cohen RG, Kamm MA: Permanent sacral nerve stimulation for treatment of functional anorectal pain: report of a case. Dis Colon Rectum 2007;50:1275–1278.

52 Dinning PG, Fuentealba SE, Kennedy ML, Lubowski DZ, Cook IJ: Sacral nerve stimulation induces pancolonic propagating pressure waves and increases defecation frequency in patients with slow-transit constipation. Colorectal Dis 2007;9:123–132.

53 Tanagho EA: Concepts of neuromodulation. Neurourol Urodyn 1993;12:487–488.

54 Jarrett ME, Mowatt G, Glazener CM, Fraser C, Nicholls RJ, Grant AM, Kamm MA: Systematic review of sacral nerve stimulation for faecal incontinence and constipation. Br J Surg 2004;91:1559–1569.

55 Jarrett ME, Varma JS, Duthie GS, Nicholls RJ, Kamm MA: Sacral nerve stimulation for faecal incontinence in the UK. Br J Surg 2004;91:755–761.

56 Carrington EV, Evers J, Grossi U, Dinning PG, Scott SM, O'Connell PR, Jones JF, Knowles CH: A systematic review of sacral nerve stimulation mechanisms in the treatment of fecal incontinence and constipation. Neurogastroenterol Motil 2014;26: 1222–1237.

57 Fowler CJ, Swinn MJ, Goodwin RJ, Oliver S, Craggs M: Studies of the latency of pelvic floor contraction during peripheral nerve evaluation show that the muscle response is reflexly mediated. J Urol 2000; 163:881–883.

58 Tjandra JJ, Lim JF, Matzel K: Sacral nerve stimulation: an emerging treatment for faecal incontinence. ANZ J Surg 2004;74:1098–1106.

59 Tan JJ, Chan M, Tjandra JJ: Evolving therapy for fecal incontinence. Dis Colon Rectum 2007;50:1950–1967.

60 Leroi AM, Michot F, Grise P, Denis P: Effect of sacral nerve stimulation in patients with fecal and urinary incontinence. Dis Colon Rectum 2001;44:779–789.

61 Matzel KE, Kamm MA, Stosser M, Baeten CG, Christiansen J, Madoff R, Mellgren A, Nicholls RJ, Rius J, Rosen H: Sacral spinal nerve stimulation for faecal incontinence: multicentre study. Lancet 2004;363:1270–1276.
62 Leroi AM, Parc Y, Lehur PA, Mion F, Barth X, Rullier E, Bresler L, Portier G, Michot F; Study Group: Efficacy of sacral nerve stimulation for fecal incontinence: results of a multicenter double-blind crossover study. Ann Surg 2005;242:662–669.
63 Vaizey CJ, Kamm MA, Roy AJ, Nicholls RJ: Double-blind crossover study of sacral nerve stimulation for fecal incontinence. Dis Colon Rectum 2000;43:298–302.
64 Tjandra JJ, Chan MK, Yeh CH, Murray-Green C: Sacral nerve stimulation is more effective than optimal medical therapy for severe fecal incontinence: a randomized, controlled study. Dis Colon Rectum 2008;51:494–502.
65 Wexner SD, Coller JA, Devroede G, Hull T, McCallum R, Chan M, Ayscue JM, Shobeiri AS, Margolin D, England M, Kaufman H, Snape WJ, Mutlu E, Chua H, Pettit P, Nagle D, Madoff RD, Lerew DR, Mellgren A: Sacral nerve stimulation for fecal incontinence: results of a 120-patient prospective multicenter study. Ann Surg 2010;251:441–449.
66 Mellgren A, Wexner SD, Coller JA, Devroede G, Lerew DR, Madoff RD, Hull T; SNS Study Group: Long-term efficacy and safety of sacral nerve stimulation for fecal incontinence. Dis Colon Rectum 2011;54:1065–1075.
67 Hull T, Giese C, Wexner SD, Mellgren A, Devroede G, Madoff RD, Stromberg K, Coller JA; SNS Study Group: Long-term durability of sacral nerve stimulation therapy for chronic fecal incontinence. Dis Colon Rectum 2013;56:234–245.
68 George AT, Kalmar K, Panarese A, Dudding TC, Nicholls RJ, Vaizey CJ: Long-term outcomes of sacral nerve stimulation for fecal incontinence. Dis Colon Rectum 2012;55:302–306.
69 Maeda Y, Lundby L, Buntzen S, Laurberg S: Outcome of sacral nerve stimulation for fecal incontinence at 5 years. Ann Surg 2014;259:1126–1131.
70 Gallas S, Michot F, Faucheron JL, Meurette G, Lehur PA, Barth X, Damon H, Mion F, Rullier E, Zerbib F, Sielezneff I, Ouaïssi M, Orsoni P, Desfourneaux V, Siproudhis L, Mathonnet M, Menard JF, Leroi AM; Club NEMO: Predictive factors for successful sacral nerve stimulation in the treatment of faecal incontinence: results of trial stimulation in 200 patients. Colorectal Dis 2011;13:689–696.
71 Roy AL, Gourcerol G, Menard JF, Michot F, Leroi AM, Bridoux V: Predictive factors for successful sacral nerve stimulation in the treatment of fecal incontinence: lessons from a comprehensive treatment assessment. Dis Colon Rectum 2014;57:772–780.
72 Duelund-Jakobsen J, Buntzen S, Lundby L, Laurberg S: Sacral nerve stimulation at subsensory threshold does not compromise treatment efficacy: results from a randomized, blinded crossover study. Ann Surg 2013;257:219–223.
73 Hotouras A, Murphy J, Thin NN, Allison M, Horrocks E, Williams NS, Knowles CH, Chan CL: Outcome of sacral nerve stimulation for fecal incontinence in patients refractory to percutaneous tibial nerve stimulation. Dis Colon Rectum 2013;56:915–920.
74 Dinning PG, Hunt LM, Arkwright JW, Patton V, Szczesniak MM, Wiklendt L, Davidson JB, Lubowski DZ, Cook IJ: Pancolonic motor response to subsensory and suprasensory sacral nerve stimulation in patients with slow-transit constipation. Br J Surg 2012;99:1002–1010.
75 Kamm MA, Dudding TC, Melenhorst J, Jarrett M, Wang Z, Buntzen S, Johansson C, Laurberg S, Rosen H, Vaizey CJ, Matzel K, Baeten C: Sacral nerve stimulation for intractable constipation. Gut 2010;59:333–340.
76 Thomas GP, Dudding TC, Rahbour G, Nicholls RJ, Vaizey CJ: Sacral nerve stimulation for constipation. Br J Surg 2013;100:174–181.
77 Fassov JL, Lundby L, Laurberg S, Buntzen S, Krogh K: A randomized, controlled, crossover study of sacral nerve stimulation for irritable bowel syndrome. Ann Surg 2014;260:31–36.
78 Faucheron JL, Voirin D, Badic B: Sacral nerve stimulation for fecal incontinence: causes of surgical revision from a series of 87 consecutive patients operated on in a single institution. Dis Colon Rectum 2010;53:1501–1507.

Prof. Anders Mellgren, MD, PhD
Division of Colon and Rectal Surgery
Department of Surgery
University of Illinois at Chicago
840 S. Wood Street, 518 E CSB, M/C 958
Chicago, IL 60612 (USA)
E-Mail afmellgr@uic.edu

Slavin KV (ed): Stimulation of the Peripheral Nervous System. The Neuromodulation Frontier.
Prog Neurol Surg. Basel, Karger, 2016, vol 29, pp 213–224 (DOI: 10.1159/000434673)

Stimulation of the Dorsal Root Ganglion

Liong Liem

Sint Antonius Hospital, Nieuwegein, The Netherlands

Abstract

Dorsal root ganglion (DRG) stimulation has recently emerged as a new neuromodulation modality that stays on the intersection of the peripheral and central nervous system. With DRG location within the spinal column and with electrodes for DRG stimulation placed through the intraspinal epidural space, it may make more sense to group DRG stimulation together with more commonly used spinal cord stimulation (SCS) rather than peripheral nerve stimulation (PNS), particularly if one agrees that the stimulation delivered to DRG partly works downstream at the spinal cord level. Based on current experience, it appears that DRG stimulation of the spinal cord is as effective as SCS in relieving various neuropathic pain syndromes including pain due to failed back surgery syndrome, complex regional pain syndromes, and chronic postsurgical pain. In addition to its efficacy, DRG stimulation of the spinal cord is associated with a lower rate of migrations and lack of positional side effects that may be seen with SCS and PNS. Here we summarize the knowledge base and clinical evidence for DRG stimulation of the spinal cord, and present hypotheses of its mechanism of action.

The dorsal root ganglion (DRG) is emerging as a valuable target for neuromodulatory treatment of chronic neuropathic pain. In DRG stimulation of the spinal cord, technological innovations make it possible to steer percutaneous epidural leads into the lateral transforaminal recess to reach the DRG. With DRG location within the spinal column and with electrodes for DRG stimulation placed through the intraspinal epidural space, it makes more sense to group DRG stimulation together with more commonly used spinal cord stimulation (SCS) rather than peripheral nerve stimulation (PNS), particularly if one agrees that the stimulation delivered to DRG actually works at the spinal cord level. DRG stimulation appears as effective as traditional SCS in relieving neuropathic pain of the trunk and/or limbs due to failed back surgery syndrome, complex regional pain syndrome, and chronic postsurgical pain, and may allow specificity of paresthesia coverage that is as precise as PNS. Importantly, it may avoid the migration and positional side effects of both of these established neuromodulation modalities. Here we summarize the knowledge base and clinical evidence for DRG stimulation, and present hypotheses for its mechanism of action connecting peripherally generated pain relief acting through central pathways.

Dorsal Root Ganglion Stimulation of the Spinal Cord: Development of the Intervention

SCS was first described in 1967 when it was used as a last-resort modality for pain relief in a patient with terminal cancer [1]. Since that time, the clinical potential of active implantable dorsal column neuromodulation devices has been recognized and there have been massive advances in the application of such technology to the field of chronic pain management. Hardware has been miniaturized and made fully implantable with wireless programmers and remote controls. Sophisticated lead design combined with complex programming algorithms and refined implantation techniques have given implanting physicians unprecedented abilities to provide pain relief for conditions that would otherwise be intractable [2–4]. A wealth of published research spanning computer modeling, preclinical animal models, and clinical trials has supported these advances.

Although the initial costs associated with the device can be steep, it is a cost-effective intervention [3, 5–7] and SCS has likely enjoyed its surge in popularity due to its provision of three important benefits. First, the effectiveness of the device can be tested prior to permanent implantation [8]. Epidurally placed leads are attached to a temporary external stimulator for several days; the permanent device is implanted only if the patient reports significant pain relief and is able to operate the device. In this way, a patient who is unlikely to improve with the intervention can be identified before proceeding with an ultimately unnecessary procedure. Second, the SCS implantation procedure is minimally invasive [9]. Leads are epidural and are placed through a percutaneous procedure. The implantable pulse generator device is housed subcutaneously. Although risks such as dural puncture do exist [10], the clinical risks associated with SCS are far lower than with open procedures such as spinal surgery. The third benefit of SCS is its reversibility [9] relative to ablative procedures; the leads and device can be removed in a minor procedure that leaves minimal scarring and no change in spinal function. These features have contributed to the movement of SCS up the 'pain ladder'. Once considered a somewhat capricious therapy of last resort, SCS is now recommended as a first-line intervention before more invasive or irreversible ablative options [4, 11, 12].

SCS is not, however, without limitations and is not a panacea; only about 3 out of 4 patients have a successful trial period and about 3 out of 4 patients who have a permanent implant report good pain relief [13]. Although pain relief is sustainable, some reduction in effectiveness over time may occur [14, 15]. A requirement of this therapy is that, through a combination of appropriate placement of the leads against the target neural tissue and programming of the active electrodes to 'sculpt' the electrical fields, the perceptible paresthesias associated with treatment must overlap with the painful regions. It is recognized that establishing paresthesias with SCS can be difficult in axial locations [16], such as the low back [17, 18] and groin [19, 20], and in distal extremities, such as the feet [21]. Additionally, as a consequence of achieving acceptable pain-paresthesia concordance, patients can experience extraneous paresthesias in nonpainful areas [22–24] that may range from merely annoying to frankly aversive. SCS is also susceptible to lead migration [10] and positional effects, in which gravitational or mechanical forces that result from movements of the body change the relative distance between the electrodes and the dorsal columns, and result in changes in the perception of stimulation [25–27].

Because of the limitations associated with SCS, other neuromodulation targets have been explored. PNS has moved neuromodulation closer to the site of pain transduction and/or transmission. Although undeniably satisfactory for a number of pain etiologies [28, 29], PNS is also prone to lead migration and can produce considerable local irritation [28]. Other investigators have modified SCS techniques to identify feasible targets in the epidural space. Nerve root stimulation has emerged as an effective therapy [30], particularly for pain in caudal dermatomal distributions [31]. As a natural extension of nerve root stimulation, isolated case reports have discussed the extreme lateral placement of leads in an attempt to recruit the DRG [16, 32]. This structure houses primary sensory neuron (PSN) somata inside vertebral foramen and is an emerging target for a number of pain treatment options [33, 34]. With the recent advent of a novel device for DRG stimulation of the spinal cord, more prospective evidence is emerging.

Device and Implantation

The Axium™ system (Spinal Modulation, Menlo Park, Calif., USA) is a constant-voltage primary-cell spinal neurostimulation device that accommodates up to four quadripolar cylindrical percutaneous leads that are placed via standard epidural loss-of-resistance methods in an antegrade approach. Leads have a slim 1-mm diameter profile and are very flexible under fluoroscopic guidance due to their external curved guidance sheath and hollow lumen. With these features, leads are especially amenable to placement near DRGs in the lateral recesses of intraspinal foramen, and conform to the exterior surface of the DRG without compressing the neural tissue. Initial testing has shown that 93% of leads could be deployed to the target foramen within 2 min of obtaining epidural access [35].

Clinical Evidence: Dorsal Root Ganglion Stimulation Treats Neuropathic Pain Across a Variety of Etiologies and Locations

DRG stimulation of the spinal cord has demonstrated effectiveness through 12 months in a number of cohorts of mixed etiologies, addressing the radicular pain of failed back surgery syndrome, complex regional pain syndrome in lower extremities, and chronic postsurgical pain [35, 36]. Analgesia specific to chronic postherniorrhaphy groin pain [20] and foot pain [37] has also been reported, suggesting that in addition to broad regional coverage, DRG-SCS is capable of achieving coverage of subdermatomal regions. Additionally, case reports involving patients with low back pain [38], postherpetic neuralgia [39], amputation/deafferentation pain [40], phantom limb pain [41], visceral pain [42], body wall pain [43], and upper extremity pain [44] have been presented. Hitherto difficult to treat because of lack of targeted paresthesia, patients with complex regional pain syndrome of the knee, a small subpopulation of the larger complex regional pain syndrome cohort, have shown good early clinical response. Similar results have been reported in postsurgical knee pain patients.

Pain-paresthesia overlap is typically established with a high degree of precision in DRG stimulation of the spinal cord, e.g. there is high concordance of painful areas with paresthesia and very little extraneous stimulation [45]. This is likely due to the recruitment of PSNs that project to the painful regions and allows subdermatomal paresthesia coverage to be established, a goal that in SCS may require complex lead design and programming [46]. Importantly, DRG stimulation paresthesia distributions are maintained over time and appear largely indifferent to changes in body position [45]. The stability of paresthesia may be due to the location of the DRG inside the bony enclosure of the vertebral foramen. This helps to brace the lead in its desired position and ensures that the DRG and lead remain largely unperturbed by flexion or movement in the highly mobile spine. The CSF layer that surrounds the DRG is another relevant factor within the stimulation milieu; because it is very thin [47], its potential role as a current sink to disperse electrical fields is limited. Thus, DRG stimulation of the spinal cord can be achieved at low amplitudes, requiring on average about 15% of the power output of a dorsal column stimulation system [35]. Given that a primary-cell SCS system may have an average battery lifetime of 3–5 years under normal use conditions [48, 49], this could represent a considerable reduction in battery-replacement procedures, along with cost and morbidity risk.

Anatomy of the Dorsal Root Ganglion

Vertebral foramina extend obliquely and caudally from the spinal canal, and nerve roots are oriented at nearly right angles relative to the spinal cord [50]. Dorsal roots pass through the vertebral foramen, and the DRG is an enlargement of the dorsal root enclosed in the dural sac [51] as it exits the vertebral column. DRGs contain PSNs which are somatotopically arranged [52] and of mixed sensory functions [34]. The DRG PSNs involved in pain are primarily of the C and Aδ type [34]. Satellite glial cells form an interconnected network involved in metabolic and functional support of these neurons [53]. PSNs are pseudounipolar – each has a single process that bifurcates to extend both peripherally and centrally [54]. Distal to the DRG, PSN dendrites coalesce to form peripheral nerves, and their terminals are the sites of tactile and pain sensory transduction. Central to the DRG, the dorsal root terminates in the dorsal horn of the spinal cord. PSN axons facilitate synaptic communication with neurons in spinal gray matter; these signals are then modified by second- and third-order neurons and by inhibitory interneurons.

Gaining Access to the Dorsal Root Ganglion

Chronic pain therapeutic interventions directed at the DRG [33, 55] include transforaminal injections of local anesthetics and/or steroids [56], dorsal root entry zone lesions [57], dorsal rhizotomy [58], ganglionectomy [59], and conventional and pulsed radiofrequency treatments [60]. Access to the DRG may be gained via an open procedure or a percutaneous approach with fluoroscopically guided cannulation [61]. Electrical neurostimulation is an emerging option for DRG-specific pain management interventions [33]. Electrode placement for nerve root stimulation [30] has typically been reported in the literature with a similarly 'outside-in' approach, such as sacral placement of intraspinal nerve root stimulators for urinary bladder voiding dysfunction [62], but also at thoracic and lumbar sites for neuropathic pain [63]. Attempts to access the DRG at thoracic levels via the spinal canal epidural space (e.g. an 'inside-out' approach) was found to be procedurally complex due to the angles involved, requiring a retrograde lead placement and custom-made curved stylets [64]. This was all but impossible at cervical levels where the intravertebral spaces are smaller [65]. For cervical DRG neurostimulation, these options proved insufficient and recruitment of the DRG could be achieved only through an extraforaminal approach [66], and was indeed referred to as PNS.

Given the issues above, a better option was needed for electrode placement at the DRG. Unfortunately, these implantation techniques have established some historical inertia implying that an extraforaminal approach is necessary and/or ideal for establishing stimulation at the DRG. They also imply that the DRG is a component of the peripheral nervous system. These assumptions, however, are an artifact of the implant approach that was necessary given the limitations of existing form factors of the neurostimulation systems at the time. With the new DRG-SCS device, these issues have been obviated. DRG neurostimulation can be readily achieved with an antegrade percutaneous approach in the spinal epidural space in a manner similar to conventional SCS and achievable by any competent implanter.

The Dorsal Root Ganglion Is a Central Nervous System Structure

Because the DRG is separated from the spinal cord by dorsal roots, and because its dendrites extend into the periphery, spinal ganglia have been categorically included in anatomical descriptions of the peripheral nervous system [67]. However, all available evidence – and the opinion of this author – supports the notion that the DRG is actually a component of the central nervous system. Like the spinal cord, DRGs are protected inside the vertebral bones. Synaptic terminals of DRG neurons extend inside the gray matter of the spinal cord. DRGs are enclosed within the dural sac [51], albeit at a uniquely permeable site of the blood-brain barrier [68]. Embryological evidence has demonstrated that DRG nociceptive neurons arise from a boundary cell progenitor line of the neural crest [69, 70] and their differentiation and migration are dependent on molecular signaling from the neural tube [71]. Thus, DRGs may be regarded as laterally translocated gray matter of the spinal cord. Satellite cells that surround PSNs in the DRG share markers with CNS astroglia [53]. Transected axons of PSNs do not regenerate into the spinal cord [72], a feature in common with other CNS neurons and unlike sensory neural structures in the periphery [73].

Electrical neurostimulation of the DRG has recently been called DRG stimulation of the spinal cord due to its similarity to the SCS procedure. Leads are placed through percutaneous epidural antegrade access in the lateral recess of the spinal canal. The electrical field of DRG stimulation of the spinal cord electrodes thus placed is biased centrally by virtue of being medial to the bifurcation of the dorsal root and the ventral root as well as orthodromic recruitment of spinal dorsal root fibers. Empirical evidence supporting the central structure and function of DRGs can be found in the paresthesias generated by stimulation of these structures. Although focal stimulation at regionally delimited areas is possible, DRG stimulation of the spinal cord can also produce diffuse paresthesias that approach dermatomal distributions [35], similar to traditional SCS. This is in contrast to PNS-generated paresthesias that are extremely focal and follow the nerve distribution [74]. Thus, DRG stimulation of the spinal cord involves recruitment of a central nervous system structure while PNS involves electrode placement at or distal to the point where the rootlets exit the dura mater and the lateral vertebral foramen.

Physiology of the Dorsal Root Ganglion in Neuropathic Pain

In neuropathic pain conditions, pain is perceived in the absence of painful stimuli. After a peripheral lesion occurs, immune responses occur immediately. At the site of the tissue damage, inflammatory signaling molecules such as prostaglandins, bradykinin, and nerve growth factors are released, leading to hypersensitivity of nociceptive free endings [75]. Inside the DRG, there is a complex cascade of immune responses, largely mediated by immune and glial cells, that dramatically modulates neural activity [76]. Macrophages and lymphocytes, typically diffusely distributed in the DRG, proliferate and surround the cell bodies of injured PSNs. Macrophages, in particular, infiltrate the covering of satellite glial cells around the PSNs and surround them [77]. Some PSN cell death occurs after nerve injury, and therefore the immune cells may remain to remove the debris [78]. Their subsequent production of inflammatory cytokines such as interleukin-1 and tumor necrosis factor [79] elicit spontaneous, repetitive action potentials in sensory afferents [80]. A proliferation of satellite glial cells also occurs; these cells release neurotrophic factors like nerve growth factors and neurotrophin-3 that are involved in the development of allodynia [81]. In neuropathic pain initiation, neurotrophins alter activity of PSNs at the transcription level, thereby altering the phenotype of the cells by changing their quantity, distribution, and/or ratio of ion channels, neurotransmitters, and receptors [82]. Shifts in ion availability in the DRG, particularly of potassium, modulate neural activity [83]. Sympathetic fibers sprout and reach DRG PSNs [84]; the increased neural connectivity may further contribute to the pathological pain. Subthreshold oscillations of PSNs also occur [85]. This may be a cross-activation due to electrical coupling of satellite glial cells via upregulated gap junctions [86] or sensitivity to changes in ion concentrations in the extracellular matrix supported by changes in ion channel expression and activity [87].

In the spinal cord, massive recruitment and activation of microglia occurs in the dorsal horn around the central terminals of the injured PSNs [88]. This releases neurotrophins, such as brain-derived neurotrophic factor, and reduces inhibitory activity typically mediated by GABA and glycine [89]. Additionally, some inhibitory interneurons undergo apoptotic cell death, reducing GABA levels in the superficial laminae of the dorsal horn [90]. Together, these changes can result in activation-dependent plasticity in PSNs and in the dorsal column of the spinal cord. Central sensitization result from cumulative temporal summation of AMPA and NMDA receptor-dependent glutamate activity [91], and can result in long-lasting or even permanent changes.

The electrophysiological consequences of peripheral injury across the pain sensory system consist of overall hyperexcitability together with disinhibition. In normal function, DRGs may have a filtering effect on incoming sensory input from the periphery; removing that filter in neuropathic pain conditions creates widespread pathological activity throughout the nervous system [92]. It has been demonstrated that pathological activity at the initiation neuropathic pain conditions originates in the DRG itself [83, 93]. Certainly, PSNs are the common elements across all sites and processes of neuropathic pain. Changes in the DRG as a result of peripheral insult-initiated inflammation are the likely source of chronic neuropathic pain conditions [82].

Proposed Analgesic Mechanisms of Dorsal Root Ganglion Stimulation of the Spinal Cord

It is established that a net increase in activity in DRG neurons drives the neural changes in neuropathic pain conditions. Ablative interventions such as ganglionectomy and dorsal root entry zone lesions achieve their effect by preventing the hyperexcitable peripheral activity from being transmitted to the spinal cord and to supraspinal sites. DRG neurostimulation may serve a similar conceptual function by actively reducing the net nociceptive input to the spinal cord; such reduction of PSN activity by field stimulation has been demonstrated in vitro [94]. Thus, DRG stimulation of the spinal cord may restore the neural filtering function of the DRG that was lost in response to peripheral injuries. This could have consequences for all downstream neural structures, including the spinal cord, intraspinal nerves, rami communicantes, and the lumbar sympathetic trunk [95].

The gate control theory, in which activation of large-diameter sensory fibers blocks the transmission of nociceptive signals in small-diameter fibers, was proposed in 1965 [96]; it is considered an underlying mechanism of action for SCS [1, 3, 9] and has been supported by recent empirical evidence [27]. However, the gate control theory may be insufficient as an explanation for the mechanism of DRG stimulation of the spinal cord. This is because DRG stimulation of the spinal cord normalizes peripheral input before it arrives at the spinal cord, making moot the challenge to preferentially recruit the dorsal fibers involved in the individual expression of the neuropathic condition. It is possible that over time DRG stimulation of the spinal cord could reverse the central pathologic plasticity and reduce central sensitization. It is also possible that, if initiated early in the neuropathic pain development cascade, DRG stimulation of the spinal cord could prevent the maladaptive plastic changes. More research is needed for this new innovation in neuromodulation.

Conclusions

With this review we have established the DRG's role in chronic neuropathic pain, and its value as a site of neurostimulation for pain treatment. DRG stimulation of the spinal cord is now technically feasible with recent implantable device innovations and the evidence to support its effectiveness is accumulating. DRG stimulation of the spinal cord is another option in the pain management physician's armamentarium for changing peripheral perception via modulation of central nervous system pathways.

Acknowledgment

The author thanks Allison Foster, PhD, an independent medical writer supported by Spinal Modulation Inc., Jeffery M. Kramer, PhD, chief scientific officer at Spinal Modulation, and Jeyakumar Subbaroyan, PhD, senior clinical research manager at Spinal Modulation, for their intellectual input in drafting the manuscript.

References

1 Shealy CN, Mortimer JT, Reswick JB: Electrical inhibition of pain by stimulation of the dorsal columns: preliminary clinical report. Anesth Analg 1967;46: 489–491.

2 Bradley K: The technology: the anatomy of a spinal cord and nerve root stimulator: the lead and the power source. Pain Med 2006;7:S27–S34.

3 Kumar K, Abbas M, Rizvi S: The use of spinal cord stimulation in pain management. Pain Manag 2012; 2:125–134.

4 Kumar K, Rizvi S: Historical and present state of neuromodulation in chronic pain. Curr Pain Headache Rep 2014;18:387.

5 Hollingworth W, Turner JA, Welton NJ, Comstock BA, Deyo RA: Costs and cost-effectiveness of spinal cord stimulation (SCS) for failed back surgery syndrome: an observational study in a workers' compensation population. Spine 2011;36:2076–2083.

6 Taylor RS, Ryan J, O'Donnell R, Eldabe S, Kumar K, North RB: The cost-effectiveness of spinal cord stimulation in the treatment of failed back surgery syndrome. Clin J Pain 2010;26:463–469.

7 Mekhail N, Wentzel DL, Freeman R, Quadri H: Counting the costs: case management implication of spinal cord stimulation treatment for failed back surgery syndrome. Prof Case Manag 2011;16:27–36.

8 Chincholkar M, Eldabe S, Strachan R, Brookes M, Garner F, Chadwisk R, Gulve A, Ness J: Prospective analysis of the trial period for spinal cord stimulation treatment for chronic pain. Neuromodulation 2011; 14:523–529.

9 Stojanovic MP, Abdi S: Spinal cord stimulation. Pain Physician 2002;5:156–166.

10 Cameron T: Safety and efficacy of spinal cord stimulation for the treatment of chronic pain: a 20-year literature review. J Neurosurg 2004;100:254–267.

11 National Institute for Health and Clinical Excellence (NICE). Spinal Cord Stimulation for Chronic Pain of Neuropathic or Ischaemic Origin; NICE Technology Appraisal Guidance 159. London, National Health Service, 2011.

12 Poree L, Krames E, Pope J, Deer TR, Levy R, Schultz L: Spinal cord stimulation as treatment for complex regional pain syndrome should be considered earlier than last resort therapy. Neuromodulation 2013;16: 125–141.

13 Kumar K, Hunter G, Demeria D: Spinal cord stimulation in treatment of chronic benign pain: challenges in treatment planning and present status, a 22-year experience. Neurosurgery 2006;58:481–496.

14 Kemler MA, De Vet HC, Barendse GA, Van Den Wildenberg FA, Van Kleef M: Effect of spinal cord stimulation for chronic complex regional pain syndrome type I: five-year final follow-up of patients in a randomized controlled trial. J Neurosurg 2008;108: 292–298.

15 Kumar K, Taylor RS, Jacques L, Eldabe S, Meglio M, Molet J, Thomson S, O'Callaghan J, Eisenberg E, Milbouw G, Buchser E, Fortini G, Richardson J, North RB: The effects of spinal cord stimulation in chronic pain are sustained: a 24-month follow-up of the prospective randomized controlled multicenter trial of the effectiveness of spinal cord stimulation. Neurosurgery 2008;63:762–770.

16 Aló KM, Yland MJ, Redko V, Feler C, Naumann C: Lumbar and sacral nerve root stimulation (NRS) in the treatment of chronic pain: a novel anatomic approach and neuro stimulation technique. Neuromodulation 1999;2:23–31.

17 Oakley JC: Spinal cord stimulation in axial low back pain: solving the dilemma. Pain Med 2006;7:S58–S63.

18 Rigoard P, Delmotte A, D'Houtaud S, Misbert L, Diallo B, Roy-Moreau A, Durand S, Royoux S, Giot JP, Bataille B: Back pain: a real target for spinal cord stimulation? Neurosurgery 2012;70:574–585.

19 Lepski G, Vahedi P, Tatagiba MS, Morgalla M: Combined spinal cord and peripheral nerve field stimulation for persistent post-herniorrhaphy pain. Neuromodulation 2013;16:84–89.

20 Schu S, Gulve A, Eldabe S, Baranidharan G, Wolf K, Demmel W, Rasche D, Sharma M, Klase D, Jahnichen G, Wahlstedt A, Nijhuis H, Liem L: Spinal cord stimulation of the dorsal root ganglion for groin pain – a retrospective review. Pain Pract 2015;15: 293–299.

21 Deer TR, Barolat G: Stimulation of the nervous system to treat neuropathic pain of the foot; in Deer TR (ed): Atlas of Implantable Therapies for Pain Management. New York, Springer, 2011, pp 81–86.

22 North RB, Kidd DH, Olin J, Sieracki JM, Farrokhi F, Petrucci L, Cutchis PN: Spinal cord stimulation for axial low back pain: a prospective, controlled trial comparing dual with single percutaneous electrodes. Spine 2005;30:1412–1418.

23 North RB, Lanning A, Hessels R, Cutchis PN: Spinal cord stimulation with percutaneous and plate electrodes: side effects and quantitative comparisons. Neurosurg Focus 1997;2:e3.

24 North R, Shipley J: Practice parameters for the use of spinal cord stimulation in the treatment of chronic neuropathic pain. Pain Med 2007;8:S200–S275.

25 Barolat G, Schwartzman R, Woo R: Epidural spinal cord stimulation in the management of reflex sympathetic dystrophy. Stereotact Funct Neurosurg 1989;53:29–39.
26 Schade CM, Schultz D, Tamayo N, Iyer S, Panken E: Automatic adaptation of neurostimulation therapy in response to changes in patient position: results of the Posture Responsive Spinal Cord Stimulation (PRS) Research Study. Pain Physician 2011;14:407–417.
27 Parker JL, Karantonis DM, Single PS, Obradovic M, Cousins MJ: Compound action potentials recorded in the human spinal cord during neurostimulation for pain relief. Pain 2012;153:593–601.
28 Slavin KV: Peripheral nerve stimulation for neuropathic pain. Neurotherapeutics 2008;5:100–106.
29 Deogaonkar M, Slavin KV: Peripheral nerve/field stimulation for neuropathic pain. Neurosurg Clin N Am 2014;25:1–10.
30 Haque R, Winfree CJ: Spinal nerve root stimulation. Neurosurg Focus 2006;21:E4.
31 Aló KM, Mckay E: Selective nerve root stimulation (SNRS) for the treatment of intractable pelvic pain and motor dysfunction: a case report. Neuromodulation 2001;4:19–23.
32 Weigel R, Capelle HH, Schmelz M, Krauss JK: Selective thoracic ganglionectomy for the treatment of segmental neuropathic pain. Eur J Pain 2012;16:1398–1402.
33 Pope JE, Deer TR, Kramer J: A systematic review: current and future directions of dorsal root ganglion therapeutics to treat chronic pain. Pain Med 2013;14:1477–1496.
34 Deer TR, Levy RM, Kramer JM: Interventional perspectives on the dorsal root ganglion as a target for the treatment of chronic pain: a review. Minim Invasive Surg Pain 2013;1:23–33.
35 Deer TR, Grigsby E, Weiner RL, Wilcosky B, Kramer JM: A prospective study of dorsal root ganglion stimulation for the relief of chronic pain. Neuromodulation 2013;16:67–72.
36 Liem L, Russo M, Huygen FJ, Van Buyten JP, Smet I, Verrills P, Cousins M, Brooker C, Levy R, Deer T, Kramer J: A multicenter, prospective trial to assess the safety and performance of the spinal modulation dorsal root ganglia neurostimulator system in the treatment of chronic pain. Neuromodulation 2013;16:471–482.
37 Wolf K: Long-term outcomes using stimulation of the dorsal root ganglion (DRG) for foot pain (poster No. 357). NANS 2013: Today's Vision, Tomorrow Reality, Las Vegas, 2013.
38 Nijhuis H, Liem L, Huygen F: A post-market cohort to assess the performance of a neurostimulator system for the management of intractable chronic back pain. Neuromodulation 2013;16:e140.
39 Klase D, Thoma R, Baranidharan G, Liem L, Patel NK, Love-Jones S, Espinet AJ, Verrills P, Schu S: Does convergence of multi-segmental afferent inputs at the spinal lamina enable treatment of postherpetic neuralgia with dorsal root ganglion (DRG) stimulation possible (poster No. 311)? NANS 2013: Today's Vision, Tomorrow Reality, Las Vegas, 2013.
40 Burger K, Moser H, Liem L, Klase D, Eldabe S: Spinal cord stimulation (SCS) of the dorsal root ganglion (DRG) in the treatment of post amputation pain. NANS 2012: From Innovation to Reality, Las Vegas, 2012, p 145.
41 Bara GA, Maciaczyk J, Slotty P, Schu S, Vesper J: Dorsal root ganglion stimulation for treatment of phantom limb pain (poster No. 420). NANS 2013: Today's Vision, Tomorrow Reality, Las Vegas, 2013.
42 Baranidharan G: Reduction in dermatomal hyperalgesia in patients with visceral pain treated with spinal cord stimulation (SCS) of the dorsal root ganglion (DRG) (poster No. 360). NANS 2013: Today's Vision, Tomorrow Reality, Las Vegas, 2013.
43 Gulve A, Eldabe S, Koneti K, Garner F, West S, King R, Chadwick R: Dorsal root ganglion stimulation for the treatment of body wall pain: Middlesbrough experience (poster No. 285). NANS 2013: Today's Vision, Tomorrow Reality, Las Vegas, 2013.
44 Liem L, Demmel W, Thoma R, Neumann H, Rasche D, Schu S: Spinal cord stimulation (SCS) of the dorsal root ganglion (DRG) for chronic pain of the upper limbs – a multi-center case series. Neuromodulation 2013;16:e141.
45 Kramer J, Liem L, Russo M, Smet I, Van Buyten JP, Huygen F: Lack of body positional effects on paresthesias when stimulating the dorsal root ganglion (DRG) in the treatment of chronic pain. Neuromodulation 2015;18:50–57.
46 Rigoard P, Desai MJ, North RB, Taylor RS, Annemans L, Greening C, Tan Y, Van den Abeele C, Shipley J, Kumar K: Spinal cord stimulation for predominant low back pain in failed back surgery syndrome: study protocol for an international multicenter randomized controlled trial (PROMISE study). Trials 2013;14:376.
47 Brierley JB: The penetration of particulate matter from the cerebrospinal fluid into the spinal ganglia, peripheral nerves, and perivascular spaces of the central nervous system. J Neurol Neurosurg Psychiatry 1950;13:203–215.
48 Geurts JW, Smits H, Kemler MA, Brunner F, Kessels AG, van Kleef M: Spinal cord stimulation for complex regional pain syndrome type I: a prospective cohort study with long-term follow-up. Neuromodulation 2013;16:523–529.

49 McAuley J, Farah N, van Gröningen R, Green C: A questionnaire-based study on patients' experiences with rechargeable implanted programmable generators for spinal cord stimulation to treat chronic lumbar spondylosis pain. Neuromodulation 2013;16: 142–146.
50 Crock HV: Normal and pathological anatomy of the lumbar spinal nerve root canals. J Bone Joint Surg Br 1981;63B:487–490.
51 Wiltse LL: Anatomy of the extradural compartments of the lumbar spinal canal. Peridural membrane and circumneural sheath. Radiol Clin North Am 2000; 38:1177–1206.
52 Puigdellivol-Sánchez A, Prats-Galino A, Ruano-Gil D, Molander C: Sciatic and femoral nerve sensory neurones occupy different regions of the L4 dorsal root ganglion in the adult rat. Neurosci Lett 1998; 251:169–172.
53 Hanani M: Satellite glial cells in sensory ganglia: from form to function. Brain Res Brain Res Rev 2005; 48:457–476.
54 Hogan QH: Labat lecture: the primary sensory neuron: where it is, what it does and why it matters. Reg Anesth Pain Med 2010;35:306–311.
55 Sapunar D, Kostic S, Banozic A, Puljak L: Dorsal root ganglion – a potential new therapeutic target for neuropathic pain. J Pain Res 2012;5:31–38.
56 Buenaventura RM, Datta S, Abdi S, Smith HS: Systematic review of therapeutic lumbar transforaminal epidural steroid injections. Pain Physician 2009;12: 233–251.
57 Aichaoui F, Mertens P, Sindou M: Dorsal root entry zone lesioning for pain after brachial plexus avulsion: results with special emphasis on differential effects on the paroxysmal versus the continuous components. A prospective study in a 29-patient consecutive series. Pain 2011;152:1923–1930.
58 Loeser JD: Dorsal rhizotomy for the relief of chronic pain. J Neurosurg 1972;36:745–750.
59 North RB, Kidd DH, Campbell JN, Long DM: Dorsal root ganglionectomy for failed back surgery syndrome: a 5-year follow-up study. J Neurosurg 1991; 74:236–242.
60 Nagda JV, Davis CW, Bajwa ZH, Simopoulos TT: Retrospective review of the efficacy and safety of repeated pulsed and continuous radiofrequency lesioning of the dorsal root ganglion/segmental nerve for lumbar radicular pain. Pain Physician 2011;14: 371–376.
61 Simopoulos TT, Kraemer J, Nagda JV, Aner M, Bajwa ZH: Response to pulsed and continuous radiofrequency lesioning of the dorsal root ganglion and segmental nerves in patients with chronic lumbar radicular pain. Pain Physician 2008;11:137–144.
62 Tanagho EA: Neuromodulation and neurostimulation: overview and future potential. Transl Androl Urol 2012;1:44–49.
63 Weigel R, Capelle HH, Krauss JK: Failure of long-term nerve root stimulation to improve neuropathic pain. J Neurosurg 2008;108:921–925.
64 Haque R, Winfree CJ: Transforaminal nerve root stimulation: a technical report. Neuromodulation 2009;12:254–257.
65 Kellner CP, Kellner MA, Winfree CJ: Spinal nerve root stimulation. Prog Neurol Surg 2011;24:180–188.
66 Lynch PJ, McJunkin T, Eross E, Gooch S, Maloney J: Case report: successful epiradicular peripheral nerve stimulation of the C2 dorsal root ganglion for postherpetic neuralgia. Neuromodulation 2011;14: 58–61.
67 Kiernan JA, Rajakumar N: Barr's The Human Nervous System: An Anatomical Viewpoint. Baltimore, Lippincott Williams & Wilkins, 2014.
68 Abram SE, Yi J, Fuchs A, Hogan QH: Permeability of injured and intact peripheral nerves and dorsal root ganglion. Anesthesiology 2006;105:146–153.
69 Hjerling-Leffler J, Marmigère F, Heglind M, Cederberg A, Koltzenburg M, Enerbäck S, Ernfors P: The boundary cap: a source of neural crest stem cells that generate multiple sensory neuron subtypes. Development 2005;132:2623–2632.
70 Maro GS, Vermeren M, Voiculescu O, Melton L, Cohen J, Charnay P, Topilko P: Neural crest boundary cap cells constitute a source of neuronal and glial cells of the PNS. Nat Neurosci 2004;7:930–938.
71 Kalcheim C, Le Douarin NM: Requirement of a neural tube signal for the differentiation of neural crest cells into dorsal root ganglia. Dev Biol 1986;116:451–466.
72 Golding J, Shewan D, Cohen J: Maturation of the mammalian dorsal root entry zone – from entry to no entry. Trends Neurosci 1997;20:303–308.
73 Raisman G: What hope for repair of the brain? Ann Neurol 1978;3:101–106.
74 Aló KM, Abramova MV, Richter EO: Percutaneous peripheral nerve stimulation. Prog Neurol Surg 2011;24:41–57.
75 Julius D, Basbaum AI: Molecular mechanisms of nociception. Nature 2001;413:203–210.
76 Scholz J, Woolf CJ: The neuropathic pain triad: neurons, immune cells and glia. Nat Neurosci 2007;10: 1361–1368.
77 Hu P, McLachlan EM: Macrophage and lymphocyte invasion of dorsal root ganglia after peripheral nerve lesions in the rat. Neuroscience 2002;112:23–38.
78 Hu P, McLachlan EM: Distinct functional types of macrophage in dorsal root ganglia and spinal nerves proximal to sciatic and spinal nerve transections in the rat. Exp Neurol 2003;184:590–605.
79 Moalem G, Tracey DJ: Immune and inflammatory mechanisms in neuropathic pain. Brain Res Rev 2006;51:240–264.

80 Sorkin LS, Xiao WH, Wagner R, Myers RR: Tumour necrosis factor-alpha induces ectopic activity in nociceptive primary afferent fibres. Neuroscience 1997; 81:255–262.
81 Zhou XF, Deng YS, Xian CJ, Zhong JH: Neurotrophins from dorsal root ganglia trigger allodynia after spinal nerve injury in rats. Eur J Neurosci 2000;12: 100–105.
82 Woolf CJ: Phenotypic modifications of primary sensory neurons: the role of nerve growth factor in the production of persistent pain. Philos Trans R Soc Lond B Biol Sci 1996;351:441–448.
83 Kajander KC, Wakisaka S, Bennett GJ: Spontaneous discharge originates in the dorsal root ganglion at the onset of a painful peripheral neuropathy in the rat. Neurosci Lett 1992;138:225–228.
84 Chung K, Lee BH, Yoon YW, Chung JM: Sympathetic sprouting in the dorsal root ganglia of the injured peripheral nerve in a rat neuropathic pain model. J Comp Neurol 1996;376:241–252.
85 Amir R, Michaelis M, Devor M: Membrane potential oscillations in dorsal root ganglion neurons: role in normal electrogenesis and neuropathic pain. J Neurosci 1999;19:8589–8596.
86 Pannese E, Ledda M, Cherkas PS, Huang TY, Hanani M: Satellite cell reactions to axon injury of sensory ganglion neurons: increase in number of gap junctions and formation of bridges connecting previously separate perineuronal sheaths. Anat Embryol (Berl) 2003;206:337–347.
87 Waxman SG, Dib-Hajj S, Cummins TR, Black JA: Sodium channels and their genes: dynamic expression in the normal nervous system, dysregulation in disease states. Brain Res 2000;886:5–14.
88 Echeverry S, Shi XQ, Zhang J: Characterization of cell proliferation in rat spinal cord following peripheral nerve injury and the relationship with neuropathic pain. Pain 2008;135:37–47.
89 Zeilhofer HU: Loss of glycinergic and GABAergic inhibition in chronic pain – contributions of inflammation and microglia. Int Immunopharmacol 2008; 8:182–187.
90 Moore KA, Kohno T, Karchewski LA, Scholz J, Baba H, Woolf CJ: Partial peripheral nerve injury promotes a selective loss of GABAergic inhibition in the superficial dorsal horn of the spinal cord. J Neurosci 2002;22:6724–6731.
91 Ji RR, Kohno T, Moore KA, Woolf CJ: Central sensitization and LTP: do pain and memory share similar mechanisms? Trends Neurosci 2003;26:696–705.
92 Woolf CJ, Salter MW: Neuronal plasticity: increasing the gain in pain. Science 2000;288:1765–1769.
93 Wall PD, Devor M: Sensory afferent impulses originate from dorsal root ganglia as well as from the periphery in normal and nerve injured rats. Pain 1983; 17:321–339.
94 Koopmeiners AS, Mueller S, Kramer J, Hogan QH: Effect of electrical field stimulation on dorsal root ganglion neuronal function. Neuromodulation 2013; 16:304–311.
95 Tsou HK, Chao SC, Wang CJ, Chen HT, Shen CC, Lee HT, Tsuei YS: Percutaneous pulsed radiofrequency applied to the L-2 dorsal root ganglion for treatment of chronic low-back pain: 3-year experience. J Neurosurg Spine 2010;12:190–196.
96 Melzack R, Wall PD: Pain mechanisms: a new theory. Science 1965;150:971–979.

Liong Liem, MD
Sint Antonius Hospital
Postbus 2500
NL–3430 EM Nieuwegein (The Netherlands)
E-Mail l.liem@antoniusziekenhuis.nl

Slavin KV (ed): Stimulation of the Peripheral Nervous System. The Neuromodulation Frontier.
Prog Neurol Surg. Basel, Karger, 2016, vol 29, pp 225–237 (DOI: 10.1159/000434674)

Regulation of Peripheral Nerve Stimulation Technology

Daniel M. Birk • Dali Yin • Konstantin V. Slavin
Department of Neurosurgery, University of Illinois at Chicago, Chicago, Ill., USA

Abstract
The number of peripheral nerve stimulation (PNS) indications, targets, and devices is expanding, yet the development of the technology has been slow because many devices used for PNS do not have formal regulatory approval. Manufacturers have not sought Food and Drug Administration (FDA) approval for PNS devices because of a perceived lack of interest amongst practitioners and patients. Without FDA approval, companies cannot invest in marketing to educate the implanters and the patients about the benefits of PNS in the treatment of chronic pain. Violation of this has resulted in governmental investigation and prosecution. Most of the PNS devices currently used to treat chronic pain are FDA approved for epidural spinal cord stimulation. Many of the complications seen in PNS surgery can be attributed to the lack of purpose-built hardware with FDA approval. Despite the lack of regulatory approval, there are insurance companies that approve PNS procedures when deemed medically necessary. As the targets and indications for PNS continue to expand, there will be an even greater need for customized technological solutions. It is up to the medical device industry to invest in the design and marketing of PNS technology and seek out FDA approval. Market forces will continue to push PNS into the mainstream and physicians will increasingly have the choice to implant devices specifically designed and approved to treat chronic peripheral nerve pain.

Peripheral nerve stimulation (PNS) technology consists of electrode contact(s) arranged on a lead that deliver electrical energy from a pulse generator to a peripheral nerve. Today, the number of PNS indications, targets, and devices is rapidly expanding, yet the development of PNS hardware and technology has been slowed by a lack of formal regulatory approval. Manufacturers have not sought United States (US) Food and Drug Administration (FDA) approval for PNS devices because of a relative lack of interest amongst practitioners and patients. Due to a perceived lack of return on investment, companies have not invested in such approval that would allow them to pursue marketing and education efforts to inform both the implanters and the patients about the benefits of PNS in the treatment of chronic pain. As a result of all this, the majority of the technology used for PNS applications in treatment of chronic pain is approved by the FDA for use in spinal cord stimulation (SCS). Many of the complications seen in PNS surgery can be attributed to the lack of purpose-built hardware with FDA approval for the treatment of chronic pain.

The goal of our paper is to introduce the reader to the current regulatory environment for PNS technology. We begin with a brief summary of the development of technology for PNS and how regulatory issues have come into play. Next, device regulation in the US, Europe, Canada, and Australia is reviewed. Then, a review of the current and future state of PNS device regulation is provided. Readers should pay particular attention to table 1, which outlines most of the currently available PNS devices and their regulatory status.

Device Evolution and Regulatory Approval

Early on in the development of PNS technology, leads were custom made in small batches. Wire leads gave way to the cuff-type leads that wrap around the nerve, thereby providing long-term stimulation [1]. Issues with cuff-type electrodes include scarring, fibrosis, and nerve constriction, as well as muscle contractions from inadvertent motor fascicle stimulation in mixed nerves. 'Cuff-type' electrodes were replaced by the 'button type', which can be sutured to the perineurium over the desired segment of the nerve circumference. Both varieties of electrode contact are associated with good outcomes, but they require surgically exposing the nerve which subjects the patient to a higher risk of complications.

Since cuff- and button-type electrodes can cause perineural fibrosis, it was suggested to use flat plate 'paddle-type' multicontact electrodes, which were serially produced and designed for SCS, placing them adjacent to the nerve and thereby avoiding this complication. Introduced in the late 1980s, the quadripolar lead was implanted under the nerve so that the four metal contacts faced the nerve [2]. The multitude of contacts allows various programming options and increases the chance of satisfactory pain relief. The use of fascia for padding between the electrode and the nerve further reduced fibrosis. Medtronic developed a lead with a mesh attached specifically for suturing to the fascia in PNS applications (OnPoint; Medtronic, Minneapolis, Minn., USA) [3]. Prior to introduction of the OnPoint lead, other flat paddle electrodes such as Resume and Symmix, both manufactured by Medtronic, were created for SCS and readily available for use in PNS. Despite all of these advantages, paddle electrode implantation still carried the added risks associated with invasive surgical exploration.

In the 1990s, the percutaneous transspinal techniques developed for SCS electrode implantation were adapted for PNS procedures in order to avoid the risks involved with dissection of the target nerve [4]. Both quadripolar and octopolar electrodes have been used for percutaneous implantation. In 1999, it was established that placing a

Table 1. Regulatory approval status of PNS systems

No.	Indication	Company	Device	USA (FDA)	Europe (CE mark)	Canada (Health Canada)	Notes
Pain							
1	Severe intractable pain	Medtronic	RF systems (X-Trel, Mattrix) with Resume II (3587A), Resume TL (3986A), and OnPoint (3987A) electrode	*	*	05/2000	True PNS system/RF systems only
2	Severe intractable pain	St. Jude Medical	RF system (Renew) with percutaneous leads (3143, 3146, 3153, 3156, 3183, 3186, 3066, 3161, 3163, 3166, 3169)	*	*		True PNS system/RF systems only
3	Chronic intractable postsurgical back pain	Medtronic	RestoreUltra, RestoreAdvanced, RestoreSensor, and PrimeAdvanced with percutaneous leads		05/2011	*	Subcutaneous nerve stimulation
4	Intractable chronic migraine	St. Jude Medical	Genesis system		09/2011		PNS of occipital nerves
5	Intractable chronic migraine	St. Jude Medical	Eon Mini system		09/2012		PNS of occipital nerves
6	Chronic intractable pain in the trunk	Boston Scientific	Precision Plus SCS system		08/2012		PNS
7	Pain due to diseases of peripheral nerves	Neurimpulse	Lightpulse 100, 100L, 102 systems		11/2010		Subcutaneous PNS
8	Chronic intractable pain	Spinal Modulation	Axium system	IDE, 08/2013	12/2011		Dorsal root ganglion stimulation
9	Acute pain of cluster headache	Autonomic Technologies	Pulsante SPG stimulation system	IDE, 07/2014	10/2012		Sphenopalatine ganglion stimulation
10	Chronic shoulder pain	SPR Therapeutics	Smartpatch PNS system		01/2013		Up to 30 days stimulation
11	Chronic migraine	CerboMed	t-VNS system		08/2012		Transcutaneous vagus nerve stimulation
12	Chronic migraine	Cephaly Technology	Cephaly TENS system	04/2014	*	11/2010	Transcutaneous trigeminal nerve stimulation
13	Chronic peripheral neuropathic pain	Algotec	Neurostimulator PENS therapy		*		PENS therapy – no implant involved
14	Chronic amputation pain	Neuros Medical	Altius implantable system	IDE, 09/2013			High frequency nerve block
15	Chronic pain of peripheral nerve origin	Bioness	StimRouter neuromodulation system	IDE, 04/2012			Implanted PNS device with external power source

Table 1. Continued

No.	Indication	Company	Device	USA (FDA)	Europe (CE mark)	Canada (Health Canada)	Notes
16	Chronic low back pain	Mainstay Medical	ReActiv8 system				Medial branch stimulation
Motor dysfunction							
17	Partial or complete respiratory insufficiency	Avery Biomedical	Mark IV breathing pacemaker	03/1998	*(1999)		Phrenic nerve stimulation
18	Need in maintenance of artificial respiration	Atrotech	Atrostim PNS V2.0 system		*		Phrenic nerve stimulation
19	Respiratory failure due to SCI	Synapse Biomedical	NeuRx diaphragm pacing system	HDE, 06/2008	11/2007	03/2013	Diaphragmal stimulation
20	Respiratory failure due to ALS	Synapse Biomedical	NeuRx diaphragm pacing system	HDE, 09/2011	11/2007		Diaphragmal stimulation
21	Obstructive sleep apnea	Inspire Medical	Inspire system	04/2014	12/2010		Hypoglossal nerve stimulation
22	Obstructive sleep apnea	ImThera Medical	Aura 6000 system	IDE, 11/2014	03/2012		Hypoglossal nerve stimulation
23	Obstructive sleep apnea	Apnex Medical	HGNS system	IDE, 08/2011			Hypoglossal nerve stimulation
Epilepsy							
24	Refractory epilepsy	Cyberonics	NCP/Demipulse/Aspire systems	*(1997)	*(1994)	08/1998	Implanted vagus nerve stimulation
25	Epilepsy	CerboMed	NEMOS system		03/2010		Transcutaneous vagus nerve stimulation
26	Epilepsy/ Lennox-Gastaut syndrome	NeuroSigma	Monarch eTNS system	HDE, 01/2015	09/2012	04/2013	Transcutaneous trigeminal nerve stimulation
Depression							
27	Treatment-resistant depression	Cyberonics	VNS system	07/2005	03/2001	04/2001	Implanted vagus nerve stimulation
28	Depression	CerboMed	NEMOS system		03/2010		Transcutaneous vagus nerve stimulation
29	Depression	NeuroSigma	Monarch eTNS system		09/2012	04/2013	Transcutaneous trigeminal nerve stimulation
Urinary/gastrointestinal dysfunction							
30	Urinary/fecal urge incontinence	Medtronic	InterStim (3023) and InterStim II (3058) neurostimulators	*(1997)	*(1994)	12/1999	Sacral nerve stimulation

Table 1. Continued

No.	Indication	Company	Device	USA (FDA)	Europe (CE mark)	Canada (Health Canada)	Notes
31	Overactive bladder/urinary retention	Medtronic	InterStim II (3058) neurostimulator	07/2006	*(2006)	*	Sacral nerve stimulation
32	Overactive bladder	Axonics	Axonics system				Sacral nerve stimulation
Hypertension/heart failure							
33	Resistant hypertension	CVRx	Rheos Baroflex/ Barostim neo hypertension therapy system	HDE, 10/2014	10/2007		Carotid sinus and nerve stimulation
34	Heart failure	CVRx	Barostim neo system		09/2014		Carotid sinus and nerve stimulation
Obesity							
35	Severe obesity	EnteroMedics	Maestro system	01/2015	03/2009		Vagus nerve block
Tinnitus							
36	Tinnitus	Micro-Transponder	Serenity system	IDE, 10/2013			Vagus nerve stimulation with paired impulses

* Asterisk denotes existence of full regulatory approval when the date of approval is unknown or unconfirmed. HDE = Humanitarian device exemption; IDE = investigational device exemption.

PNS electrode in the proximity of the occipital nerve is as effective, and easier to implant, as the wrap-around cuff-type electrodes in treating occipital neuralgia [5]. Since then, percutaneous PNS approaches have been used to treat multiple pain syndromes including migraine headaches, cluster headaches, supraorbital neuralgia, back pain, and other syndromes throughout the body including fibromyalgia [6–12].

Modern electrode leads used for PNS in the treatment of pain are either the percutaneous cylindrical or flat paddle types, and they come in various sizes. Percutaneous electrodes manufactured by three major neuromodulation technology companies [Medtronic, St. Jude Medical (St. Paul, Minn., USA; formerly Advanced Neuromodulation Systems, Plano, Tex., USA), and Boston Scientific (Marlborough, Mass., USA; formerly Advanced Bionics, Valencia, Calif., USA)] have been used successfully for PNS. Paddle electrodes remain an accepted technology and are used for stimulating large nerves as well as for greater occipital nerve stimulation. They stimulate in a unidirectional manner and have a lower incidence of migration, but they also require invasive surgical exposure for implantation.

Cuff-type electrode technology remains in use for vagus nerve stimulators for refractory epilepsy and treatment-resistant depression (Cyberonics, Houston, Tex., USA), and in phrenic nerve stimulation systems for diaphragmal pacing in treatment-resistant respiratory failure (Avery Biomedical Devices, Commack, N.Y., USA).

The number of contacts and leads incorporated into PNS system design is determined by the electrical generator technology. Early generators used radio frequency (RF)-coupled systems with an implanted receiver and external generator and control unit. The advantages of RF systems are the ability to deliver high-power complex stimulation and easy recharging with household batteries, but they also demand more patient participation.

Despite requiring interval battery replacement surgery, the fully implantable pulse generators (IPG) used for SCS were more appealing to the PNS patient. RF-coupled devices are rarely used anymore except for breathing pacemakers. Interestingly, RF-coupled systems remain the only devices that are FDA approved for PNS in the treatment of chronic pain. Although fully implantable systems need costly interval battery replacement surgery, patients and their physicians consistently choose this approach because the need for external attachments is limited and the patients may swim or shower at will without worrying about poor contact between the antenna and receiver [13]. The RF devices are still listed in the catalogues and this helps maintain the clinical indication of PNS for chronic pain for marketing and educational purposes.

IPG technology has undergone substantial evolution. The first generation accommodated four contacts and powered a single quadripolar lead. Later iterations could accommodate eight contacts and allowed for multiple stimulation programs. More recent IPGs have the capacity for 16, or even 32, contacts and the patient may recharge them on their own without undergoing additional surgery.

The latest devices also boast a smaller profile, which makes them particularly well suited for PNS. Boston Scientific developed a miniaturized rechargeable microstimulation device called Bion, which was tested for several PNS indications including urinary incontinence and severe headaches. The Bion device is small and cylindrical in shape, making implantation more straightforward. Unfortunately, this device is no longer available. A different miniaturized device, Freedom 4, manufactured by Stim-Wave (Miami Beach, Fla., USA), has recently been approved for SCS use and could be an excellent option for PNS applications.

Beyond electrodes, generators, and receivers, most PNS systems also incorporate extension cables, splitters, and anchors to hold the wires in place and prevent migration. There are also other necessary device accessories such as insertion needles, stylets, guide wires, introducers, passers, dissecting tools, and wrenches. All of these ancillary devices are approved for SCS and used off-label for PNS implantation.

In combination, these technologies have enabled surgeons to treat a variety of neuropathic pain syndromes. As the PNS neuromodulation community has grown, so have reports of complications such as erosion, migration, and disconnection. Although surgeons have refined their implantation techniques to reduce complications, many complications are attributable to problems with using technology designed for use in a different part of the body, specifically the spinal epidural space.

Today, most of the devices used for PNS in the treatment of chronic pain are still designed, approved, and marketed exclusively for SCS, which accounts for a large number of PNS complications. Due to low interest amongst the majority of practitioners, manufacturers have not obtained FDA approval for use of the implantable generators for PNS. According to the manufacturer's manuals, the only devices specifically approved for PNS in treatment of pain are the practically obsolete RF systems by Medtronic and St. Jude Medical, and the only electrode specifically designed and approved for PNS in the treatment of pain is the paddle with integrated mesh made by Medtronic. Poor predictability and lack of testability have also slowed growth of the technique in general.

Overview of Medical Device Regulation in the United States

Medical devices comprise a large category of tools and equipment that range from simple bandages to complex MRI machines. Broadly defined, a medical device is a thing intended to diagnose, cure, treat, or prevent a disease that affects the structure or function of the body. It must not accomplish its effect via chemical reaction or through its own metabolization, like a pharmaceutical agent. According to the Federal Food, Drug, and Cosmetic Act (FD&C), the FDA requires 'reasonable assurance of safety and effectiveness' of devices before marketing is permitted. The FDA has three classes of medical devices. Class I are low risk (bandages, drapes), and class II are mild-to-moderate risk (catheters, hearing aids). Peripheral nerve stimulators are usually designated as class III devices due to the high risks associated with their use.

All three classes are subject to the FDA's General Controls and there are additional controls for class II and III devices. Most class I devices are exempt from the FDA's premarket notification 510(k) process. Most class II devices determined to be a moderate risk require premarket notification 510(k) and most class III devices require premarket approval (PMA). Therefore, as high-risk devices, PNS generators are granted initial approval through the PMA pathway.

In general, 510(k) prenotification is required for devices that are substantially equivalent to existing technologies and PMA approval is required for devices involving new technological concepts. If the device is substantially equivalent to any 510(k)s already cleared by the FDA, then the applicant should submit a 510(k). If no such equivalent product can be found, the applicant should submit a PMA.

The FDA defines a humanitarian use device (HUD) as one that is intended to benefit patients by treating or diagnosing a condition that affects fewer than 4,000 individuals in the US per year. Since the manufacturer's return on investment may not exceed the costs in this population, the HUD provision is an incentive for the development of devices for these small patient populations. To obtain approval for an HUD, the FDA requires a humanitarian device exemption application. This is similar to the PMA pathway, but it does not require the same rigorous proof of effectiveness. The FDA will verify that the HUD does not pose a significant risk of illness or injury and that the health benefits outweigh the risks. Devices approved for humanitarian use may only be implanted at centers with an institutional review board for approval and supervision.

The FDA will allow an investigational device exemption so that an investigational device may be used in a clinical study. These studies are done to gather safety and effectiveness data to support PMA. Obtaining an investigational device exemption requires a plan approved by an institutional review board, informed consent from patients, labeling specifying investigational use only, monitoring of the study, and mandatory reporting to the FDA.

Marketing a medical device in the US involves many controls and both premarket and postmarket requirements. Premarket requirements include classifying the device, choosing the correct premarket submission, preparing and submitting the appropriate information, and finally listing the device and registering the establishment that will manufacture and distribute it. Postmarket requirements include instituting tracking systems and reporting device malfunctions, serious injuries, or deaths. There are also postmarket surveillance studies and postapproval studies that the FDA may require when they grant PMA or an exemption for a humanitarian or investigational device. All devices must be registered with the FDA via the Unified Registration and Listing System (FURLS).

Premarket Notification

Premarket notification is accomplished by submitted a 510(k) application to the FDA. This is a premarket petition submitted to the FDA to demonstrate that the medical device is safe and effective as well as substantially equivalent to a current legally marketed device. An establishment cannot commercially distribute the device until the FDA provides a letter of substantial equivalence. The 510(k) submission will contain a comparison to one or more similar devices on the US market to establish substantial equivalence.

With the current FDA system, initial acceptance is not based on a substantive review of the information provided but on administrative criteria. Any deviation from the checklist should be accompanied by a rationale. Only once the acceptance review is completed does the FDA conduct a substantive review to determine substantial equivalence of the device. The preliminary acceptance checklist questions for a traditional 510(k) are as follows:

(1) Is the product a device [per section 201(h) of the FD&C Act] or a combination product [per Title 21 Code of Federal Regulations 3.2(e)] with a device constituent part subject to review in a 510(k)?
(2) Is the application with the appropriate center?
(3) If a Request for Designation (RFD) was submitted for the device or combination product with a device constituent part and assigned to your center, identify the RFD No. and confirm the following:

a. Is the device or combination product the same as that presented in the RFD submission?
b. Are the indications for use of the device or combination product identified in the 510(k) the same as those identified in the RFD submission?

(4) Is this device type eligible for a 510(k) submission?
(5) Is there a pending PMA for the same device with the same indications for use?
(6) If clinical studies have been submitted, is the submitter the subject of an Application Integrity Policy?

Premarket Approval

The safety and effectiveness of class III medical devices are reviewed during the PMA process. Class III devices are defined as those that sustain human life, are of substantial importance in preventing impairment of human health, or which present a potential, unreasonable risk of illness or injury. Many peripheral nerve stimulator technologies will be categorized as class III devices. Due to the inherent risks of this class of devices, there is a more rigorous process to obtain marketing clearance as outlined in section 515 of the FD&C Act.

The PMA must contain sufficient and valid scientific evidence to assure the device is safe and effective for its intended use. The applicant is often the inventor or developer and later the manufacturer of the device. During the review, the FDA may hold a public meeting to review the PMA. After approval or denial, a notice is published on the Internet announcing the data on which the decision is based and providing an opportunity for other parties to petition the decision within 30 days. Regulations for PMA may be found in Title 21 Code of Federal Regulations Part 814, Premarket Approval. If a device fails to meet PMA requirements, it is considered adulterated under section 501(f) of the FD&C Act and cannot be marketed.

PMA data requirements encompass technical data sections for nonclinical laboratory studies and clinical investigations. Nonclinical laboratory studies may include data on microbiology, toxicology, immunology, biocompatibility, stress, wear, shelf life, and other laboratory or animal tests. Clinical data includes study protocols, safety and efficacy data, adverse reactions and complications, device failures and replacements, patient information, patient complaints, statistical analyses, and more. Applicants should pay attention to study design and conduct and ensure proper data analyses, coherent presentations, and sound conclusions.

The PMA review has several components including the initial administrative review and a limited scientific review to assess completeness. Then, the FDA conducts an in-depth scientific, regulatory, and quality system review. Approval is contingent on a draft of the final labeling and on the condition that the applicant submits a copy of the final printed labeling to the FDA before any marketing activity begins [14, 15].

Overview of Medical Device Regulation in the European Union

Since the 1990s, the European Union (EU) has dictated requirements to market a medical device in any of the EU member countries. Approved devices earning a Conformité Européenne (CE) mark in any member country can be marketed in all the EU states. Devices are categorized into four classes (I, IIa, IIb, and III) depending on the device's risk profile. Each country has a governing body called a 'competent authority', which oversees device regulation in that nation. Devices deemed to be low risk are reported to the competent authority, who may inspect and review standards and technical aspects of the device. For higher risk or more complicated devices like PNS ones, independent companies called 'notified bodies' are assigned to oversee evaluation and approval.

Regardless of the regulatory environment, PNS devices are generally considered to be complex and higher risk. Therefore, the manufacturer of a PNS device in Europe must select a designated notified body to oversee performance and reliability testing. A device will usually be approved if it performs as intended so that the benefits outweigh the risks involved with its use.

During postmarket surveillance, manufactures report adverse events to the competent authorities. The competent authority, but not the public, has access to the European Databank on Medical Devices (EUDAMED), which stores data related to the manufacturer, clinical studies, and postmarket events.

Unlike with the FDA, which prioritizes public health and device safety, the EU system is primarily intended to facilitate trade and coordinate manufacturing, safety, and environmental standards amongst decentralized groups. The EU competent authorities complete a performance-based analysis requiring proof that a device functions as intended. Unlike the FDA, there is less transparency and the review of the notified bodies is not made public. The EU system offers patients the benefit of earlier access to some higher risk devices when compared to patients in the US [15, 16].

Medical Device Regulation in Canada and Australia

In Canada, the Medical Devices Bureau of the Therapeutic Products Directorate (TPD) is the regulatory body responsible for monitoring and evaluating the safety, effectiveness and quality of medical devices. As in the US and the EU, the Canadian system entails a combination of premarket review, postapproval surveillance, and quality systems in the manufacturing process. In Canada, medical devices are categorized as class I, II, III, or IV based on the risks associated with their use including the degree of invasiveness, degree of contact with the patient, energy transmission hazard, and the consequences of device failure. Devices falling into class II, III, or IV require a medical device license. PNS devices fall into classes III and IV and therefore require a Health Canada License before marketing can begin. In addition, the license must be renewed annually [17].

In Australia, the Department of Health and Ageing oversees the Therapeutic Goods Administration (TGA), which regulates medical devices. Within the TGA, the Office of Devices Authorisation is responsible for premarket regulation of medical devices. The Office of Product Review, in turn, handles postmarket regulation. As in the US and the EU, medical devices are classified according to the level of potential risk to the patient. Higher risk classification necessitates additional controls and oversight. One strategy employed in Australia to reduce the regulatory burden on industry is to negotiate agreements with other international regulators. This can result in early acceptance after recognition of regulatory decisions made in other countries [18].

Current Status of Peripheral Nerve Stimulation Device Regulation

Table 1 summarizes the current status of PNS device regulation worldwide as of early 2015. Although this is not an exhaustive tabulation of all devices used for PNS, it includes those that are most commonly used. Many PNS procedures for chronic pain are performed with devices that are not specifically approved for this indication. Most of the time, devices approved for SCS are used for PNS in the treatment of chronic pain. Those electrodes and devices that are specifically approved for PNS, such as the RF systems, are rarely used anymore. These include OnPoint, Resume, and Symmix electrodes and RF receivers Mattrix and X-Trel (all from Medtronic), and electrode leads and the Renew RF receiver (St. Jude Medical).

Devices used for PNS have different regulatory approval status in different national jurisdictions. Many neurostimulators are approved for PNS in treating chronic pain in Europe and Australia, but not in the US. Some devices, such as the Lightpulse PNS system (Neurimpulse, Rubano, Italy), are only approved for use in Europe and are not marketed in the US. The Medtronic and Boston Scientific devices have a CE mark for PNS in treatment of back and/or trunk pain, and the St. Jude Medical IPGs (EON and Genesis) have received the CE mark approval for the treatment of chronic migraine headaches. All of these systems are FDA approved for SCS and are used off-label in the US in the setting of PNS.

Other devices are approved in multiple international markets and include the Cyberonics VNS Therapy System, which is approved in the EU, US, Canada, and Japan for the treatment of medically refractory epilepsy.

As of February 2015, the FDA has not cleared any implantable PNS device for headache management or for occipital neuralgia. Use of these devices for craniofacial pain is still on an off-label basis.

Future of Peripheral Nerve Stimulation Device Regulation

The field of peripheral nerve neuromodulation is on the cusp of exponential growth with an expanding number of indications, scientific understanding, and devices on the horizon. For the time being, PNS devices are used on an off-label basis, but this promises to change in the future. As the popularity of PNS amongst patients and providers grows, there will be better opportunities to collect scientific data on the safety, efficacy, and cost-effectiveness of PNS devices. With increased demand and better data, manufacturers will finally have an incentive to seek regulatory approval. Neuromodulation companies will also accelerate their efforts to market PNS devices and to educate both patients and providers about their use.

There is a great need for devices specifically tailored to PNS. For instance, there is a need for a PNS paddle electrode that can be inserted through a percutaneous needle [19], but this is just one example of the myriad ways the technology should be specifically designed for PNS parameters.

Despite the lack of regulatory approval from FDA, there are some insurance companies with a policy of approving PNS procedures when deemed medically necessary. Their criteria of appropriateness may include pain isolated to a single nerve, pain refractory to medical management, favorable psychological evaluation, a successful trial, and diagnostic confirmation with nerve blocks [20]. While this is good news for patients with chronic peripheral nerve pain, the lack of regulatory approval prevents device companies from legal marketing, promotion, and physician education when it comes to PNS. Violation of this results in governmental investigation and prosecution: it was recently reported that Medtronic has agreed to pay a fine of USD 2.8 million to the FDA for promoting off-label use of SCS devices for PNS [21].

It remains to be seen whether all this will motivate industry to invest in research, design, and marketing of FDA-approved PNS technology. As the targets and indications for PNS expand, so does the need for more advanced and customized technological solutions. Market forces will continue to push PNS into the mainstream and physicians will increasingly be able to implant devices specifically designed and approved for PNS indications.

References

1 Van Calenbergh F, Gybels J, Van Laere K, Dupont P, Plaghki L, Depreitere B, Kupers R: Long term clinical outcome of peripheral nerve stimulation in patients with chronic peripheral neuropathic pain. Surg Neurol 2009;72:330–335.

2 Racz GB, Browne T, Lewis R Jr: Peripheral stimulator implant for treatment of causalgia caused by electrical burns. Tex Med 1988;84:45–50.

3 Mobbs RJ, Blum P, Rossato R: Mesh electrode for peripheral nerve stimulation. J Clin Neurosci 2003;10:476–477.

4 Urban BJ, Nashold BS Jr: Combined epidural and peripheral nerve stimulation for relief of pain. Description of technique and preliminary results. J Neurosurg 1982;57:365–369.

5 Weiner RL, Reed KL: Peripheral neurostimulation for control of intractable occipital neuralgia. Neuromodulation 1999;2:217–221.

6 Popeney CA, Aló KM: Peripheral neurostimulation for the treatment of chronic, disabling transformed migraine. Headache 2003;43:369–375.
7 Johnson MD, Burchiel KJ: Peripheral stimulation for treatment of trigeminal postherpetic neuralgia and trigeminal posttraumatic neuropathic pain: a pilot study. Neurosurgery 2004;55:135–141; discussion 141–142.
8 Weiner RL: Occipital neurostimulation (ONS) for treatment of intractable headache disorders. Pain Med 2006;7:S137–S139.
9 Slavin KV, Burchiel KJ: Use of long-term nerve stimulation with implanted electrodes in the treatment of intractable craniofacial pain. J Neurosurg 2000;92:576.
10 Magis D, Allena M, Bolla M, De Pasqua V, Remacle JM, Schoenen J: Occipital nerve stimulation for drug-resistant chronic cluster headache: a prospective pilot study. Lancet Neurol 2007;6:314–321.
11 Ordia J, Vaisman J: Subcutaneous peripheral nerve stimulation with paddle lead for treatment of low back pain: case report. Neuromodulation 2009;12:205–209.
12 Thimineur M, De Ridder D: C2 area neurostimulation: a surgical treatment for fibromyalgia. Pain Med 2007;8:639–646.
13 Slavin KV: Epidural spinal cord stimulation: indications and technique; in Schulder M (ed): Handbook of Functional and Stereotactic Surgery. New York, Marcel Dekker, 2002, pp 417–430.
14 US Food and Drug Administration: Overview of Device Regulation. http://www.fda.gov/MedicalDevices/DeviceRegulationandGuidance/Overview/default.htm (accessed on February 11, 2015).
15 Kramer D, Shuai X, Kesselheim A: Regulation of medical devices in the United States and European Union. N Engl J Med 2012;366:848–855.
16 European Commission: Medical Devices. http://ec.europa.eu/growth/sectors/medical-devices/ (accessed on February 11, 2015).
17 Health Canada: Safe Medical Devices in Canada. http://www.hc-sc.gc.ca/dhp-mps/md-im/activit/fs-fi/meddevfs_matmedfd-eng.php (accessed on February 11, 2015).
18 Therapeutic Goods Administration: Australian Regulatory Guidelines for Medical Devices (ARGMD). https://www.tga.gov.au/publication/australian-regulatory-guidelines-medical-devices-argmd (accessed on February 11, 2015).
19 Gofeld M, Hanlon JG: Ultrasound-guided placement of a paddle lead onto peripheral nerves: surgical anatomy and methodology. Neuromodulation 2014;17:48–53.
20 Blue Cross Blue Shield of Kansas: Implanted Peripheral Nerve Stimulator (PNS) for Pain Control. http://www.bcbsks.com/CustomerService/Providers/MedicalPolicies/policies/policies/ImplantedPeripheralNerveStimulator_PainControl_2015-02-10.pdf (accessed on February 11, 2015).
21 Spencer J: Medtronic to pay $2.8 million to settle off-label promotion chargers. Star Tribune. February 7, 2015. http://m.startribune.com/business/291053531.html.

Daniel M. Birk, MD
Department of Neurosurgery, University of Illinois at Chicago
912 South Wood Street, M/C 799, Rm. 451N
Chicago, IL 60612 (USA)
E-Mail dmbirk@uic.edu

Author Index

Abdunnur, S.V. 64
Amar, A.P. 20
Apuzzo, M.L.J. 20
Attenello, F. 20

Banakhar, M. 192
Birk, D.M. 225
Boller, A.-M. 200

Cameron, T. 1
Carlson, J.D. 139
Cukiert, A. 39

Deer, T.R. 139
Dodick, D.W. 117

Eljamel, S. 53

Fang, Z.-P. 158

Green, A.L. 117

Hassouna, M. 192

Kim, D.H. 64

Lengele, B. 94
Liem, L. 213
Liu, C. 20
Lunsford, L.D. VII

Mellgren, A. 200
Mwenge, G.B. 94

Nordenstam, J. 200

Parker, J.L. 1
Perryman, L.T. 168
Pope, J.E. 139

Rodenstein, D. 94
Rombaux, P. 94
Rosenberg, W.S. 139
Russo, M. 127

Schoenen, J. 106
Schwedt, T.J. 117
Slavin, K.V. IX, 83, 139, 225
Soin, A. 158

Tronnier, V.M. 29

Van Buyten, J.-P. 76
Velasco, J. 158
Verrills, P. 127

Yearwood, T.L. 168
Yin, D. 83, 225

Subject Index

ALS, *see* Amyotrophic lateral sclerosis
Altius Electric Nerve Block, extremity pain management 151, 152
Amputation, *see* Postamputation pain
Amyotrophic lateral sclerosis (ALS), phrenic nerve stimulation therapy 75
Anxiety, vagus nerve stimulation therapy 24
Arm pain, *see* Extremity pain
Avery Laboratories devices 3, 4, 65
Avery Mark IV Breathing Pacemaker System 65–67

Back pain, *see* Low back pain
Baroreflex activation therapy (BAT) 85, 86, 89, 90
BAT, *see* Baroreflex activation therapy
Bion device 7–9
Botulin toxin
  chronic migraine management 118
  overactive bladder management 197

Callosotomy, vagus nerve stimulation therapy outcomes versus vagus nerve stimulation in Lennox-like syndrome 47–49
Carotid sinus/nerve stimulation
  anatomy 84
  animal studies 88, 89
  baroreflex mechanism 84
  devices 86–88
  heart failure 90
  prospects for study 90, 91
  rationale 84, 85
  resistant hypertension
    clinical features 83, 84
    stimulation outcomes 89
  surgical technique 87
CH, *see* Cluster headache
Cluster headache (CH), sphenopalatine ganglion stimulation therapy
  efficacy 111, 112
  mechanism of action 112, 113
  overview 109, 110
  safety 112
  technique 110
Congenital central hypoventilation syndrome, phrenic nerve stimulation therapy 68
Constipation, sacral nerve stimulation therapy 202, 208
Continuous positive airway pressure (CPAP)
  hypoglossal nerve stimulation outcome
    comparison 102–104
  sleep apnea management 98
CPAP, *see* Continuous positive airway pressure
Cranioacial pain syndromes, classification 77

Depression, vagus nerve stimulation therapy
  dosing 55
  informed consent 55
  major depression
    complications 60, 61
    outcomes 56–60
    patient criteria 55, 56
  overview 24, 53, 54
Dorsal root ganglion (DRG), stimulation therapy
  analgesia mechanisms 219, 220
  anatomy 216–218
  devices 215
  historical perspective 214
  implantation 215, 217
  neuropathic pain
    physiology 218, 219
    trials 216
  overview 213, 214

spinal cord stimulation comparison 213–215, 218
wireless stimulation for failed back surgery syndrome-related lumbar radiculitis 186, 187
DRG, *see* Dorsal root ganglion

Epilepsy, vagus nerve stimulation therapy
evidence-based medicine analysis
adverse events 43, 44
outcomes 42–45
study design 40–42
historical perspective 21
Lennox-Gastaut syndrome 45–49
Lennox-like syndrome 45–49
overview 40
reflex eating seizure 50, 51
Extremity pain
peripheral nerve stimulation
devices
Altius Electric Nerve Block 151, 152
Freedom 4 and 8 Stimulators 152, 153, 156
MicroPulse 153
SmartPatch 153
StimRouter 151, 155
long-term follow-up 148–150
outcomes 153–155
paddle insertion 150, 151
paddle lead peripheral nerve stimulation 144–148
percutaneous peripheral nerve stimulation 141–144
prospects 156
treatment overview 139–141

Failed back surgery syndrome-related lumbar radiculitis, dorsal root ganglion wireless stimulation 186, 187
Fecal incontinence, sacral nerve stimulation therapy 201, 202, 204–208
Food and Drug Administration, *see* Regulatory approval, peripheral nerve stimulation devices
Freedom 4 and 8 Stimulators, extremity pain management 152, 153, 156
Frequency-urgency syndrome, sacral neuromodulation therapy 195

Gasserian ganglion stimulation
cranioacial pain syndrome classification 77
historical perspective 78
outcomes 81
rationale 78
technique 79–81

Headache, *see* Cluster headache; Migraine
Heart failure, carotid sinus stimulation 90
HFAC block, *see* High-frequency alternating current block
HGNS, *see* Hypoglossal nerve stimulation
High-frequency alternating current (HFAC) block, postamputation pain management
implantation technique 162–164
outcomes 166
overview 160
parameter settings 164, 166
patient selection 163, 164
Humanitarian use device, *see* Regulatory approval, peripheral nerve stimulation devices
Hypertension, *see* Carotid sinus/nerve stimulation
Hypoglossal nerve stimulation (HGNS)
breathing circuit 96, 97
sleep apnea
clinical trials 99–102
continuous positive airway pressure outcome comparison 102–104
overview 97, 98
tongue anatomy and function 94–96

IBS, *see* Irritable bowel syndrome
Interstitial cystitis, sacral neuromodulation therapy 196
Investigational device exemption, *see* Regulatory approval, peripheral nerve stimulation devices
Irritable bowel syndrome (IBS), sacral nerve stimulation therapy 208

Leg pain, *see* Extremity pain
Lennox-Gastaut syndrome (LGS), vagus nerve stimulation therapy for seizure 45–49
Lennox-like syndrome (LLS), vagus nerve stimulation therapy for seizure 45–49
LGS, *see* Lennox-Gastaut syndrome
LLS, *see* Lennox-like syndrome
Low back pain, peripheral nerve field stimulation
advantages 136, 137
applications 128

complications 136
lead depth 131–133
outcomes
analgesia use 135
functional outcomes 135, 136
pain indices 132, 134
patient satisfaction 135
patient selection 129
principles 128–130
pulse generator implantation 131
trial procedure and programming 130, 131

Major depression, *see* Depression
Medical Implant Communication Services (MICS), radiofrequency band 169
MicroPulse, extremity pain management 153
MICS, *see* Medical Implant Communication Services
Migraine
chronic migraine
conventional therapy 118, 119
features 117, 118
occipital nerve stimulation therapy
case series 120, 121
overview 119, 120
prospective randomized crossover study 121, 122
prospects for study 124
randomized sham-controlled clinical trials 122, 123
sphenopalatine ganglion stimulation therapy 113, 114
Multiple sclerosis, sacral neuromodulation therapy 195

Narcolepsy, vagus nerve stimulation therapy 25
NCP, *see* Neurocybernetic Prosthesis
Neurocybernetic Prosthesis (NCP) 20, 25
Neurovascular headache, *see* Sphenopalatine ganglion

OAB, *see* Overactive bladder
Obesity, vagus nerve stimulation therapy 24
Obstructive sleep apnea
anatomy 97
continuous positive airway pressure therapy 98
epidemiology 97, 98
hypoglossal nerve stimulation
clinical trials 99–102
continuous positive airway pressure outcome comparison 102–104
Occipital nerve stimulation (ONS), chronic migraine management
case series 120, 121
overview 119, 120
prospective randomized crossover study 121, 122
prospects for study 124
randomized sham-controlled clinical trials 122, 123
ONS, *see* Occipital nerve stimulation
Overactive bladder (OAB), sacral neuromodulation therapy 195, 197

Peripheral nerve fiber
anatomy 11
distance versus threshold stimulation current 12
fiber diameter and current 13, 14
stimulation parameters 12
stimulus current versus stimulus amplitude 13
types 170
Peripheral nerve field stimulation
back pain management, *see* Low back pain
peripheral nerve stimulation comparison 140
Peripheral nerve stimulation (PNS)
amputation patients, *see* Postamputation pain
back pain, *see* Low back pain
carotid sinus and nerve stimulation, *see* Carotid sinus/nerve stimulation
dorsal root ganglion, *see* Dorsal root ganglion
extracellular potential at node of Ranvier 13
extremities, *see* Extremity pain
historical perspective
devices
early devices 1–3
second-generation devices 3–5
overview 1, 2
percutaneous leads 5–7
hypoglossal nerve, *see* Hypoglossal nerve stimulation
ideal device features 15–17
implantable devices 7–9

limitations of technology 9, 10
occipital nerve, *see* Occipital nerve stimulation
phrenic nerve, *see* Phrenic nerve stimulation
regulatory approval of devices, *see* Regulatory approval, peripheral nerve stimulation devices
sacral nerve, *see* Sacral neuromodulation
sphenopalatine ganglion, *see* Sphenopalatine ganglion
system elements 16
trigeminal nerve, *see* Gasserian ganglion stimulation
vagus nerve, *see* Vagus nerve stimulation
wireless stimulation, *see* Wireless stimulation
Phrenic nerve stimulation
Avery Mark IV Breathing Pacemaker System 65–67
historical perspective 64, 65
indications 67, 68
outcomes 74
prospects 74, 75
surgical technique
cervical technique 70–72
complications 73
follow-up care 73
presurgical evaluation 68, 69
thoracoscopic technique 69, 70
PNS, *see* Peripheral nerve stimulation
Polio, phrenic nerve stimulation therapy 75
Postamputation pain
epidemiology 159
pathophysiology 159
peripheral neuromodulation therapy
high-frequency electrical conduction block
implantation technique 162–164
outcomes 166
overview 160
parameter settings 164, 166
patient selection 163, 164
modes 160
Premarket approval, *see* Regulatory approval, peripheral nerve stimulation devices
Premarket notification, *see* Regulatory approval, peripheral nerve stimulation devices
Pulse generators
implantable pulse generators 171, 172
implantation, *see specific nerves*
radiofrequency pulse generator 171
regulation, *see* Regulatory approval, peripheral nerve stimulation devices
transcutaneous electrical nerve stimulation 170, 171
wireless pulse generation, *see* Wireless stimulation

Reflex eating seizure, *see* Epilepsy
Regulatory approval, peripheral nerve stimulation devices
approval status of devices by country 227–229, 235
Australia 234, 235
Canada 234, 235
European Union 235
overview 225, 226
prospects 236
United States
Food and Drug Administration 225, 226, 231–234, 236
historical perspective 226, 230, 231
humanitarian use device 231
investigational device exemption 232
legislation 231, 232
premarket approval 231, 233
premarket notification 231–233

Sacral neuromodulation (SNM)
genitourinary problems
applications
frequency-urgency syndrome 195
interstitial cystitis 196
multiple sclerosis 195
overactive bladder 195, 197
spinal cord injury 195
children 197
contraindications 197
controversial issues 197
historical perspective 192, 193
internal pulse generator implantation 194, 195
percutaneous nerve evaluation 193
sexual function effects 196
stage one test 194
stimulation for bowel disorders
complications 209
constipation 202, 208
fecal incontinence 201, 202, 204–208
historical perspective 203

implant techniques 203, 204
irritable bowel syndrome 208
mechanism of action 203
overview 200
patient selection 206
SCI, *see* Spinal cord injury
SCS, *see* Spinal cord stimulation
Seizure, *see* Epilepsy
Sleep apnea, *see* Obstructive sleep apnea
SmartPatch, extremity pain management 153
SNM, *see* Sacral neuromodulation
SPG, *see* Sphenopalatine ganglion
Sphenopalatine ganglion (SPG)
anatomy and physiology 107
cluster headache and stimulation therapy
efficacy 111, 112
mechanism of action 112, 113
overview 109, 110
safety 112
technique 110
history of study 106, 107
migraine and stimulation therapy 113, 114
neurovascular headache role 107–109
prospects for stimulation therapy 114, 115
Spinal cord injury (SCI)
phrenic nerve stimulation therapy 67, 68, 74
sacral neuromodulation therapy 195
Spinal cord stimulation (SCS)
back pain 127, 137
dorsal root ganglion stimulation comparison 213–215, 218
limitations 140, 141, 215
StimRouter, extremity pain management 151, 155

Tongue, *see* Hypoglossal nerve stimulation
Topiramate, chronic migraine management 118
Trigeminal neuralgia, *see* Gasserian ganglion stimulation; Wireless stimulation

Vagus nerve stimulation (VNS)
anatomy and physiology 21–23
anti-inflammatory effects 25, 26
historical perspective 21
indications
anxiety 24
depression, *see* Depression
epilepsy, *see* Epilepsy
narcolepsy 25
obesity 24
overview 20
surgical techniques
anesthesiology 29, 30
complications 36
laryngoscopy evaluation 30
revisions 35
right-sided implantation 35
skin-to-skin procedure 30–35
VNS, *see* Vagus nerve stimulation

Wireless stimulation
applications
failed back surgery syndrome-related lumbar radiculitis 186, 187
sites for neuromodulation 179–184
trigeminal neuralgia 184–186
device design, placement, and function 175–177
external pulse generator
controller 178
features 177, 178
overview 168–170
prospects
lead design 188
market 190
miniaturization 191
novel applications 188, 189
programming 188
traditional system comparison 178, 179
trends 173, 174
wireless system criteria 172, 173